D1519836

Epigenetics and Human Health

Series Editors
Prof. Dr. Robert Feil
Institute of Molecular Genetics
CNRS and University of Montpellier
1919 route de Mende
34293 Montpellier Cedex 5
France

PD Dr. Mario Noyer-Weidner
Institute of Biology
Free University of Berlin
Altensteinstr. 6
14195 Berlin
Germany

Prof. Dr. Jörn Walter
Universität des Saarlandes
Naturwissenschaftlich-Technische Fakultät III
FR 8.3 Biowissenschaften/Genetik/Epigenetik
Postfach 151150
66041 Saarbrücken
Germany

Arturas Petronis • Jonathan Mill
Editors

Brain, Behavior and Epigenetics

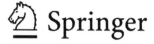 Springer

Editors
Arturas Petronis MD, PhD
Centre for Addiction and Mental
Health
The Krembil Family Epigenetics
Laboratory
College Street 250
M5T 1R8 Toronto, Ontario
Canada
arturas_petronis@camh.net

Jonathan Mill PhD
King's College London
Institute of Psychiatry
De Crispigny Park
SE5 8AF London
United Kingdom
j.mill@iop.kcl.ac.uk

ISSN 2191-2262   e-ISSN 2191-2270
ISBN 978-3-642-17425-4   e-ISBN 978-3-642-17426-1
DOI 10.1007/978-3-642-17426-1
Springer Heidelberg Dordrecht London New York

Library of Congress Control Number: 2011929222

Cover design: SPi Publisher Services

Printed on acid-free paper

Springer is part of Springer Science+Business Media (www.springer.com)

Preface by the Series Editors

Brain, Behaviour and Epigenetics is the second volume of a new Springer book series on *Epigenetics and Human Health*, edited by Robert Feil (University of Montpellier, France), Mario Noyer-Weidner (University of Berlin, Germany) and Jörn Walter (University of Saarbrücken, Germany).

With Arturas Petronis and Jonathan Mill the series has attracted two editors to this volume with a long-standing record in this emerging biomedical field. They both direct brain- and disease-oriented research programs at the Centre for Addiction and Mental Health in Toronto (Canada) and at the Kings College in London (UK), respectively. In the 14 chapters of their book they have gathered comprehensive articles ranging from basic molecular regulation in the brain to memory formation and psychiatric disorders.

The series adds to Springer's growing interest in the field of epigenetics and its many links to human health – both in the biological and clinical context. The aim of the book series is to introduce new epigenetic topics and concepts with relevance to human disease and to present them in a broad interdisciplinary context. Along this line the series aims to address both clinicians and basic scientists. We very much hope you will enjoy this volume and the series and find them useful for your professional endeavours.

May 2011

Robert Feil
Mario Noyer-Weidner
Jörn Walter

Preface to the Volume

Biomedical research in the first decade of the twenty-first century has been marked by a rapidly growing interest in epigenetics. The reasons for this are numerous, but primarily it stems from the mounting realization that research programs focused solely on DNA sequence variation, despite their breadth and depth, are unlikely to address all fundamental aspects of human biology. Some questions are evident even to nonbiologists. How does a single zygote develop into a complex multicellular organism composed of dozens of different tissues and hundreds of cell types, all genetically identical but performing very different functions? Why do monozygotic twins, despite their stunning external similarities, often exhibit significant differences in personality and predisposition to disease? If environmental factors are solely the cause of such variation, why are similar differences also observed between genetically identical animals housed in a uniform environment? These are not necessarily new questions. More than half a century ago, Conrad H. Waddington, an insightful British developmental biologist, developed a theoretical framework to explain how identical genotypes could produce a wide collection of phenotypes over the course of development, defining epigenetics as the developmental processes "connecting" a cell's genotype to its phenotype. Even before Waddington, the term *epigenesis* was used several centuries ago to conceptualize how, starting from a uniform material, every individual acquires new forms that emerge gradually over time.

Over the last couple of decades, epigenetics has undergone a significant metamorphosis from an abstract developmental theory to a very dynamic and rapidly developing branch of molecular biology. Waddington's concept of an "epigenetic landscape" linked to phenotype has materialized into the study of complex combinations of DNA and histone modifications, together acting to coordinate various genetic functions in the cell. These modifications can be heritable, both mitotically and meiotically, but do not involve changes in the DNA sequence. Contemporary epigenetics investigates DNA methylation and hydroxymethylation, in addition to a plethora of histone modifications that together play a critical role in a variety of regulatory processes within the nucleus. Epigenetic processes primarily regulate gene expression, controlling the tissue-specific orchestration of gene activity that ultimately accounts for the development of multicellular organisms. They also have a number of other important genomic functions including the suppression of retroelements, the instigation of X chromosome inactivation in females and a role in meiotic and mitotic recombination and chromosomal segregation.

Epigenetic studies in various species – from *Escherichia coli* and yeast to animals and humans – are now underway, highlighting how epigenetic regulation is critically important for the normal functioning of the genome. Cells can operate normally only if both DNA sequence and epigenetic components of the genome function properly. In other words, the cell needs both the DNA "hardware" and the epigenetic "software." Furthermore, epigenetic factors and the DNA sequence do not necessarily operate in isolation. Some DNA sequence variants can influence local epigenetic profiles, for example, via processes such as allele-specific DNA methylation. Likewise, epigenetic modifications can predispose certain nucleotides to be more mutagenic than others; for example, methylated cytosines are prone to spontaneous deamination and conversion to thymines.

Epigenetic information varies among cells of the same tissue, across the cells of different tissues, and also between individuals. Epigenetic changes may be rapid and short-lived (e.g., the cyclical changes observed in response to the circadian rhythm) or highly stable once established (e.g., the maintenance of tissue and cell type specificity). Despite the extremely fast growth in epigenetic research over the last decade, we are only just beginning to understand the full complexity of the epigenome. We are still mapping the epigenetic landscape of the cell, uncovering new epigenetic mechanisms, and novel roles for epigenetic processes. Recent years, for instance, have seen the recognition about the importance of noncoding RNA and RNA-mediated epigenetic gene regulation, as well as physical interactions among genes in three-dimensional space within the nucleus.

The recent advent of high-throughput genomic approaches, first via the application of microarrays and more recently via next generation sequencing, has enabled a technological quantum leap in molecular epigenetic studies; epigenome-wide mapping experiments can now be feasibly performed at unprecedented resolution. The term "epigenome" is used to describe the complex distribution of epigenetic modifications across the entire genome in a specific cell or cell population. As in genome-wide association studies, scans of epigenomes will soon become a routine procedure in experimental laboratories. Large-scale epigenomic mapping projects initiated by the NIH, European Science Foundation, and other major funding agencies have already mapped numerous layers of epigenomic information using these latest technologies. Hopefully, this effort will result in a global, integrated view of different cellular states. Unlike the human genome, mapping the epigenome is an open-end project: each cell in each individual may have a distinct epigenome that reflects its developmental state, environmental exposures, stochastic effects, among numerous other multidirectional effects that form the epigenetic uniqueness of each cell, each tissue, and each individual.

The focus of this volume is behavioral and brain epigenetics, representing a novel a frontier in neurobiological and psychiatric research. One of the primary objectives of behavioral epigenetics is to understand the molecular basis of various brain functions (e.g., memory, cognition, homeostasis, and adaptation to new environments). Of particular interest is the putative role of epigenetic dysfunction in brain pathology and mental illness. While epigenetic factors have been intensively investigated in the malignant transformation of cells in cancer, similar processes may be highly relevant to various complex non-Mendelian diseases. Epigenetic mechanisms – often more efficiently than genetic ones – are able to integrate a number of apparently unrelated clinical, epidemiological, and molecular data into a new theoretical framework. Putative epigenetic misregulation is consistent with various epidemiological, clinical, and molecular features in complex diseases, including most psychiatric disorders. It is apparent that the dysregulation of gene activity and deviations from a normal expression pattern can be as detrimental to a cell as mutant DNA sequences resulting in dysfunctional proteins. It is important to note that epigenetic changes that are partially both inherited and acquired can be the primary disease causes, rather than just one of numerous secondary or further downstream epiphenomena.

Another pertinent question is how exposure to a wide scope of environmental factors, such as toxins, drugs of abuse, infection, nutrition, and stress can affect epigenetic regulation in the brain that ultimately translate into alterations in behavior. Epigenetic studies will provide new insights into the interface between the environment and the genome, and the mechanisms by which exposures at key points in development may mediate long-term effects on behavior. Some epigenetic changes are transient, whereas others may be relatively stable and persist much longer. Some chromatin changes are mitotically heritable and can affect somatic tissues, whereas others may even be inherited through meiosis and affect subsequent generations.

This volume represents a compilation of our current understanding about the key aspects of epigenetic processes in the brain and their role in behavior. The chapters in this book bring together some of the leading researchers in the field of behavioral epigenetics. They explore many of the epigenetic processes that operate or may be operating to mediate neurobiological functions in the brain and describe how perturbations to these systems may play a key role in mediating behavior and the origin of brain diseases. Akbarian et al. analyze the mechanisms by which epigenetic factors, such as covalent histone modifications, can contribute to dysregulation of gene expression in schizophrenia. Another chapter dedicated to schizophrenia, by Grayson and colleagues, summarizes their detailed epigenetic analysis of genes encoding reelin and glutamate decarboxylase 67. Theoretical evidence, with some preliminary experimental findings, that bipolar disorder is a promising candidate for epigenetic and epigenomic studies is summarized by Kato. The epigenetics and disease theme is further elaborated by Labonté and Turecki, who discuss the complex relationship between adverse life events and social stress, on the one hand, and major depression and suicidal behavior on the other, exploring the putative role of molecular epigenetic factors. Malaspina et al. provide epidemiological evidence that paternal age, toxin exposure, and psychological stressors may increase the risk for mental disease and suggest that these environmental hazards can be indirectly uncovered using epigenetic strategies, both in humans and animal models. The theme of epidemiological epigenetics in psychiatric diseases is elaborated by Susser et al., who discuss how prenatal famine and childhood ethnic minority status is associated with higher degree of psychopathology. Craig et al. discuss the complex epigenetic regulation of the X chromosome and its impact on human behavioral phenotypes. Crespi, in a theoretical *tour de force*, attempts to link parent–offspring conflict, attachment theory, and genomic imprinting. The numerous roles of genomic imprinting, a classical epigenetic mechanism, in brain and behavior studies are overviewed by Isles and Wilkinson. The intriguing observations about the epigenetic effects of social experiences occurring during infancy, and its role in the establishment and maintenance of environmental programming are summarized in two chapters, one by Curley and Champagne and a second by Weaver. Finally, three chapters by Labrie, Estevez and Abel, and Reul et al. discuss evidence that epigenetic mechanisms can play a critical role in synaptic plasticity, learning, and memory.

Despite significant progress in molecular epigenetic research and its enormous potential, there are still considerable challenges to overcome before we can fully understand the role of epigenetic processes in brain function and behavior. For instance, what comprises a "normal" brain epigenome and what is the degree of tissue and cellular specificity of epigenetic landscapes in the brain? How do the multiple layers of epigenetic information interact and change over time? How common is meiotic epigenetic heritability and what role it may play in complex psychiatric disease? To what extent is the epigenome plastic and malleable in response to environmental influences? This volume demonstrates that such questions can now be explored in an experimental molecular biology laboratory. While the community is only just starting to acknowledge the importance of epigenetic processes in the brain, there is no doubt that numerous breakthrough discoveries in brain and behavioral epigenetics will be made in the decades to come.

Toronto, Canada   Arturas Petronis
London, UK   Jonathan Mill

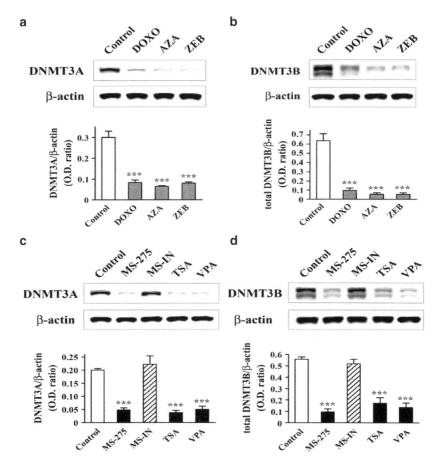

Fig. 2.5 DNMT and HDAC inhibitors decrease DNMT3A and DNMT3B protein levels. Western blot analyses of DNMT3A and DNMT3B proteins were performed using nuclear extracts prepared from control cells and cells treated with either DNMT inhibitors (**a** and **b**) or HDAC inhibitors (**c** and **d**). For assays with DNMT inhibitors, cells were treated with 250 nM DOXO (48 h), 5 μM AZA (48 h), or 500 μM ZEB (48 h followed by 48-h incubation with untreated medium). HDAC inhibitor treatments were performed as follows: 5 μM MS-275 (48 h), 5 μM MS-IN (48 h), 0.3 μM TSA (24 h), and 5 mM VPA (24 h). In all cases (**a–d**), representative Western blots are shown (*upper panels*) together with the graphs depicting the ratio of the DNMT3A or DNMT3B (both isoforms) band over the area of the β-actin band (*lower panels*). Data represent the mean ± S.E.M. of three independent experiments. ***$p < 0.001$ vs. control group (one-way ANOVA followed by Bonferroni test). Reprinted (Kundakovic et al. 2007) with permission of the American Society for Pharmacology and Experimental Therapeutics

DNMT and HDAC inhibitors was also associated with the downregulation of two other DNMT enzymes, DNMT3A and DNMT3B, in nuclei of NT-2 cells (Fig. 2.5). Figure 2.5a shows the effects of DNMT inhibitors on DNMT3A protein levels, while Fig. 2.5c shows the same for various HDAC inhibitors. Similarly, Fig. 2.5b shows the results obtained using selected DNMT inhibitors on DNMT3B protein with comparable results using various HDAC inhibitors shown below (Fig. 2.5d). The inactive enantiomer of MS-275 had no effect on the level of either protein.

2.8   Epigenetic Drugs Facilitate the Dissociation of DNMT-Containing Repressor Complexes from Reelin and *GAD67* Promoters

Our studies provide evidence that all three DNMT proteins, DNMT1, DNMT3A, and DNMT3B, might participate in the formation of transcriptional repressor complexes at the *reelin* and *GAD67* promoters (Fig. 2.6). These complexes also include MeCP2 and HDAC1 proteins. Our data support the concept that treatment with DNMT inhibitors (Kundakovic et al. 2009) and HDAC inhibitors (Fig. 2.6) results in the dissociation of all three DNMT proteins, together with MeCP2 and HDAC1, from both promoters. Increased local histone acetylation was also observed, implying that both classes of drugs facilitate the relaxation of chromatin

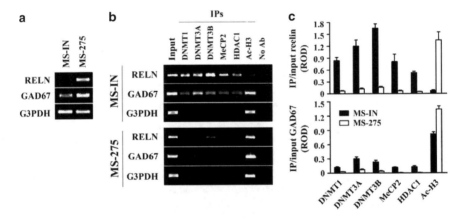

Fig. 2.6 Reelin and GAD67 gene activation is accompanied by dissociation of repressor complexes from the corresponding promoters. NT-2 cells were treated with either 5 μM of HDAC inhibitor MS-275 or 5 μM of its inactive stereoisomer MS-IN for 48 h. (**a**) RT-PCR analysis confirmed that reelin and GAD67 mRNAs were induced by MS-275 compared to MS-IN treatment. (**b**) The corresponding chromatin preparations were immunoprecipitated with DNMT1, DNMT3A, DNMT3B, MeCP2, HDAC1, and Ac-H3 antibodies (IPs). Nonimmunoprecipitated samples were used as negative controls (No Ab). DNA isolated from inputs, Ips, and control samples were PCR-amplified using primers specific for the reelin, GAD67, and G3PDH promoter regions. Relative optical densities (RODs) of the bands derived from ethidium bromide-stained gels were quantified. (**c**) Graphs show the results (mean ± S.E.M. of three independent experiments) of semiquantitative analysis of the occupancy of DNMT1, DNMT3A, DNMT3B, MeCP2, HDAC1, and Ac-H3 on the reelin (*upper panel*) and GAD67 (*lower panel*) promoters in MS-IN- and MS-275-treated cells, normalized to input DNA (each comparison MS-IN vs. MS-275 showed a statistical significance of at least $p < 0.05$, *t*-test). Reprinted (Kundakovic et al. 2007) with permission of the American Society for Pharmacology and Experimental Therapeutics

surrounding the *reelin* and *GAD67* promoters. In addition, each inhibitor reduces total nuclear DNMT enzyme activity and facilitates a reduction in DNA methylation in the same *reelin* and *GAD67* promoter regions that are associated with changes in chromatin structure (Kundakovic et al. 2009). These data imply that the formation of the repressor complexes is likely DNA-methylation dependent. Furthermore, we suggest that promoter demethylation might not be required for a slight to moderate induction of *reelin* and *GAD67* transcription, but is likely relevant for maximal activation of these two promoters.

2.9   Discussion

Results from our studies provide evidence that the human *reelin* and *GAD67* promoters are coordinately regulated through epigenetic mechanisms and also suggest an underlying molecular mechanism to understand this regulation. Our data imply that both promoters are negatively regulated through methylation-dependent recruitment of transcriptional repressor complexes containing DNMT1, DNMT3A, DNMT3B, MeCP2, and HDAC1 proteins. These complexes reduce the transcriptional activity of the promoters by shifting the surrounding chromatin into a more compact state, thus resulting in decreased transcription factor accessibility (Fig. 2.7). While our data are directly applicable to the epigenetic regulation of the *reelin* and *GAD67* promoters in neuronal progenitor cells, an increasing body of evidence suggests that similar regulatory mechanisms are operative in adult GABAergic neurons (Costa et al. 2004, 2006; Szyf et al. 2008).

Further, this study gives new insight into the molecular mechanisms that underlie the downregulation of reelin and *GAD67* mRNAs in the brains of SZ. It has been reported that the reductions in reelin and GAD67 transcripts correlate with increased DNMT1 and HDAC1 expression in the same GABAergic neurons (Hayes 1989; Ruzicka et al. 2007; Benes et al. 2007). Therefore, we propose that the upregulation of DNMT1 mRNA could promote downregulation of the *reelin* and *GAD67* genes by inducing promoter hypermethylation (Abdolmaleky et al. 2005; Chen et al. 2002; Grayson et al. 2005) and increased binding of DNMT1- and HDAC1-containing corepressor complexes to the reelin and *GAD67* promoters. According to our data, these complexes most likely also contain additional DNMTs (DNMT3A and DNMT3B) and MeCP2 and other proteins as well. However, further studies with postmortem human brains will be necessary to confirm this hypothesis.

Additionally, we would like to suggest a new approach for the treatment of SZ that focuses on the reactivation of mRNA expression profiles that are downregulated due to modifications in the epigenome. We report that treatment of neuronal progenitor cells with various DNMT and HDAC inhibitors leads to a robust induction of reelin and GAD67 mRNAs. Furthermore, we demonstrate that both classes of epigenetic drugs target DNMT1 and HDAC1, which are aberrantly expressed in SZ (Fig. 2.7). These drugs downregulate DNMT1 and directly or indirectly inhibit the repressor activity of HDAC1. Moreover, the same drugs induce

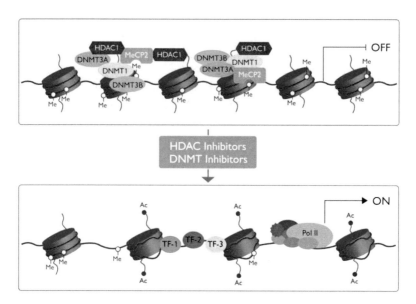

Fig. 2.7 Hypothetical model for promoter activation by HDAC and DNMT inhibitors. For simplicity, promoters are shown as either silent (repressed – OFF) or fully active (ON). The transcriptionally inactive chromatin structure surrounding the indicated promoter region (*upper panel*) is the consequence of cytosine methylation and subsequent recruitment of repressor proteins, including DNMT1, DNMT3A, DNMT3B, MeCP2, and HDAC1 (most likely others, also). The downregulation of DNMT proteins (by DNMT inhibitors and HDAC inhibitors), together with the inhibition of HDAC enzymatic activity and the decrease in MeCP2 expression (in the case of the HDAC inhibitors), results in dissociation of these repressor complexes. This leads to DNA demethylation, histone acetylation, and a relaxation of the chromatin surrounding the respective regulatory regions (*lower panel*). The more open chromatin configuration allows the recruitment of specific transcription factors (TFs), such as Sp1 and the general transcriptional machinery (*gray shapes*) to the promoters. Collectively, this results in the drug-induced epigenetic changes leading to promoter activation (as we have proposed for the reelin and GAD67 genes)

changes in the methylation status of the CpG-island-containing reelin promoter that is hypermethylated in the brains of SZ patients (Veldic et al. 2004, Abdolmaleky et al. 2005, Grayson et al. 2005). Therefore, these data provide a mechanistic rationale for our hypothesis that HDAC inhibitors and DNMT inhibitors used either individually or in combination may represent a novel pharmacological approach for correcting reelin and GAD67 mRNA levels, and the GABAergic deficits associated with SZ (Guidotti et al. 2005; Levenson 2007).

A recent study examined alterations in GABA-related mRNAs in the PFC of subjects with SZ (Hashimoto et al. 2008). Reduced mRNA levels corresponding to presynaptic regulators of GABA function, numerous neuropeptides, and GABA-A receptor subunits were detected. In addition, studies show that the downregulation of NMDA receptors in GABA neurons could be the consequence of a primary epigenetic defect (Belforte et al. 2010). These data are consistent with the GABA deficit hypothesis proposed by us (Guidotti et al. 2005) and others (Lewis et al. 2005;

Benes et al. 2007). Additional work will identify which mRNAs are activated by various HDACs, in which brain regions and in which neurons. As the collection of these compounds increases, it should not be too long before researchers are able to design these drugs to target subclasses of HDACs showing selective expression patterns in the desired brain regions (Broide et al. 2007).

Preliminary data in rodents support the notion that MS-275 crosses the blood–brain barrier and increases histone acetylation in the frontal cortex of treated animals (Simonini et al. 2006). However, a recent pharmacokinetic study using positron emission tomography (PET) showed that MS-275 exhibits poor brain penetration (Hooker et al. 2010). So while the levels of MS-275 that cross into the brain may be sufficient for some assays, this issue needs additional clarification in terms of new drug design. Increasing attention is being paid to various HDAC inhibitors in the context of therapeutic intervention for certain cancers. It seems prudent that a similar approach may prove beneficial in reactivating genes that are downregulated as a consequence of promoter hypermethylation, as we have suggested occurs in SZ (Grayson et al. 2010). For example, in addition to *reelin* and *GAD67*, the promoter corresponding to the NMDA receptor subunit 2A is embedded in a CpG island and is downregulated in the postmortem cortex of SZ subjects (Woo et al. 2005, 2008). Interestingly, this reduced expression is in parvalbumin-expressing neurons of the cortex that also contain GAD67 and reelin (Noh et al. 2005). Clearly, the glutamatergic input onto cortical GABA interneurons plays a key role in determining synaptic GABA release onto efferent pyramidal neurons. This suggests that the two major conceptual schools that characterize the dysfunctional neural circuits that define SZ may contribute to an integrated hypothesis. That is, glutamatergic hypofunction and GABAergic hypofunction are linked provided they function at the level of the same cortical GABA neurons. Thus, it is possible that drugs acting at the level of chromatin remodeling could induce each of the mRNAs downregulated in SZ, thereby correcting the GABA neuron deficits. As such, by increasing the GABA interneuron content of GAD67, reelin, and NMDA receptor subunits, relevant neurons may more appropriately respond to uncompromised afferent NMDA receptor stimulation by releasing more GABA.

Acknowledgments We would like to dedicate this work to the memory of our friend and colleague, Dr. Erminio Costa, University of Illinois at Chicago, who died November 28, 2009.

References

Abdolmaleky HMK, Cheng A, Russo CL, Smith SV, Faraon M, Wilcox R, Shafa SJ, Glatt G, Nguyen JF, Ponte S, Thiagalingam TMT (2005) Hypermethylation of the reelin (RELN) promoter in the brain of schizophrenic patients: a preliminary report. Am J Med Genet B Neuropsychiatr Genet 134:60–66

Akbarian S, Kim JJ, Potkin SG, Hagman JO, Tafazzoli A, Bunney WE, Jones EG (1995) Gene expression for glutamic acid decarboxylase is reduced without loss of neurons in prefrontal cortex of schizophrenics. Arch Gen Psychiatry 52:258–266

Belforte JE, Zsiros V, Sklar ER, Jiang Z, Yu G, Quinlan Li Y, Nakazawa EMK (2010) Postnatal NMDA receptor ablation in corticolimbic interneurons confers schizophrenia-like phenotypes. Nat Neurosci 13:76–83

Benes J, Vincent SL, Alsterberger G, Bird ED, San Giovanni JP (1992) Increased GABAergic receptor binding in superficial layers of cingulate cortex in schizophrenia. J Neurosci 12: 924–929

Benes FM, Lim B, Matzilevich D, Walsh JP, Subburaju S, Minns M (2007) Regulation of the GABA cell phenotype in hippocampus of schizophrenics and bipolars. Proc Natl Acad Sci USA 104:10164–10169

Breese CR, Lee MJ, Adams CE, Sullivan B, Logel J, Gillen KM, Marks MJ, Collins AC, Leonard S (2000) Abnormal regulation of high affinity nicotinic receptors in subjects with schizophrenia. Neuropsychopharmacology 23:351–364

Broide RS, Redwine JM, Aftahi N, Yound W, Bloom FE, Winrow CJ (2007) Distribution of histone deacetylases 1-11 in the rat brain. J Mol Neurosci 31:47–58

Chen Y, Sharma RP, Costa RH, Costa E, Grayson DR (2002) On the epigenetic regulation of the human reelin promoter. Nucleic Acids Res 30:2930–2939

Conn PJ, Lindsley CW, Jones CK (2008) Activation of metabotropic glutamate receptors as a novel approach for the treatment of schizophrenia. Trends Pharmacol Sci 30:25–31

Costa E, Davis J, Grayson DR, Guidotti A, Pappas GD, Pesold C (2001) Dendritic spine hypoplasticity and downregulation of reelin and GABAergic tone in schizophrenia vulnerability. Neurobiol Dis 8:723–742

Costa E, Davis JM, Dong E, Grayson DR, Guidotti A, Tremolizzo L, Veldic M (2004) A GABAergic cortical deficit dominates schizophrenia pathophysiology. Crit Rev Neurobiol 16:1–23

Costa E, Dong E, Grayson DR, Ruzicka WB, Simonini MV, Veldic M, Guidotti A (2006) Epigenetic targets in GABAergic neurons to treat schizophrenia. Adv Pharmacol 54: 95–117

Costa E, Dong E, Grayson DR, Guidotti A, Ruzicka WB, Veldic M (2007) Reviewing the role of DNA (cytosine-5) methyltransferase overexpression in the cortical GABAergic dysfunction associated with psychosis vulnerability. Epigenetics 2:29–36

D'Arcangelo G, Miao GG, Chen SC, Soares HD, Morgan JI, Curran T (1995) A protein related to extracellular matrix proteins deleted in the mouse mutant reeler. Nature 376:292–293

Fatemi SH, Earle JA, McMenomy T (2000) Reduction in Reelin immunoreactivity in hippocampus of subjects with schizophrenia, bipolar disorder and major depression. Mol Psychiatry 5:654–663

Gonzalez-Burgos G, Lewis DA (2008) GABA neurons and the mechanisms of network oscillations: implications for understanding cortical dysfunction in schizophrenia. Schizophr Bull 34: 944–961

Gray JA, Roth BL (2007) The pipeline and future of drug development in schizophrenia. Mol Psychiatry 12:904–922

Grayson DR, Jia X, Chen Y, Sharma RP, Mitchell CP, Guidotti A, Costa E (2005) Reelin promoter hypermethylation in schizophrenia. Proc Natl Acad Sci USA 102:9341–9346

Grayson DR, Kundakovic M, Sharma RP (2010) Is there a future for HDAC inhibitors in the pharmacotherapy of psychiatric disorders? Mol Pharmacol 77(2):126–135

Guidotti A, Auta J, Davis JM, Dwivedi Y, Gerevini VD, Impagnatiello F, Pandey G, Pesold C, Sharma R, Uzunov DP, Costa E (2000) Decrease in reelin and glutamic acid decarboxylase$_{67}$ (GAD$_{67}$) expression in schizophrenia and bipolar disorder, a postmortem brain study. Arch Gen Psychiatry 57:1061–1069

Guidotti A, Auta J, Davis JM, Dong E, Grayson DR, Veldic M, Zhang X, Costa E (2005) GABAergic dysfunction in schizophrenia: a new treatment on the horizon. Psychopharmacology (Berl) 180:191–205

Guidotti A, Ruzicka W, Grayson DR, Veldic M, Davis J, Costa E (2007) S-Adenosyl methionine and DNA-methyltransferase-1 overexpression in psychosis. Neuroreport 18:57–60

Hashimoto T, Arion D, Unger T, Maldonado-Aviles JG, Morris HM, Volk DW, Mirnics K, Lewis DA (2008) Alterations in GABA-related transcriptome in the dorsolateral prefrontal cortex of subjects with schizophrenia. Mol Psychiatry 13:147–161

Hayes SG (1989) Long-term use of valproate in primary psychiatric disorders. J Clin Psychiatry 50:35S–39S

Hayman S (2008) A glimmer of light for neuropsychiatric disorders. Nature 455:890–893

Hooker JM, Kim SW, Alexoff D, Xu Y, Shea C, Reid A, Volkow N, Fowler JS (2010) Histone deacetylase inhibitor MS-275 exhibits poor brain penetration: pharmakokinetic studies of [^{11}C] MS-275 using positron emission tomography. ACS Chem Neurosci 1:65–73

Homayoun H, Moghaddam B (2007) NMDA receptor hypofunction produces opposite effects on prefrontal cortex interneurons and pyramidal neurons. J Neurosci 27:11496–11500

Howes OD, Kapur S (2009) The dopamine hypothesis of schizophrenia: version III-the final common pathway. Schizophr Bull 35:549–562

Impagnatiello F, Guidotti A, Pesold C, Dwivedi Y, Caruncho H, Pisu MG, Uzunov DP, Smalheiser NR, Davis JM, Pandey GN, Pappas GD, Tueting P, Sharma RP, Costa E (1998) A decrease of reelin expression as a putative vulernability factor in schizophrenia. Proc Natl Acad Sci USA 95:15718–15723

Kundakovic M, Chen Y, Costa E, Grayson DR (2007) DNA methyltransferase inhibitors coordinately induce expression of the human reelin and glutamic acid decarboxylase 67 genes. Mol Pharmacol 71:644–653

Kundakovic M, Chen Y, Guidotti A, Grayson DR (2009) The reelin and GAD67 promoters are activated by epigenetic drugs that facilitate the disruption of local repressor complexes. Mol Pharmacol 75:342–354

Levenson JM, Qiu S, Weeber EJ (2008) The role of reelin in adult synaptic function and the genetic and epigenetic regulation of the reelin gene. Biochim Biophys Acta 1779:433–431

Lewis DA, Hashimoto T, Volk DW (2005) Cortical inhibitory neurons and schizophrenia. Nat Rev Neurosci 6:312–324

Lieberman JA, Bymaster FP, Meltzer HY, Deutch AY, Duncan GE, Marx CE, Aprille JR, Dwyer DS, Li XM, Mahadik SP, Duman RS, Porter JH, Modica-Napolitano JS, Newton SS, Csernansky JG (2008) Antipsychotic drugs, comparison in animal models of efficacy, neurotransmitter regulation, and neuroprotection. Pharmacol Rev 60:358–403

Lisman JE, Coyle JT, Green RW, Javitt DC, Benes FM, Heckers S, Grace AA (2008) Circuit-based framework for understanding neurotransmitter and risk gene interactions in schizophrenia. Trends Neurosci 31:234–242

Mellios N, Huang HS, Baker SP, Galdzicka M, Ginns E, Akbarian S (2009) Molecular determinants of dysregulated GABAergic gene expression in the prefrontal cortex of subjects with schizophrenia. Biol Psychiatry 65:1006–1014

Mill J, Tang T, Kaminsky Z, Khare T, Yazdanpanah S, Bouchard L, Jia P, Assadzadeh A, Flanagan J, Schumacher A, Wang SC, Petronis A (2008) Epigenomic profiling reveals DNA-methylation changes associated with major psychosis. Am J Hum Genet 82:696–711

Noh JS, Sharma RP, Veldic M, Salvacion AA, Jia X, Chen Y, Costa E, Guidotti A, Grayson DR (2005) DNA methyltransferase 1 regulates reelin mRNA expression in mouse primary cortical cultures. Proc Natl Acad Sci USA 102:1749–1754

Poulter MO, Du L, Weaver IC, Palkovits M, Faludi G, Merali Z, Szyf M, Anisman H (2008) GABAA receptor promoter hypermethylation in suicide brain, implications for the involvement of epigenetic processes. Biol Psychiatry 64:645–652

Ptak C, Petronis A (2008) Epigenetics and complex disease: from etiology to new therapeutics. Annu Rev Toxicol 48:257–276

Ruzicka WB, Zhubi A, Veldic M, Grayson DR, Costa E, Guidotti A (2007) Selective epigenetic alteration of layer I GABAergic neurons isolated from prefrontal cortex of schizophrenia patients using laser-assisted microdissection. Mol Psychiatry 12:385–397

Satta R, Maloku E, Zhubi A, Pibiri F, Hajos M, Costa E, Guidotti A (2008) Subcutaneous nicotine decreases DNMT1 expression and GAD67 promoter methylation in selected populations of mouse telencephalic GABAergic neurons. Proc Natl Acad Sci USA 105:16356–16361

Simonini MV, Camargo LM, Dong E, Maloku E, Veldic M, Costa E, Guidotti A (2006) The benzamide MS-275 is a potent, long-lasting brain region-selective inhibitor of histone deacetylases. Proc Natl Acad Sci USA 103:1587–1592

Soghomonian JJ, Martin DL (1998) Two isoforms of glutamate decarboxylase: why? Trends Pharmacol Sci 19:500–505

Szyf M, McGowan P, Meaney MJ (2008) The social environment and the epigenome. Environ Mol Mutagen 49:46–60

Tremolizzo L, Carboni G, Ruzicka WB, Mitchell CP, Sugaya I, Tueting P, Sharma RP, Grayson DR, Costa E, Guidotti A (2002) An epigenetic mouse model for molecular and behavioral neuropathologies related to schizophrenia vulnerability. Proc Natl Acad Sci USA 99:17095–17100

Tremolizzo L, Doueiri MS, Dong E, Grayson DR, Davis J, Pinna G, Tueting P, Rodriguez-Menendez V, Costa E, Guidotti A (2005) Valproate corrects the schizophrenia-like epigenetic behavioral modifications induced by methionine in mice. Biol Psychiatry 57:500–509

Van Emburgh BO, Robertson KD (2008) DNA methyltransferases and methyl CpG binding proteins as multifunctional regulators of chromatin structure and development in mammalian cells. In: Tost J (ed) Epigenetics, Kaister. Academic, Norwich, UK, pp 23–62

Veldic M, Caruncho HJ, Liu WS, Davis J, Satta R, Grayson DR, Guidotti A, Costa E (2004) DNA-methyltransferase 1 mRNA is selectively overexpressed in telencephalic GABAergic interneurons of schizophrenia brains. Proc Natl Acad Sci USA 101:348–353

Veldic M, Guidotti A, Maloku E, Davis JM, Costa E (2005) In psychosis, cortical interneurons overexpress DNA-methyltransferase 1. Proc Natl Acad Sci USA 102:2152–2157

Veldic M, Kadriu B, Maloku E, Agis-Balboa RC, Guidotti A, Davis JM, Costa E (2007) Epigenetic mechanisms expressed in basal ganglia GABAergic neurons differentiate schizophrenia from bipolar disorder. Schizophr Res 91:51–61

Woo TUW, Walsh JP, Benes FP (2005) Density of glutamic acid decarboxylase 67 messenger RNA-containing neurons that express the N-methyl-D-aspartate receptor subunit NR2A in the anterior cingulate cortex in schizophrenia and bipolar disorder. Arch Gen Psychiatry 61: 649–657

Woo TUW, Kim AM, Viscidi E (2008) Disease-specific alterations in glutamatergic neurotransmission on inhibitory interneurons in the prefrontal cortex in schizophrenia. Brain Res 1218: 267–277

Wyatt RJ, Termini BA, Davis JM (1971) Biochemical and sleep studies of schizophrenia. A review of the literature 1960–1970. Schizophr Res 4:10–44

Zhubi A, Veldic M, Puri NV, Kadriu B, Caruncho H, Loza I, Sershen H, Lajtha A, Smith RC, Guidotti A, Davis JM, Costa E (2009) An upregulation of DNA-methyltransferase 1 and 3a expressed in telencephalic GABAergic neurons of schizophrenia patients is also detected in peripheral blood lymphocytes. Schizophr Res 111:115–122

Chapter 3
Possible Roles of DNA Methylation in Bipolar Disorder

Tadafumi Kato

Abstract Although the role of DNA sequence-based factors is implicated in bipolar disorder (BPD), traditional genetic approaches have not been very productive in the identification of causative genes. As a result, other approaches, such as epigenetics, should also be considered in the search for the molecular basis of BPD. Genomic imprinting has been suggested to play a role in disease development, as the risk of BPD acquisition in the offspring partially depends on the sex of the disease-transmitting parent. In addition, higher parental age is associated with an increased risk of BPD in the offspring, which suggests that age-dependent alteration of DNA methylation might be involved in the etiopathogenesis of the condition. Molecular effects of drugs also support the role of epigenetics; valproate, a histone deacetylase inhibitor, is effective in the treatment of mania. Consistent with the epigenetic theory of psychiatric disease, studies of monozygotic twins discordant for BPD revealed the DNA methylation differences between siblings. Additional studies support that DNA methylation patterns at certain genes are altered in the brain tissues of bipolar disease patients. Collectively, these findings suggest that the epigenetic studies may improve our understanding of the etiology and pathogenesis of BPD.

Keywords Bipolar disorder · Epigenetics · Monozygotic twins

3.1 Introduction

Bipolar disorder (BPD) is characterized by recurrent episodes of mania and depression, affecting around 1% of the population and causing severe psychosocial dysfunction. Mounting evidence, especially from twin studies, suggests that genetic

T. Kato

Laboratory for Molecular Dynamics of Mental Disorders, RIKEN Brain Science Institute, Hirosawa 2-1, Wako, Saitama 351-0198, Japan
e-mail: kato@brain.riken.jp

A. Petronis and J. Mill (eds.), *Brain, Behavior and Epigenetics*,
Epigenetics and Human Health, DOI 10.1007/978-3-642-17426-1_3,
© Springer-Verlag Berlin Heidelberg 2011

factors contribute to this disorder. Classical studies that focused on the identification of DNA sequence-based factors have yielded inconsistent results. More recently, genome-wide association studies were performed in a large number of BPD patients and controls, and several promising candidate genes such as *ANK3* (ankyrin G) and *CACNA1C* (L-type voltage-dependent calcium channel, alpha 1C subunit) (Ferreira et al. 2008) and single nucleotide polymorphism (SNPs) at 3p21.1 were suggested (McMahon et al. 2010); however, the odds ratios of these SNPs were less than 1.5, suggesting only a modest contribution to the etiology of BPD. In addition to common DNA polymorphisms, the role of rare variations is gaining attention, for example, rare variants of *ABCA13* [ATP-binding cassette (ABC) transporter] have been suggested to confer a risk of BPD and schizophrenia (Knight et al. 2009). Progress in next generation sequencing will soon enable whole genome – or at least the exome – sequencing in a large group of patients and controls. Such innovation will accelerate the search for rare mutations related to the disease, but it is not known such studies will fully explain the molecular basis of BPD. Epigenetic studies may shed a new light on the origin of BPD and other psychiatric diseases and significantly advance our understanding of the molecular basis of BPD, schizophrenia, autism, among numerous other brain diseases. Petronis (2003) has suggested that epigenetics may play a role in BPD based on the non-Mendelian features of this disease, such as discordance in monozygotic (MZ) twins, the critical age for susceptibility to the disease, clinical differences in males and females, and major fluctuations of the disease course. A number of epigenetic mechanisms may be involved in BPD, including partial epigenetic instability in somatic cells and epigenetic divergence in monozygotic twins, parental origin-dependent epigenetic regulation (genomic imprinting), skewed X-chromosome inactivation, inherited and acquired epigenetic misregulation of genes expressed in the brain, and several others. Some of the epigenetic studies in BPD are discussed below, and a summary is provided in Table 3.1.

3.2 Epigenetic Studies of BPD

3.2.1 Monozygotic Twins

Kuratomi et al. (2008) searched for DNA methylation differences between two MZ twins discordant for BPD using methylation-sensitive representational difference analysis. Bisulfite sequencing analysis confirmed that DNA methylation was altered in four genes, which became the focus of further investigation. Among the four genes, *SMS* (spermine synthase) showed epigenetic differences in female subjects in a case-control study, but the direction of the change was contrary to the finding in the twins (Kuratomi et al. 2008). The gene for peptidylprolyl isomerase E-like (*PPIEL*) showed DNA methylation differences consistent both in the twins discordant for BPD and unrelated individuals affected with BP II

Table 3.1 Main findings of DNA methylation studies in BPD

First author (year)	Tissue	Experimental technique	Findings
Dempster et al. (2006)	Brain (cerebellum) (15 BPD, 15 controls, 15 SZ, 15 MDD)	Bisulfite modification and pyrosequencing	No methylation difference of soluble isoform of *COMT*
Abdolmaleky et al. (2006)	Brain (frontal lobe) (35 BPD, 35 + 5 controls, 35 + 5 SZ)	Methylation specific PCR	*MB-COMT* is hypomethylated in BPD
Tamura et al. (2007)	Brain (forebrain) (35 BPD, 35 controls, 35 SZ)	Methylation-sensitive restriction enzymes and real-time PCR	Lack of correlation between the levels of DNA methylation in *RELN* and age in BPD
Kuratomi et al. (2008)	Lymphoblastoid cells (1 discordant MZ twin pair, 16 BPI, 7 + 14 BPII, 18 controls)	MS-RDA, bisulfite sequencing, pyrosequencing	PPIEL is differentially methylated in MZ twins discordant for BPD. PPIEL is hypomethylated in BP II disorder
Rosa et al. (2008)	Blood and buccal swabs (63 female MZ twin pairs)	Methylation-sensitive restriction enzymes and (nonquantitative) PCR	Discordant female BPD twins showed greater methylation differences between two X-chromosomes than concordant twin pairs
Mill et al. (2008)	Brain (frontal cortex) (35 BPD, 35 controls, 35 SZ). Sperm (20 BPD, 20 controls)	Epigenomic profiling by DNA microarray, bisulfite modification, pyrosequencing	DNA methylation was altered in a number of genes, but all were sex specific. No DNA methylation changes in the sperm of BPD patients
Bromberg (2009)	Peripheral blood leukocytes (49 BPD, 27 controls)	Cytosine-extension assay	Leukocyte global DNA methylation did not differ between BPD and controls

COMT the gene for catechol-*O*-methyltransferase, *MB-COMT* the gene for membrane-bound-COMT, *MS-RDA* methylation sensitive representational difference analysis, *SZ* schizophrenia, *BPD* bipolar disorder, *BP I disorder* bipolar I disorder, *BP II disorder* bipolar II disorder, *MDD* major depressive disorder, *MZ* monozygotic twins

disorder compared with controls. In the human brain, *PPIEL* is highly expressed in the pituitary gland and the substantia nigra. In another twin study, X-chromosome inactivation patterns were investigated in DNA samples from blood and/or buccal epithelial cells in a sample of 63 female MZ twin pairs concordant or discordant for BD or schizophrenia, as well as healthy MZ controls (Rosa et al. 2008). Female twins discordant for BPD showed greater DNA methylation differences in both maternal and paternal X alleles than the concordant twin pairs, which suggests that differential skewing of X-chromosome inactivation may contribute to BPD in females and the potential involvement of X-linked loci in the disorder.

3.2.2 Parental Origin Effects and Genomic Imprinting

Decades ago, it was noted that father-to-son transmission of BPD is a rare event (Winokur and Tanna 1969), and initially, this was interpreted as X-linked inheritance. McMahon and colleagues (1995) provided a new interpretation for the parental origin effects in BPD, suggesting that the disease may be transmitted by genomically imprinted genes or that transmission was related to maternal effects due to mitochondrial DNA. In the case of genomic imprinting, only one of the two inherited alleles (maternal or paternal) is expressed, while the other allele is suppressed by DNA methylation and other epigenetic mechanisms. Consequently, diseases induced by mutations in imprinted genes follow a complex inheritance pattern. Although a mutant allele is transmitted from a parent, the offspring will not express the disease if the mutated gene is imprinted (Kato et al. 1996). Linkage analysis can be performed by considering the parent-of-origin of segregating DNA markers, and several earlier studies showed that BPD is linked to chromosome 18 only when the parent-of-origin effect was considered (Gershon et al. 1996). To date, the parent-of-origin effect has been utilized several times in linkage analyses of BPD; however, detection of imprinted BPD genes is a challenging task. Recent studies of parental origin-dependent differences in gene expression in the brain demonstrated that genomic imprinting is a common and far more complex phenomenon than the "on–off" type regulation of a small group of classical imprinted genes (Gregg et al. 2010). The latter study showed that most of the imprinted genes exhibit quantitative rather than qualitative differences in expression of maternal and paternal alleles. In addition, parental origin effects are highly variable across different brain regions and dependent on the developmental stage (Gregg et al. 2010).

3.2.3 Postmortem Brain Studies

Studies of DNA methylation in postmortem brain samples from BPD patients and controls showed differences in several candidate genes, such as *COMT* (catechol-*O*-methyltransferase) (Abdolmaleky et al. 2006, Dempster et al. 2006) and Reelin (Tamura et al. 2007), but it remains unknown if these changes are causal to BPD or if they were induced by compensatory brain mechanisms, treatment, or some other disease-related factors. Thus far, only one study performed a comprehensive microarray-based search for DNA methylation differences in the postmortem brains from BPD and schizophrenia patients ($N = 105$, brain samples from the Stanley Medical Research Foundation) (Mill et al. 2008). In this study, the enriched unmethylated genomes were interrogated on 12K CpG island microarrays, which revealed DNA methylation differences in many genes with both brain- and nonspecific functions. Aberrant DNA methylation was detected in the genes involved in glutamatergic and GABAergic neurotransmission pathways, as well as in genes related to brain development in both BPD and schizophrenia females. Epigenetic differences were also observed at loci involved in stress response in male BPD patients. In addition to the locus- and gene-specific comparisons, the network analysis revealed a lower degree of DNA methylation modularity in the germline of male BPD patients (0.33) compared with the unaffected controls (0.47), which suggests that epigenetic dysfunction in BPD may involve a large group of genes and even whole nuclear compartments.

3.2.4 Miscellaneous Findings Relevant to the Epigenetic Hypothesis in BPD

Another possible epigenetic mechanism of BPD involves abnormal DNA methylation that impairs the suppression of retroelements, such as long interspersed nuclear elements (*LINEs*) (Kan et al. 2004). *LINE*1 is a repetitive sequence in the mammalian genome with more than 500,000 copies, and this sequence comprises about 17% of the human genome. Full length *LINE*1 is about 6 kb long, containing open reading frames encoding an RNA-binding protein and a protein with endonuclease and reverse-transcriptase activities that enables *LINE* elements to transpose (Cordaux and Batzer 2009). Studying human postmortem brains, Coufal and colleagues (2009) recently reported that *LINE*1 can transpose in human neural progenitor cells, and that CpG sites at the 5' untranslated region of *LINE*1 showed lower DNA methylation in fetal brain samples compared with skin samples. Since DNA methylation is thought to be one of the mechanisms that inactivate retrotransposons, deficiencies in *LINE*1 methylation in the brain may lead to increased de novo retrotransposition and, therefore, disruption of coding DNA sequences.

Higher paternal and maternal ages at conception were detected in the recent BPD studies (Menezes et al. 2010). Among several other interpretations, the effects of parental age may be explained by age-related epigenetic changes in the germline (Flanagan et al. 2006). Age-dependent aberrations in DNA methylation may be one of the risk factors for major psychiatric disease in the offspring (Perrin et al. 2007).

The role of DNA methylation in BPD is further supported by the fact that some drugs used to effectively treat this condition are epigenetic modifiers. Valproate, a mood stabilizer, acts in many ways to alleviate symptoms of BPD; in addition to numerous other effects, valproate inhibits class I histone deacetylases (HDAC) (Phiel et al. 2001) and alters DNA methylation through histone acetylation (Detich et al. 2003). Furthermore, *S*-adenosyl methionine (SAM), a methyl donor in the methylation of various targets, including DNA (Rydberg and Lindahl 1982), was shown to facilitate the switch from depression to elevated mood state in an open trial of intravenous and oral SAM (Carney et al. 1989), which also argues for the involvement of epigenetic factors in mood regulation.

3.3 Future Directions

The study of putative epigenetic misregulation in BPD has only just begun. Some findings provide potentially important insight into the etiology of BPD, but further studies will be required to elucidate the possible role of DNA methylation. Development of microarrays specifically dedicated to DNA methylation mapping is of significant value in the whole DNA methylome studies (Feinberg 2010). Furthermore, genome-wide DNA methylation analysis at the single base-pair level is now possible using next-generation sequencing technology (Lister et al. 2009). In addition to the methylation at CpG sites, non-CpG sites have also been reported to be methylated in embryonic stem cells (Lister et al. 2009). The role of such non-CpG methylation in neural stem cells is currently unknown and requires further investigation.

Several new phenomena have recently been reported, and may prove relevant to BPD. In addition to the methylated cytosine (the fifth base pair), the sixth base pair, hydroxymethylcytosine was found to be enriched in the brain (Kriaucionis and Heintz 2009). Though the functional relevance of hydroxymethylcytosine is not known, it would be of great interest to study its role in the postmortem brain of patients affected with BPD. By considering an additional regulatory mechanism in the brain, the etiology of BPD and other diseases could potentially become more apparent.

Epigenetics is a rapidly growing, cutting-edge area of molecular biology. We hope that epigenetic strategies and approaches will help to uncover the inherited and acquired basis of BPD.

References

Abdolmaleky HM, Cheng KH, Faraone SV et al (2006) Hypomethylation of MB-COMT promoter is a major risk factor for schizophrenia and bipolar disorder. Hum Mol Genet 15:3132–3145

Bromberg A, Bersudsky Y, Levine J, et al (2009) Global leukocyte DNA methylation is not altered in euthymic bipolar patients. J Affect Disord 118:234–239

Carney MW, Chary TK, Bottiglieri T et al (1989) The switch mechanism and the bipolar/unipolar dichotomy. Br J Psychiatry 154:48–51

Cordaux R, Batzer MA (2009) The impact of retrotransposons on human genome evolution. Nat Rev Genet 10:691–703

Coufal NG, Garcia-Perez JL, Peng GE et al (2009) L1 retrotransposition in human neural progenitor cells. Nature 460:1127–1131

Dempster EL, Mill J, Craig IW et al (2006) The quantification of COMT mRNA in post mortem cerebellum tissue: diagnosis, genotype, methylation and expression. BMC Med Genet 7:10

Detich N, Bovenzi V, Szyf M (2003) Valproate induces replication-independent active DNA demethylation. J Biol Chem 278:27586–27592

Feinberg AP (2010) Genome-scale approaches to the epigenetics of common human disease. Virchows Arch 456:13–21

Ferreira MA, O'Donovan MC, Meng YA et al (2008) Collaborative genome-wide association analysis supports a role for ANK3 and CACNA1C in bipolar disorder. Nat Genet 40: 1056–1058

Flanagan JM, Popendikyte V, Pozdniakovaite N et al (2006) Intra- and interindividual epigenetic variation in human germ cells. Am J Hum Genet 79:67–84

Gershon ES, Badner JA, Detera-Wadleigh SD et al (1996) Maternal inheritance and chromosome 18 allele sharing in unilineal bipolar illness pedigrees. Am J Med Genet 67:202–207

Gregg C, Zhang J, Weissbourd B, Luo S, Schroth GP, Haig D, Dulac C (2010) High-resolution analysis of parent-of-origin allelic expression in the mouse brain. Science 329(5992):643–648

Kan PX, Popendikyte V, Kaminsky ZA et al (2004) Epigenetic studies of genomic retroelements in major psychosis. Schizophr Res 67:95–106

Kato T, Winokur G, Coryell W et al (1996) Parent-of-origin effect in transmission of bipolar disorder. Am J Med Genet 67:546–550

Knight HM, Pickard BS, Maclean A et al (2009) A cytogenetic abnormality and rare coding variants identify ABCA13 as a candidate gene in schizophrenia, bipolar disorder, and depression. Am J Hum Genet 85:833–846

Kriaucionis S, Heintz N (2009) The nuclear DNA base 5-hydroxymethylcytosine is present in Purkinje neurons and the brain. Science 324:929–930

Kuratomi G, Iwamoto K, Bundo M et al (2008) Aberrant DNA methylation associated with bipolar disorder identified from discordant monozygotic twins. Mol Psychiatry 13:429–441

Lister R, Pelizzola M, Dowen RH et al (2009) Human DNA methylomes at base resolution show widespread epigenomic differences. Nature 462:315–322

McMahon FJ, Stine OC, Meyers DA et al (1995) Patterns of maternal transmission in bipolar affective disorder. Am J Hum Genet 56:1277–1286

McMahon FJ, Akula N, Schulze TG et al (2010) Meta-analysis of genome-wide association data identifies a risk locus for major mood disorders on 3p21.1. Nat Genet 42:128–131

Menezes PR, Lewis G, Rasmussen F et al (2010) Paternal and maternal ages at conception and risk of bipolar affective disorder in their offspring. Psychol Med 40:477–485

Mill J, Tang T, Kaminsky Z et al (2008) Epigenomic profiling reveals DNA-methylation changes associated with major psychosis. Am J Hum Genet 82:696–711

Perrin MC, Brown AS, Malaspina D (2007) Aberrant epigenetic regulation could explain the relationship of paternal age to schizophrenia. Schizophr Bull 33:1270–1273

Petronis A (2003) Epigenetics and bipolar disorder: new opportunities and challenges. Am J Med Genet C Semin Med Genet 123C:65–75

Phiel CJ, Zhang F, Huang EY et al (2001) Histone deacetylase is a direct target of valproic acid, a potent anticonvulsant, mood stabilizer, and teratogen. J Biol Chem 276:36734–36741

Rosa A, Picchioni MM, Kalidindi S et al (2008) Differential methylation of the X-chromosome is a possible source of discordance for bipolar disorder female monozygotic twins. Am J Med Genet B Neuropsychiatr Genet 147B:459–462

Rydberg B, Lindahl T (1982) Nonenzymatic methylation of DNA by the intracellular methyl group donor S-adenosyl-L-methionine is a potentially mutagenic reaction. EMBO J 1:211–216

Tamura Y, Kunugi H, Ohashi J et al (2007) Epigenetic aberration of the human REELIN gene in psychiatric disorders. Mol Psychiatry 12(519):593–600

Winokur G, Tanna VL (1969) Possible role of X-linked dominant factor in manic depressive disease. Dis Nerv Syst 30:89–94

Chapter 4
The Epigenetics of Depression and Suicide

Benoit Labonté and Gustavo Turecki

Abstract Major depression and suicide, which is its most severe outcome, are common problems that represent a major burden in our society. The relationship among early life adversity, depression, and suicide has already been well demonstrated, however, the molecular mechanisms mediating this relationship still remain poorly understood. From rat studies, we have recently gained major insight into some of the genomic processes that modify behavior, which result from early social environmental experiences. These processes, collectively referred to as epigenetics, are defined by chemical modifications taking place around the DNA molecule that alter the coding capacity of a gene. Accordingly, this is believed to represent an interface through which the environment can act upon our genome to modify gene expression and behavior. As such, epigenetic alterations induced by environmental factors, such as early life adversity and social stress, are found in the brain of humans and rats. In this chapter, we review the evidence in favor of epigenetic factors playing a role in depression and suicide. Animal and human postmortem studies reporting epigenetic alterations in the brain following environmental insults are discussed to generate a global scheme of epigenetic modifications, which are believed to be involved in the pathophysiology of depressive disorders and suicidality.

Keywords Depression · DNA methylation · Early-life adversity · Environment · Epigenetics · Histone modifications · Suicide

B. Labonté
McGill Group for Suicide Studies, Douglas Hospital, McGill University, Montreal, QC, Canada

G. Turecki (✉)
McGill Group for Suicide Studies, Douglas Hospital, McGill University, Montreal, QC, Canada
and
Department of Neurology and Neurosurgery, McGill University, Douglas Hospital 6875 Lasalle Blvd, Montreal, QC H3H1R3, Canada
e-mail: gustavo.turecki@mcgill.ca

A. Petronis and J. Mill (eds.), *Brain, Behavior and Epigenetics,*
Epigenetics and Human Health, DOI 10.1007/978-3-642-17426-1_4,
© Springer-Verlag Berlin Heidelberg 2011

4.1 The Burden of Depression and Suicide

Mood disorders, also known as affective disorders, are common conditions characterized by mood dysregulation and neurovegetative dysfunction (Akiskal 1995). Major depressive disorder (MDD), commonly referred to as major depression, may or may not be recurrent and represents one of the most important and common types of mood disorder. One-year prevalence estimates for MDD range between 6.4 and 10.1% (Robins and Price 1991; Regier et al. 1988; Weissman et al. 1982; Kessler et al. 2005a, b). Consequently, MDD ranks first among the most significant causes of disability and premature death, and as such, imposes a continual economic burden on society. For example, in the USA, the direct and indirect costs are estimated at $44 billion/year (Lopez and Murray 1998). The greatest loss to our society, however, is the associated mortality of MDD related to suicide. Between 50 and 70% of suicide completers die during an episode of MDD (Arsenault-Lapierre et al. 2004; Cavanagh et al. 2003), and prospective follow-up studies of MDD suggest that between 7 and 15% of these patients will die by suicide (Angst et al. 1992, 1999, 2002; Blair-West et al. 1999).

4.2 Early Life Adversity, Major Depression, and Suicide Risk

MDD and suicide are complex phenomena believed to result from the interaction of several factors. These include neurobiological (Mann 2003; Ernst et al. 2009a) and genetic factors (Brezo et al. 2008a), which increase individual predisposition to depression and suicide; psychological and personality traits such as impulsivity and negative affect (McGirr and Turecki 2007; Yen et al. 2009); demographic variables (Kwok and Shek 2008); and early life adversity (Brezo et al. 2008b; Fergusson et al. 2008).

Among risk factors, childhood abuse [sexual (CSA), physical (CPA)] and parental neglect are among the strongest predictors of depressive disorders (Molnar et al. 2001; Arnow 2004) and suicide (Evans et al. 2005; Santa Mina and Gallop 1998). In particular, CSA is associated with earlier age of onset of depression, chronic course, and more severe depressive outcome (Gladstone et al. 2004; Dinwiddie et al. 2000; Jaffee et al. 2002). Moreover, history of CSA increases the odds of suicidal behavior up to 12 times (Molnar et al. 2001; Bensley et al. 1999). Although less consistently, CPA and neglect in childhood are also found to modify the risk for depression onset, course, severity, and associated suicidality (Evans et al. 2005; Widom et al. 2007; Ystgaard et al. 2004). The detrimental long-term consequences of childhood adversity extend beyond MDD and suicidality. In addition to being associated with these phenotypes, childhood abuse has also been found to influence the risk of other psychiatric conditions and to predict increased comorbidity (Gladstone et al. 2004; Mullen et al. 1993, 1996; Jumper 1995). While personality traits and psychological adjustment difficulties may be possible mediators (Johnson et al. 1999a, b; Finkelhor and Browne 1985), there is a clear major predictor effect between history of early life adversity, MDD, and suicidality, which is independent of family psychopathological background (Nelson et al. 2002).

4.3 Early Life Adversity and Negative Mental Health Outcomes: Molecular Mechanisms

As discussed above, the relationship between childhood adversity, major depression, and suicide is supported by substantial theoretical and empirical work. It is generally assumed that adversity during childhood impacts proper psychological development and induces maladaptive patterns of behavioral responses, which, in turn, are associated with pervasive interpersonal difficulties, enhanced reactivity to stress, and an increased risk of psychopathology. However, the molecular mechanisms that account for these relationships are poorly understood. The critical question is: "How do events occurring in childhood influence the risk of becoming depressed and dying by suicide many years later?" or alternatively stated: "What long-lasting molecular mechanisms take place as a result of the adverse life experience that could be associated with increased risk for depression and suicide?" Recently, there has been growing evidence suggesting that the genome may respond to other types of environmental stimuli, beyond those of a chemical and physical nature, through epigenetic processes. Accordingly, there is mounting evidence suggesting that our genome responds to the social environment as much as it does to the physical environment, and that the basic molecular mechanism of this response is through epigenetic modifications (see Tables 4.1 and 4.2). As such, it is possible to hypothesize that epigenetic mechanisms may account, at least in part, for the regulation of behavior as a response to environmental adversity.

Epigenetics refers to the regulation of gene expression via DNA methylation (Klose and Bird 2006), histone modifications (Kouzarides 2007), and more recently, posttranscriptional mechanisms such as microRNA (Schratt 2009a, b). Generally, it has been suggested that DNA methylation directs transcriptional repression (Klose and Bird 2006). At the chromatin level, high histone acetylation and some types of histone methylation have been associated with active transcription (Kouzarides 2007). With increasing amounts of evidence suggesting that epigenetic mechanisms may be involved in the modification of gene expression induced by environmental factors, epigenetics is now believed to be one of the molecular processes induced as a response to environmental challenges. In this sense, epigenetics may be conceptualized as the means by which our cells adapt to particular cellular and environmental conditions.

Despite the complexity and the heterogeneity of depressive disorders, common functional and physiological alterations have been consistently reported in the brain of depressed and suicide subjects. For instance, stress regulatory systems

Table 4.1 Summary of published studies assessing epigenetic components in the animal's brain following environmental insults

Studies	Brain regions	Genes	Findings
Weaver et al. (2004)	Hippocampus	GR	↑ Methylation in NGFI-A binding site within GR promoter in the hippocampus of low LG/ABN pups
			Cross-fostering reinstated normal methylation levels
			↓ H3K9 acetylation levels in low LG/ABN pups
			TSA treatment reinstated promoter methylation, H3K9 acetylation, NGFI-A binding and GR1$_7$ expression
Murgatroyd et al. (2009)	Hypothalamus [paraventricular nucleus (PVN)]	AVP	↑ AVP expression correlated with hypomethylation at five sites within AVP enhancer following early life maternal separation in 6 weeks, 3 months, and 1 year mice
			↓ MeCP2 binding to AVP enhancer associated with higher AVP expression in 10 days old stress mice
Tsankova et al. (2006)	Hippocampus	BDNF	↓ Expression of BDNF transcripts (III and IV) following chronic social stress in mice
			No effect of promoter methylation on BDNF expression
			↑ H3K27 methylation in the promoter region of transcripts III and IV
			↓ HDAC5 levels associated with ↑ H3 acetylation and ↑ H3K4 methylation in the promoter of transcripts III and IV following imipramine treatment in chronically stressed mice
Roth et al. (2009)	PFC	BDNF	↓ Expression of BDNF transcripts (IV and IX) in the PFC of maternally maltreated rats
			↑ Promoter (III and IX) methylation in the PFC of maternally maltreated rats

[hypothalamic-pituitary–adrenal (HPA) axis, polyamines], cell signaling molecules [ribosomal RNA (rRNA)], brain-derived neurotrophic factor (BDNF), neurotrophic tyrosine kinase receptor (trkB), quaking (QKI) and neurotransmitters [gamma-aminobutyric acid (GABA)], and reelin and serotonin (5-HT) have all been suggested to be involved in depression and suicide. Indeed, altered expression of genes and proteins involved in the regulation of these systems has been reported in the brains of depressed and suicide subjects, and similar alterations have also been reported in the brains of animal models. With the growing interest in epigenetics, numerous studies suggest that these alterations could be due to epigenetic modifications. The following sections will review these findings.

Table 4.2 Summary of published studies assessing epigenetic components in postmortem brains of suicide completers

Studies	Brain regions	Genes	Findings
McGowan et al. (2009)	Hippocampus	GR	↑ Methylation in NGFI-A binding site within GR promoter in the hippocampus of suicide completers with history of abuse
			↓ Expression of GR in the hippocampus of suicide completers with history of abuse
McGowan et al. (2008)	Hippocampus	rRNA	Overall hypermethylation of rRNA promoter in the hippocampus of suicide completers with history of abuse
			↓ Expression of rRNA gene in the hippocampus of suicide completers with history of abuse
Ernst et al. (2009b)	Frontal cortex	TrkB-T1	↑ Methylation in two sites within the promoter of TrkB-T1 in the frontal cortex of suicide completers
			↓ Expression of TrkB-T1 in the frontal cortex of suicide completers
Ernst et al. (2009c)	Frontal cortex	TrkB-T1	↑ H3K27 methylation in the frontal cortex of suicide completers
			Negative correlation between H3K27 methylation levels and TrkB-T1 expression in the frontal cortex of suicide completers
Poulter et al. (2008)	Frontopolar cortex (FPC) Hippocampus Amygdala Brain stem	GABA$_A$ α1 DNMT1 DNMT3a DNMT3b	*FPC*: ↓ Expression of DNMT1 mRNA in suicide completers
			↑ Expression of DNMT3b mRNA and protein levels in suicide completers
			↑ Methylation at two sites in the promoter region of GABAA receptor subunit α1 in suicide completers
			Limbic system: ↓ Expression of DNMT1 and DNMT3b mRNA levels in suicide completers
			Brain stem: ↓ Expression of DNMT3b mRNA in suicide completers
Grayson et al. (2005)	Occipital cortex	Reelin, GAD67	↑ Methylation in CREB binding sites within reelin promoter in the occipital cortex of schizophrenia subjects

(*continued*)

Table 4.2 (continued)

Studies	Brain regions	Genes	Findings
Tamura et al. (2007)	Forebrain	Reelin	↑ Methylation at three sites within reelin promoter in the forebrain of schizophrenia subjects ↓ Expression of reelin mRNA in the forebrain of schizophrenia subjects
Fiori and Turecki (2010)	PFC	SMOX, SMS	No effects of promoter's methylation in SMOX and SMS on expression levels
Fiori and Turecki (unpublished)	PFC	SAT1	Negative correlation between promoter's methylation levels and expression of SAT1
De Luca et al. (2009)	PFC	5-HT2A	↓ Methylation in the promoter region of 5-HT2A receptor associated with a C-allele (trend) in the PFC of suicide completers ↑ Methylation in the promoter region of 5-HT2A receptor associated with a C-allele in leukocytes of suicide attempters
Klempan et al. (2009b)	Frontal cortex	QKI	No difference in methylation pattern between suicide completers and controls

4.4 Stress Regulatory Systems

4.4.1 Hypothalamic-Pituitary–Adrenal Axis

The HPA axis is the stress regulatory system (Pariante and Lightman 2008). When facing stressors, corticotropin-releasing factor (CRF) and vasopressin (AVP) are released from the hypothalamus. CRF and AVP induce the release of adrenocorticotropic hormone (ACTH) and proopiomelanocortin (POMC) from the pituitary gland into the blood, which reach the adrenal cortex and stimulate release of glucocorticoids – cortisol in humans and corticosterone in rodents. Glucocorticoids then act at each level of the HPA axis to regulate the stress response by decreasing the release of CRF, AVP, POMC, and ACTH. The locus of regulation of the HPA axis lies in the hippocampus, where glucocorticoids bind glucocorticoid receptors (GR) and induce an inhibitory feedback on the activation of the HPA axis to return the activity of the stress response back to basal levels.

Hyperactivity of the HPA axis is a common feature in depressed patients and childhood abuse victims. High levels of salivary, plasma, and urine glucocorticoids have been reported in depressed patients (Nemeroff and Vale 2005). Similarly, higher ACTH and cortisol levels have been reported in victims of childhood abuse following stress and dexamethasone (DEX) challenges (Heim et al. 2000, 2008). HPA axis hyperactivity is thought to be related to attenuated feedback inhibition that is normally induced by endogenous glucocorticoids at the different levels of the HPA axis. In the hippocampus, this is, in part, due to the binding of glucocorticoids to their receptor. Accordingly, rat pups raised by low licking and grooming (LG) mothers have altered the HPA axis negative feedback (Liu et al. 1997), coinciding with lower glucocorticoid receptor (GR) mRNA hippocampal levels (Liu et al. 1997), and exhibit depressive-like behavior during adulthood (Francis et al. 1999). Similarly, suicide completers with a history of childhood abuse have lower GR levels in the hippocampus (McGowan et al. 2009). Consequently, reduced levels of GR in the hippocampus of depressed patients and abuse victims could be responsible for the blunted and maladaptive responses to stress in those patients.

The GR gene is preceded by 14 noncoding exons in humans and by 10 in rats (Turner and Muller 2005; McCormick et al. 2000). These noncoding exons possess multiple transcription factor binding sites and exhibit highly variable methylation patterns (Turner et al. 2008), suggesting that they might be involved in the regulation of GR expression in different tissues. The noncoding exon 1_F and its rat homologue 1_7 are specific to the hippocampus (Turner and Muller 2005) and possess a number of canonical and noncanonical binding sites for the neural growth factor inducible A (NGFI-A) transcription factor, which is expected to play a major role in GR hippocampal expression (Meaney 2001). Accordingly, it was hypothesized that promoter hypermethylation could be responsible for the down-regulation of GR in the hippocampus of rats raised by low LG/ABN mothers and in suicide completers with a history of abuse. As a matter of fact, DNA methylation in $GR1_7$ in rats and 1_F in human promoters was shown to be elevated in both pups raised by low LG/ABN mothers (Weaver et al. 2004) and abused suicide completers (McGowan et al. 2009). Importantly, hypermethylation was found mainly within the NFGI-A-binding sites, suggesting that it could repress the binding of this transcription factor to its cognate DNA sequence and decrease the transcription of this gene. Indeed, NGFI-A was shown to significantly increase the transcriptional activity of $GR1_F$ promoter, while artificial methylation at its binding site decreases this activity, even in the presence of NGFI-A (McGowan et al. 2009).

NGFI-A has been previously shown to recruit the histone acetylase CREB-binding protein, CBP (Weaver et al. 2007). Hypermethylation within the NGFI-A-binding site could repress both the NGFI-A binding and the recruitment of CBP to the promoter of GR. This is supported by the fact that lower H3K9 acetylation and NGFI-A levels in the GR 1_7 promoter region were found in low LG/ABN pups (Weaver et al. 2004). Interestingly, cross-fostering pups from low LG/ABN mothers to high LG/ABN mothers during the first week of life was sufficient to reinstate basal methylation values, suggesting that these modifications can be reversed. Moreover, pharmacological challenge with the histone deacetylase inhibitor TSA raised H3K9 acetylation levels, restored methylation levels, increased NGFI-A binding in GR 1_7 promoter, and returned GR expression to basal levels in the hippocampus. It is also noteworthy that the treated rats were less reactive to stressful conditions.

Early life stress also affects other components of the HPA axis. Recently, it has been shown that earlylife infant–maternal separation in mice induces a long-lasting increase in corticosterone secretion accompanied by increased expression of POMC and AVP in the paraventricular nucleus (PVN) of the hypothalamus. These physiological modifications were also associated with stress-coping behavioral alterations (Murgatroyd et al. 2009). The AVP gene in mice is composed of three coding exons located on chromosome 20 at locus 20p13. Four CpG islands have been identified throughout the gene, one of which is found in the intergenic region separating the neighboring tail-to-tail-oriented *Avp* and oxytocin genes, and is known to include an enhancer region in the first 2.1 kb proximal to the *Avp* gene, which is important for *Avp* expression (Gainer et al. 2001).

The regulation of *Avp* expression in stressed mice has recently been shown to involve a dual epigenetic mechanism (Murgatroyd et al. 2009). Hypomethylation at $5'$ sites within the enhancer was strongly correlated with higher *Avp* mRNA expression in 6-week- to 1-year-old stressed mice compared with controls. In this sense, treatment with the demethylating agent 5-azacytidine decreased methylation levels and increased *Avp* expression in cell lines; the deletion of the enhancer almost completely abolished transcriptional activity in reporter assays. These observations are consistent with the repressive role of DNA methylation on transcriptional activity; however, no methylation difference was observed at 10 days. Interestingly, these sites were shown to be putative binding sites for the methylated CpG-binding protein, MeCP2, and, despite the repressive role of MeCP2 on transcription, increased expression of *Avp* was reported. Nevertheless, it has been previously suggested that neuronal depolarization might trigger Ca^{2+}/calmodulin-dependent protein kinase II (CaMKII) phosphorylation of MeCP2, causing its dissociation from putative targets (Chen et al. 2003; Zhou et al. 2006). In fact, higher CaMKII immunoreactivity and phosphorylated MeCP2 levels were found in *Avp*-expressing neurons in the PVN of 10-day-old stressed mice, suggesting that activity-induced phosphorylation of MeCP2 decreases its binding to the *Avp* enhancer and increases the expression of *Avp*. This effect can be mimicked by a site-specific hypomethylation in the enhancer of *Avp* induced by early life stress, which could be responsible for the long-lasting increased *Avp* expression in the PVN of those mice. These results suggest that alterations in DNA methylation found outside of the promoter might also be involved in physiological and behavioral modifications induced by environmental factors.

4.4.2 Polyamine System

The polyamines are important ubiquitous aliphatic molecules known to be involved in cellular function, including growth, division, and signaling cascades (Gilad and Gilad 2003; Minguet et al. 2008); but also in stress responses, both at the cellular and behavioral level (Rhee et al. 2007; Fiori and Turecki 2008). These polyamines include putrescine, spermidine, spermine, and agmatine (Moinard et al. 2005). Moreover, polyamine-associated molecules, including the polyamine oxidase (PAO), spermine synthase (SMS), spermidine/spermine *N*-acetyltransferases (SAT1,2), ornithine decarboxylase (ODC), and ornithine aminotransferase (OAT), are also involved in the polyamine system.

Many lines of evidence suggest that the polyamine system might be involved in MDD and suicide. For example, chronic unpredictable stress in rats decreases the expression of putrescine, spermidine, and spermine in the hippocampus (Genedani et al. 2001). Agmatine and putrescine have also been shown to induce antidepressant and anxiolytic effects in rodents through a mechanism thought to involve NMDA receptors (Zomkowski et al. 2002, 2006; Gong et al. 2006). In humans, agmatine and PAO levels were shown to be increased in the plasma and serum of depressed patients and were normalized following chronic bupropion and electroconvulsive therapy (ECT) treatment (Dahel et al. 2001; Halaris et al. 1999). Moreover, the expression of SMS, SAT1 and -2, and OAT has been shown to be altered in the limbic system of suicide completers with a history of depressive disorders (Sequeira et al. 2006, 2007). It is interesting to note that the polyamine system is also reactive to stressors (Gilad and Gilad 2003) – acute stressors have been shown to increase ODC activity and putrescine and agmatine levels in the brain of rodents, while chronic stress increases ODC activity and putrescine, spermine, and spermidine levels (Gilad and Gilad 2003; Aricioglu et al. 2003). Furthermore, the emergence of the characteristic adult polyamine stress response is correlated with the cessation of the hyporesponsive period of the HPA axis system (Gilad et al. 1998).

Given the alterations in the polyamine gene expression reported in the brains of suicide completers with a history of depression, the methylation patterns of particular polyamine genes were recently assessed. Promoter methylation was found to be negatively correlated with the expression of *SAT1* (Fiori et al. unpublished results), although not with the gene for spermine oxidase (*SMOX*) and *SMS* (Fiori and Turecki 2010). Moreover, no association was found between H3K27me3 modification in the promoter region of SMS and SMOX and suicide completion or expression of these genes in BA 8/9. These findings suggest that epigenetic alterations in the promoter region of genes involved in the polyamine synthesis do not play a major role in suicidal behavior, although they may partly explain why polyamine gene expression is decreased in the brain of suicide completers.

4.5 Cell Signaling

4.5.1 Ribosomal RNA

The rRNA is the principal component of the ribosome. Its role is to decode the mRNA into amino acids and to provide enzymatic activity allowing the right amino acid to be added to the synthesized polypeptides. Consequently, rRNA is a bottleneck structure for protein synthesis, allowing the right proteins to be synthesized depending on the needs of the cell.

The rRNA promoter is composed of two regulatory regions, namely the upstream control element (UCE) and the core promoter that binds the upstream binding factor (UBF) (Haltiner et al. 1986; Learned et al. 1986; Ghoshal et al. 2004). The expression of rRNA genes has been shown to be epigenetically regulated both in mice (Santoro and Grumm 2001) and humans (Ghoshal et al. 2004; Brown and Szyf 2007). In mice, the recruitment of transcription repressors has been suggested to induce chromatin modifications leading to methylation of a single CpG found within UBF-binding sites in the UCE. This is thought to prevent UBF from binding to its cognate sequence and to decrease rRNA expression (Santoro and Grumm 2001). In humans, despite the fact that the CpG density in both promoter regions differ from mice (Ghoshal et al. 2004; Santoro and Grumm 2001), rRNA expression has nevertheless been shown to be epigenetically regulated (Brown and Szyf 2007). Indeed, the active portion of the rRNA promoter associated with Pol I has been shown to be completely unmethylated, while the inactive portion is almost fully methylated (Brown and Szyf 2007).

Recently, the epigenetic regulation of rRNA expression was studied in the hippocampus of suicide completers with a history of childhood abuse (McGowan et al. 2008). Analysis of the methylation pattern in the rRNA promoter (core promoter and UCE) revealed hypermethylation on 21 out of 26 CpGs, and was associated with low rRNA expression in the hippocampus of abused suicide completers compared with controls. In other words, abused subjects showed increased overall promoter methylation compared with controls, which exhibited consistently low levels of methylation. From a mechanistic point of view, it could be hypothesized that promoter hypermethylation represses the interaction of transcription factors with the DNA sequence and consequently decreases the transcriptional activity of RNA polymerase.

It should be noted that these epigenetic alterations were restricted to the hippocampus, since no group difference in rRNA methylation pattern was found in the cerebellum, a brain region that has not been primarily associated with MDD or suicide. Moreover, among the abused suicide completers, the assessment of genome-wide methylation levels did not reveal any methylation differences, further suggesting that this epigenetic alteration was specific to the hippocampus.

4.5.2 Brain-Derived Neurotrophic Factor

Neurotrophic factors have consistently emerged as candidate molecules in the neurobiology of suicide. Neurotrophins are involved in neuronal survival and plasticity, and they are found throughout the brain, including the limbic system, where emotional behaviors are processed. Their alteration could underlie, at least in part, changes in plasticity observed in the brains of suicide completers as well as the defective affect observed in depressive patients. While the major neurotrophic factors include nerve growth factor (NGF), neurotrophin 3 and 4 (NT-3/4), fibroblast growth factor (FGF), and BDNF, the latter has received most of the attention concerning the potential implication of neurotrophic factors in MDD and suicide.

In humans, low serum and brain *BDNF* mRNA levels were found in patients with major depression (Brunoni et al. 2008; Dwivedi et al. 2003; Pandey et al. 2008), and in addition, these levels were found to be reversible by antidepressant treatment (Chen et al. 2001; Sen et al. 2008; Matrisciano et al. 2009). Depressive-like behaviors have also been reported in mice following BDNF depletion (Chan et al. 2006). In rats, chronic stress and persistent pain have been shown to reduce *BDNF* expression in the hippocampus (Gronli et al. 2006; Duric and McCarson 2005), an effect that was counteracted by antidepressant treatment (Duric and McCarson 2006; Rogoz et al. 2005; Xu et al. 2006).

Recently, the epigenetic state of *Bdnf* was assessed in mice (Tsankova et al. 2006) and rats (Roth et al. 2009). In both species, the Bdnf gene has been shown to contain nine 5′ noncoding first exons with their own promoter coding for the same protein (Aid et al. 2007). The alternative splicing of these exons specifies the tissue in which *Bdnf* is expressed (Aid et al. 2007). In mice, chronic social stress was shown to decrease the expression of two specific *Bdnf* transcripts (III and IV) in the hippocampus (Tsankova et al. 2006). Similarly, lower *Bdnf* mRNA expression has been reported in the PFC of maltreated rats (Roth et al. 2009). Although similar, these transcriptional alterations were shown to be induced by different epigenetic mechanisms. In mice, low hippocampal Bdnf levels were related to higher H3K27 methylation levels in the promoter regions transcripts III and IV, while DNA hypermethylation was found in the promoter of transcripts IV and IX of maltreated rats. Interestingly, site-specific hypermethylation in maltreated rats was reported for exon IX immediately after the maltreatment regimen, while exon IV methylation gradually increased to reach significantly altered levels only at adulthood. These findings suggest that chronic stress might alter different epigenetic mechanisms than those altered by maternal maltreatment in rodents: the first leading to the compaction of chromatin in its heterochromatic state and the second blocking the binding of transcription factors to DNA both alterations decreasing transcription of BDNF.

The effect of chronic stress on *Bdnf* transcription in mice was shown to be reversed by chronic treatment with the tricyclic antidepressant imipramine, but via an indirect pathway (Tsankova et al. 2006). Indeed, chronic imipramine treatment did not reinstate H3K27 basal methylation levels, but rather decreased HDAC5 levels in the hippocampus of chronically stressed mice. This was associated with higher hippocampal levels of H3 acetylation and H3K4me in the area of *Bdnf* III and IV promoters, with both modifications related to transcriptional activation (Kouzarides 2007). Taken together, these results suggest the existence of a compensatory mechanism in the reinstatement of basal Bdnf levels by chronic imipramine treatment following chronic stress.

4.5.3 Tropomyosin-Related Kinase B

Tropomyosin-related kinase B (TRKB) receptor is a transmembrane receptor with high affinity for BDNF, which has been consistently linked to mood disorders and suicide (Dwivedi et al. 2003, 2009; Duman and Monteggia 2006; Kim et al. 2007). For example, microarray studies have reported lower *TRKB* expression in the PFC of depressed subjects (Aston et al. 2005; Nakatani et al. 2006), and antidepressant treatment has been shown to increase its expression in cultured astrocytes (Mercier et al. 2004).

The TRKB gene is found on chromosome 9 at locus q22.1 and has five splice variants; splice variant b T1 or TRKB-T1 is an astrocytic truncated form of TRKB lacking catalytic activity (Rose et al. 2003). Recently, a subset of suicide completers with low levels of TRKB-T1 expression in the PFC were identified (Ernst et al. 2009b). Such a pattern of expression is expected to increase predispositions to suicidal behaviors.

Analysis of the methylation pattern in the promoter of those low TRKB-T1 expressors revealed two sites where methylation levels were higher in suicide completers compared with controls. The methylation pattern at those two sites was negatively correlated with the expression of TRKB-T1 in the low expression subset of suicide completers. These results were specific to the PFC, since no significant difference was found in the cerebellum. Moreover, enrichment of H3K27 methylation associated with TRKB-T1 promoter has been reported in the same subjects (Ernst et al. 2009c). This suggests that the astrocytic variant of TRKB may be under the control of epigenetic mechanisms involving histone modifications and DNA methylation, and that these epigenetic changes are involved in suicidal behavior. These findings also support the involvement of an astrocytic component in suicide. Further studies will be necessary to identify other genes expressed in astrocytes that may be altered in suicide.

4.5.4 Quaking

In the brain, quaking (QKI) is expressed specifically in oligodendrocytes and is thought to be involved in cell development and myelination processes (Ebersole et al. 1996; Zhao et al. 2006). QKI expression was reported to be decreased in schizophrenia subjects, independent of neuroleptic treatment (Aberg et al. 2006; Aston et al. 2004). More recently, its expression was also shown to be reduced in cortical regions from suicide completers (Klempan et al. 2009a).

QKI gene in human is located on chromosome 6q26 and undergoes extensive splicing leading to different isoforms, each differing in the 3' region but all exhibiting a common 5' region (Li et al. 2002; Siomi et al. 1993). It has been recently shown that alterations in methylation were not involved in the decreased cortical expression of QKI. Indeed, methylation was very low in the promoter region of both suicide completers and controls, which suggests that other mechanisms may be responsible for the modified expression of QKI in suicide completers (Klempan et al. 2009b). On the other hand, since the promoter region investigated was relatively small, it remains possible that other sites within the promoter control the expression of QKI. It is also possible that the altered expression of this gene is related to posttranslational mechanisms, such as microRNA.

4.6   Neurotransmitters and Their Receptors

4.6.1   GABA

GABA is the main inhibitory neurotransmitter in the brain – it is ubiquitous and acts as a modulator of neuronal activity. It has been frequently suggested that the GABAergic system is involved in suicide (Brezo et al. 2008a; Mann 1998), for instance, the expression of numerous GABA receptor subunits has been shown to be altered in both the PFC, frontopolar cortex (FPC) and limbic system of suicide and depressed subjects (Sequeira et al. 2007; Klempan et al. 2009a; Merali et al. 2004; Poulter et al. 2008). Decreased expression of $GABA_A$ receptor subunits $\alpha 1$, $\alpha 3$, $\alpha 4$, and δ was reported in the FPC of suicide completers compared with controls (Merali et al. 2004). Moreover, higher density of GABA neurons was reported in several brain areas, including the hippocampus in MDD suicide subjects vs. controls (Bielau et al. 2007). In contrast, these findings have been challenged by another group reporting lower density of GABA neurons in the dorsolateral PFC of MDD suicide subjects compared with controls (Rajkowska et al. 2007).

Lower expression of $GABA_A$ receptor subunit $\alpha 1$ in the FPC of suicide completers has been correlated with promoter hypermethylation (Poulter et al. 2008). Indeed, hypermethylation was reported at two specific CG sites within the promoter and the transcription start site (TSS) regions in suicide completers compared with controls. Being responsible for the addition of methyl groups to DNA, it was hypothesized that aberrant activity of DNA methyltransferases (DNMT) could be responsible for the increase in methylation reported in the promoter of the $GABA_A$ receptor $\alpha 1$ subunit. Accordingly, a significant negative correlation between DNMT3b and methylation levels in the promoter of the $\alpha 1$ subunit was reported in suicide completers (Poulter et al. 2008). Given the role of DNMT3b in de novo methylation, these findings suggest that DNMT3b could be responsible for the increased methylation found in the promoter of $GABA_A$ receptor subunit $\alpha 1$ in suicide completers. Moreover, one of the hypermethylated sites is a putative binding site for CREB (Kang et al. 1994). All together, these findings suggest that modifications in the epigenetic machinery occurring in suicide brains could generate alterations in DNA methylation patterns. Consequently, this could block the binding of transcription factors to regulatory regions and repress the expression of genes involved in fundamental neuronal processes. This suggests that histone modifications and DNA methylation might be altered in the brain of suicide completers with schizophrenia, however, it is also possible that such alterations might be found only in a subpopulation of schizophrenia subjects with a particular predisposition to commit suicide.

4.6.2   Reelin

Reelin is a protein selectively expressed in GABAergic neurons in the cortex, hippocampus, and cerebellum (Ikeda and Terashima 1997; Pesold et al. 1998), with a major role in synaptic plasticity, learning, and memory formation (Weeber et al. 2002; Beffert et al. 2006; D'Arcangelo 2005). In the cortex and hippocampus, reelin is released from the dendritic spines of glutamatergic neurons and promotes binding and phosphorylation of NMDA receptors. This results in increased protein synthesis within dendritic spines and neuronal signaling (Dong et al. 2003).

The reelin gene maps to chromosome 7q21–22, spans through 450 kb and is composed of 65 exons (Chen et al. 2002). Its promoter region is GC – rich (75%), expanding from 1,200 bp upstream to about 200 bp downstream of the TSS (Grayson et al. 2006). A 50% reduction of reelin mRNA (Guidotti et al. 2000) and an increase in DNMT1 expression (Veldic et al. 2004) were previously reported in *postmortem* brains of schizophrenia and patients with bipolar disorder, including suicide completers. In the occipital cortex, this has been associated with site-specific hypermethylation in reelin's promoter (two sites) and in the first exon following the TSS (one site) (Grayson et al. 2005), both regions with putative CREB-binding site. Similarly, Tamura et al. (2007) found a significant negative correlation between reelin expression and methylation level at three different CG sites in reelin's promoter.

4.6.3   Serotonin

The serotonergic system has been associated with MDD and suicidality (Brezo et al. 2008a; Mann 1998), with lower concentration, binding, neurotransmission, and reuptake of serotonin and its metabolites representing risk markers for suicidality and MDD (Cronholm et al. 1977; Bhagwagar and Cowen 2008). Particular attention has been given to the 5-HT$_{2A}$ receptor gene as being a major candidate in association studies of suicidal behavior (Du et al. 2001). The 5-HT$_{2A}$ receptor gene polymorphism T102C has been extensively studied and the CC genotype has been previously associated with higher scores in the Hamilton depression scale HAMD (Du et al. 2000), suicidal ideation (Du et al. 2000), and suicidal attempts (Arias et al. 2001), however, these findings failed to be replicated by other groups (Vaquero-Lorenzo et al. 2008; Li et al. 2006). The C allele does not alter the amino acid sequence, although it may modify the secondary structure of mRNA (Arranz et al. 1995) and thus generates less transcriptionally active mRNA than the T allele (Polesskaya and Sokolov 2002). Moreover, the C allele has been associated with lower 5-HT$_{2A}$ receptor binding in postmortem suicide brains (Turecki et al. 1999).

Recently, De Luca et al. (2009) investigated C allele methylation levels in suicide and control subjects with schizophrenia, based on the hypothesis that the 102T/C polymorphism might directly influence 5-HT$_{2A}$ mRNA levels through methylation of the C allele. A trend toward lower C allele methylation levels in the PFC of suicide completers compared with controls was initially reported. On the other hand, hypermethylation was found in leukocytes from patients with a history of lifetime suicide attempts. These findings suggest that methylation levels of the C allele may be different in individuals who have committed suicide than in those who are planning or attempting suicide. The same group previously showed that the C/T allele expression ratio was significantly smaller in the PFC of suicide subjects compared with controls (De Luca et al. 2007). With their latest results, the authors suggest that the 102C allele may generate a repressor binding site, which would explain lower steady mRNA level of the C allele. Thus, methylation at this particular site could abolish the repressiveness of this site by blocking the binding of the repressor to its cognate sequence, thereby increasing 102C allele expression in the PFC of suicide subjects with schizophrenia (De Luca et al. 2009); however, functional studies are required to validate this hypothesis.

4.7 Concluding Remarks

Although we have increased our knowledge concerning the role of epigenetic factors in depressive disorders and suicide over the last few years, we are still far from understanding how environmental events induce specific alterations at the level of DNA, mRNA, and proteins. For now, strong direct experimental evidence in rats and indirect retrospective evidence in humans support the fact that environmental factors could alter the epigenetic mechanisms that govern expression of genes thought to be involved in the control of important neuronal processes, which, in turn, are associated with behavioral changes. The majority of studies performed to date have explored candidate genes hypothesized to be involved in the pathophysiology of major depression and suicide, but, while these studies are important, they are limited in scope. Consequently, the time has come to examine epigenetic alterations on a large scale. For instance, genome-wide high throughput comparative hybridization arrays, large scale genome-based "deep" sequencing and ChIP-based methods assessing histone modifications are now available. These large-scale studies will open the door to the systematic investigation of epigenetic effects that may be involved in suicide risk and allow the future development of novel and more targeted therapeutic strategies.

References

Aberg K, Saetre P, Lindholm E, Ekholm B, Pettersson U, Adolfsson R, Jazin E (2006) Human QKI, a new candidate gene for schizophrenia involved in myelination. Am J Med Genet B Neuropsychiatr Genet 141B:84–90

Aid T, Kazantseva A, Piirsoo M, Palm K, Timmusk T (2007) Mouse and rat BDNF gene structure and expression revisited. J Neurosci Res 85:525–535

Akiskal HS (1995) Developmental pathways to bipolarity: are juvenile-onset depressions pre-bipolar? J Am Acad Child Adolesc Psychiatry 34:754–763

Angst J, Degonda M, Ernst C (1992) The Zurich Study: XV. Suicide attempts in a cohort from age 20 to 30. Eur Arch Psychiatry Clin Neurosci 242:135–141

Angst J, Angst F, Stassen HH (1999) Suicide risk in patients with major depressive disorder. J Clin Psychiatry 60(Suppl 2):57–62, discussion 75–56, 113–116

Angst F, Stassen HH, Clayton PJ, Angst J (2002) Mortality of patients with mood disorders: follow-up over 34-38 years. J Affect Disord 68:167–181

Arias B, Gasto C, Catalan R, Gutierrez B, Pintor L, Fananas L (2001) The 5-HT(2A) receptor gene 102T/C polymorphism is associated with suicidal behavior in depressed patients. Am J Med Genet 105:801–804

Aricioglu F, Regunathan S, Piletz JE (2003) Is agmatine an endogenous factor against stress? Ann N Y Acad Sci 1009:127–132

Arnow BA (2004) Relationships between childhood maltreatment, adult health and psychiatric outcomes, and medical utilization. J Clin Psychiatry 65(Suppl 12):10–15

Arranz M, Collier D, Sodhi M, Ball D, Roberts G, Price J, Sham P, Kerwin R (1995) Association between clozapine response and allelic variation in 5-HT2A receptor gene. Lancet 346:281–282

Arsenault-Lapierre G, Kim C, Turecki G (2004) Psychiatric diagnoses in 3275 suicides: a meta-analysis. BMC Psychiatry 4:37

Aston C, Jiang L, Sokolov BP (2004) Microarray analysis of postmortem temporal cortex from patients with schizophrenia. J Neurosci Res 77:858–866

Aston C, Jiang L, Sokolov BP (2005) Transcriptional profiling reveals evidence for signaling and oligodendroglial abnormalities in the temporal cortex from patients with major depressive disorder. Mol Psychiatry 10:309–322

Beffert U, Durudas A, Weeber EJ, Stolt PC, Giehl KM, Sweatt JD, Hammer RE, Herz J (2006) Functional dissection of Reelin signaling by site-directed disruption of Disabled-1 adaptor binding to apolipoprotein E receptor 2: distinct roles in development and synaptic plasticity. J Neurosci 26:2041–2052

Bensley LS, Van Eenwyk J, Spieker SJ, Schoder J (1999) Self-reported abuse history and adolescent problem behaviors. I. Antisocial and suicidal behaviors. J Adolesc Health 24:163–172

Bhagwagar Z, Cowen PJ (2008) 'It's not over when it's over': persistent neurobiological abnormalities in recovered depressed patients. Psychol Med 38:307–313

Bielau H, Steiner J, Mawrin C, Trubner K, Brisch R, Meyer-Lotz G, Brodhun M, Dobrowolny H, Baumann B, Gos T, Bernstein HG, Bogerts B (2007) Dysregulation of GABAergic neurotransmission in mood disorders: a postmortem study. Ann N Y Acad Sci 1096:157–169

Blair-West GW, Cantor CH, Mellsop GW, Eyeson-Annan ML (1999) Lifetime suicide risk in major depression: sex and age determinants. J Affect Disord 55:171–178

Brezo J, Klempan T, Turecki G (2008a) The genetics of suicide: a critical review of molecular studies. Psychiatr Clin North Am 31:179–203

Brezo J, Paris J, Vitaro F, Hebert M, Tremblay RE, Turecki G (2008b) Predicting suicide attempts in young adults with histories of childhood abuse. Br J Psychiatry 193:134–139

Brown SE, Szyf M (2007) Epigenetic programming of the rRNA promoter by MBD3. Mol Cell Biol 27:4938–4952

Brunoni AR, Lopes M, Fregni F (2008) A systematic review and meta-analysis of clinical studies on major depression and BDNF levels: implications for the role of neuroplasticity in depression. Int J Neuropsychopharmacol 11:1169–1180

Cavanagh JT, Carson AJ, Sharpe M, Lawrie SM (2003) Psychological autopsy studies of suicide: a systematic review. Psychol Med 33:395–405

Chan JP, Unger TJ, Byrnes J, Rios M (2006) Examination of behavioral deficits triggered by targeting Bdnf in fetal or postnatal brains of mice. Neuroscience 142:49–58

Chen B, Dowlatshahi D, MacQueen GM, Wang JF, Young LT (2001) Increased hippocampal BDNF immunoreactivity in subjects treated with antidepressant medication. Biol Psychiatry 50:260–265

Chen Y, Sharma RP, Costa RH, Costa E, Grayson DR (2002) On the epigenetic regulation of the human reelin promoter. Nucleic Acids Res 30:2930–2939

Chen WG, Chang Q, Lin Y, Meissner A, West AE, Griffith EC, Jaenisch R, Greenberg ME (2003) Derepression of BDNF transcription involves calcium-dependent phosphorylation of MeCP2. Science 302:885–889

Cronholm B, Asberg M, Montgomery S, Schalling D (1977) Suicidal behaviour syndrome with low CSF 5-HIAA. Br Med J 1:776

D'Arcangelo G (2005) Apoer2: a reelin receptor to remember. Neuron 47:471–473

Dahel KA, Al-Saffar NM, Flayeh KA (2001) Polyamine oxidase activity in sera of depressed and schizophrenic patients after ECT treatment. Neurochem Res 26:415–418

De Luca V, Likhodi O, Kennedy JL, Wong AH (2007) Differential expression and parent-of-origin effect of the 5-HT2A receptor gene C102T polymorphism: analysis of suicidality in schizophrenia and bipolar disorder. Am J Med Genet B Neuropsychiatr Genet 144B:370–374

De Luca V, Viggiano E, Dhoot R, Kennedy JL, Wong AH (2009) Methylation and QTDT analysis of the 5-HT2A receptor 102C allele: analysis of suicidality in major psychosis. J Psychiatr Res 43:532–537

Dinwiddie S, Heath AC, Dunne MP, Bucholz KK, Madden PA, Slutske WS, Bierut LJ, Statham DB, Martin NG (2000) Early sexual abuse and lifetime psychopathology: a co-twin-control study. Psychol Med 30:41–52

Dong E, Caruncho H, Liu WS, Smalheiser NR, Grayson DR, Costa E, Guidotti A (2003) A reelin-integrin receptor interaction regulates Arc mRNA translation in synaptoneurosomes. Proc Natl Acad Sci USA 100:5479–5484

Du L, Bakish D, Lapierre YD, Ravindran AV, Hrdina PD (2000) Association of polymorphism of serotonin 2A receptor gene with suicidal ideation in major depressive disorder. Am J Med Genet 96:56–60

Du L, Faludi G, Palkovits M, Bakish D, Hrdina PD (2001) Serotonergic genes and suicidality. Crisis 22:54–60

Duman RS, Monteggia LM (2006) A neurotrophic model for stress-related mood disorders. Biol Psychiatry 59:1116–1127

Duric V, McCarson KE (2005) Hippocampal neurokinin-1 receptor and brain-derived neurotrophic factor gene expression is decreased in rat models of pain and stress. Neuroscience 133:999–1006

Duric V, McCarson KE (2006) Effects of analgesic or antidepressant drugs on pain- or stress-evoked hippocampal and spinal neurokinin-1 receptor and brain-derived neurotrophic factor gene expression in the rat. J Pharmacol Exp Ther 319:1235–1243

Dwivedi Y, Rizavi HS, Conley RR, Roberts RC, Tamminga CA, Pandey GN (2003) Altered gene expression of brain-derived neurotrophic factor and receptor tyrosine kinase B in postmortem brain of suicide subjects. Arch Gen Psychiatry 60:804–815

Dwivedi Y, Rizavi HS, Zhang H, Mondal AC, Roberts RC, Conley RR, Pandey GN (2009) Neurotrophin receptor activation and expression in human postmortem brain: effect of suicide. Biol Psychiatry 65:319–328

Ebersole TA, Chen Q, Justice MJ, Artzt K (1996) The quaking gene product necessary in embryogenesis and myelination combines features of RNA binding and signal transduction proteins. Nat Genet 12:260–265

Ernst C, Mechawar N, Turecki G (2009) Suicide neurobiology. Prog Neurobiol

Ernst C, Deleva V, Deng X, Sequeira A, Pomarenski A, Klempan T, Ernst N, Quirion R, Gratton A, Szyf M, Turecki G (2009b) Alternative splicing, methylation state, and expression profile of tropomyosin-related kinase B in the frontal cortex of suicide completers. Arch Gen Psychiatry 66:22–32

Ernst C, Chen ES, Turecki G (2009c) Histone methylation and decreased expression of TrkB.T1 in orbital frontal cortex of suicide completers. Mol Psychiatry 14:830–832

Evans E, Hawton K, Rodham K (2005) Suicidal phenomena and abuse in adolescents: a review of epidemiological studies. Child Abuse Negl 29:45–58

Fergusson DM, Boden JM, Horwood LJ (2008) Exposure to childhood sexual and physical abuse and adjustment in early adulthood. Child Abuse Negl 32:607–619

Finkelhor D, Browne A (1985) The traumatic impact of child sexual abuse: a conceptualization. Am J Orthopsychiatry 55:530–541

Fiori LM, Turecki G (2008) Implication of the polyamine system in mental disorders. J Psychiatry Neurosci 33:102–110

Fiori LM, Turecki G (2010) Genetic and epigenetic influence on expression of spermine synthase and spermine oxidase in suicide completers. Int J Neuropsychopharmacol 13(6):725–736. Epub 2010 Jan 11

Francis D, Diorio J, Liu D, Meaney MJ (1999) Nongenomic transmission across generations of maternal behavior and stress responses in the rat. Science 286:1155–1158

Gainer H, Fields RL, House SB (2001) Vasopressin gene expression: experimental models and strategies. Exp Neurol 171:190–199

Genedani S, Saltini S, Benelli A, Filaferro M, Bertolini A (2001) Influence of SAMe on the modifications of brain polyamine levels in an animal model of depression. Neuroreport 12: 3939–3942

Ghoshal K, Majumder S, Datta J, Motiwala T, Bai S, Sharma SM, Frankel W, Jacob ST (2004) Role of human ribosomal RNA (rRNA) promoter methylation and of methyl-CpG-binding protein MBD2 in the suppression of rRNA gene expression. J Biol Chem 279:6783–6793

Gilad GM, Gilad VH (2003) Overview of the brain polyamine-stress-response: regulation, development, and modulation by lithium and role in cell survival. Cell Mol Neurobiol 23:637–649

Gilad GM, Gilad VH, Eliyayev Y, Rabey JM (1998) Developmental regulation of the brain polyamine-stress-response. Int J Dev Neurosci 16:271–278

Gladstone GL, Parker GB, Mitchell PB, Malhi GS, Wilhelm K, Austin MP (2004) Implications of childhood trauma for depressed women: an analysis of pathways from childhood sexual abuse to deliberate self-harm and revictimization. Am J Psychiatry 161:1417–1425

Gong ZH, Li YF, Zhao N, Yang HJ, Su RB, Luo ZP, Li J (2006) Anxiolytic effect of agmatine in rats and mice. Eur J Pharmacol 550:112–116

Grayson DR, Jia X, Chen Y, Sharma RP, Mitchell CP, Guidotti A, Costa E (2005) Reelin promoter hypermethylation in schizophrenia. Proc Natl Acad Sci USA 102:9341–9346

Grayson DR, Chen Y, Costa E, Dong E, Guidotti A, Kundakovic M, Sharma RP (2006) The human reelin gene: transcription factors (+), repressors (-) and the methylation switch (+/-) in schizophrenia. Pharmacol Ther 111:272–286

Gronli J, Bramham C, Murison R, Kanhema T, Fiske E, Bjorvatn B, Ursin R, Portas CM (2006) Chronic mild stress inhibits BDNF protein expression and CREB activation in the dentate gyrus but not in the hippocampus proper. Pharmacol Biochem Behav 85:842–849

Guidotti A, Auta J, Davis JM, Di-Giorgi-Gerevini V, Dwivedi Y, Grayson DR, Impagnatiello F, Pandey G, Pesold C, Sharma R, Uzunov D, Costa E (2000) Decrease in reelin and glutamic acid decarboxylase67 (GAD67) expression in schizophrenia and bipolar disorder: a postmortem brain study. Arch Gen Psychiatry 57:1061–1069

Halaris A, Zhu H, Feng Y, Piletz JE (1999) Plasma agmatine and platelet imidazoline receptors in depression. Ann N Y Acad Sci 881:445–451

Haltiner MM, Smale ST, Tjian R (1986) Two distinct promoter elements in the human rRNA gene identified by linker scanning mutagenesis. Mol Cell Biol 6:227–235

Heim C, Newport DJ, Heit S, Graham YP, Wilcox M, Bonsall R, Miller AH, Nemeroff CB (2000) Pituitary-adrenal and autonomic responses to stress in women after sexual and physical abuse in childhood. J Am Med Assoc 284:592–597

Heim C, Mletzko T, Purselle D, Musselman DL, Nemeroff CB (2008) The dexamethasone/corticotropin-releasing factor test in men with major depression: role of childhood trauma. Biol Psychiatry 63:398–405

Ikeda Y, Terashima T (1997) Expression of reelin, the gene responsible for the reeler mutation, in embryonic development and adulthood in the mouse. Dev Dyn 210:157–172

Jaffee SR, Moffitt TE, Caspi A, Fombonne E, Poulton R, Martin J (2002) Differences in early childhood risk factors for juvenile-onset and adult-onset depression. Arch Gen Psychiatry 59: 215–222

Johnson JG, Cohen P, Skodol AE, Oldham JM, Kasen S, Brook JS (1999a) Personality disorders in adolescence and risk of major mental disorders and suicidality during adulthood. Arch Gen Psychiatry 56:805–811

Johnson WB, Lall R, Bongar B, Nordlund MD (1999b) The role of objective personality inventories in suicide risk assessment: an evaluation and proposal. Suicide Life Threat Behav 29: 165–185

Jumper SA (1995) A meta-analysis of the relationship of child sexual abuse to adult psychological adjustment. Child Abuse Negl 19:715–728

Kang I, Lindquist DG, Kinane TB, Ercolani L, Pritchard GA, Miller LG (1994) Isolation and characterization of the promoter of the human GABAA receptor alpha 1 subunit gene. J Neurochem 62:1643–1646

Kessler RC, Chiu WT, Demler O, Merikangas KR, Walters EE (2005a) Prevalence, severity, and comorbidity of 12-month DSM-IV disorders in the National Comorbidity Survey Replication. Arch Gen Psychiatry 62:617–627

Kessler D, Sharp D, Lewis G (2005b) Screening for depression in primary care. Br J Gen Pract 55:659–660

Kim YK, Lee HP, Won SD, Park EY, Lee HY, Lee BH, Lee SW, Yoon D, Han C, Kim DJ, Choi SH (2007) Low plasma BDNF is associated with suicidal behavior in major depression. Prog Neuropsychopharmacol Biol Psychiatry 31:78–85

Klempan TA, Sequeira A, Canetti L, Lalovic A, Ernst C, ffrench-Mullen J, Turecki G (2009a) Altered expression of genes involved in ATP biosynthesis and GABAergic neurotransmission in the ventral prefrontal cortex of suicides with and without major depression. Mol Psychiatry 14:175–189

Klempan TA, Ernst C, Deleva V, Labonte B, Turecki G (2009b) Characterization of QKI gene expression, genetics, and epigenetics in suicide victims with major depressive disorder. Biol Psychiatry 66:824–831

Klose RJ, Bird AP (2006) Genomic DNA methylation: the mark and its mediators. Trends Biochem Sci 31:89–97

Kouzarides T (2007) Chromatin modifications and their function. Cell 128:693–705

Kwok SY, Shek DT (2008) Socio-demographic correlates of suicidal ideation among Chinese adolescents in Hong Kong. Int J Adolesc Med Health 20:463–472

Learned RM, Learned TK, Haltiner MM, Tjian RT (1986) Human rRNA transcription is modulated by the coordinate binding of two factors to an upstream control element. Cell 45:847–857

Li ZZ, Kondo T, Murata T, Ebersole TA, Nishi T, Tada K, Ushio Y, Yamamura K, Abe K (2002) Expression of Hqk encoding a KH RNA binding protein is altered in human glioma. Jpn J Cancer Res 93:167–177

Li D, Duan Y, He L (2006) Association study of serotonin 2A receptor (5-HT2A) gene with schizophrenia and suicidal behavior using systematic meta-analysis. Biochem Biophys Res Commun 340:1006–1015

Liu D, Diorio J, Tannenbaum B, Caldji C, Francis D, Freedman A, Sharma S, Pearson D, Plotsky PM, Meaney MJ (1997) Maternal care, hippocampal glucocorticoid receptors, and hypothalamic-pituitary-adrenal responses to stress. Science 277:1659–1662

Lopez AD, Murray CC (1998) The global burden of disease, 1990–2020. Nat Med 4:1241–1243

Mann JJ (1998) The neurobiology of suicide. Nat Med 4:25–30

Mann JJ (2003) Neurobiology of suicidal behaviour. Nat Rev Neurosci 4:819–828

Matrisciano F, Bonaccorso S, Ricciardi A, Scaccianoce S, Panaccione I, Wang L, Ruberto A, Tatarelli R, Nicoletti F, Girardi P, Shelton RC (2009) Changes in BDNF serum levels in patients with major depression disorder (MDD) after 6 months treatment with sertraline, escitalopram, or venlafaxine. J Psychiatr Res 43:247–254

McCormick JA, Lyons V, Jacobson MD, Noble J, Diorio J, Nyirenda M, Weaver S, Ester W, Yau JL, Meaney MJ, Seckl JR, Chapman KE (2000) 5′-heterogeneity of glucocorticoid receptor messenger RNA is tissue specific: differential regulation of variant transcripts by early-life events. Mol Endocrinol 14:506–517

McGirr A, Turecki G (2007) The relationship of impulsive aggressiveness to suicidality and other depression-linked behaviors. Curr Psychiatry Rep 9:460–466

McGowan PO, Sasaki A, Huang TC, Unterberger A, Suderman M, Ernst C, Meaney MJ, Turecki G, Szyf M (2008) Promoter-wide hypermethylation of the ribosomal RNA gene promoter in the suicide brain. PLoS One 3:e2085

McGowan PO, Sasaki A, D'Alessio AC, Dymov S, Labonte B, Szyf M, Turecki G, Meaney MJ (2009) Epigenetic regulation of the glucocorticoid receptor in human brain associates with childhood abuse. Nat Neurosci 12:342–348

Meaney MJ (2001) Maternal care, gene expression, and the transmission of individual differences in stress reactivity across generations. Annu Rev Neurosci 24:1161–1192

Merali Z, Du L, Hrdina P, Palkovits M, Faludi G, Poulter MO, Anisman H (2004) Dysregulation in the suicide brain: mRNA expression of corticotropin-releasing hormone receptors and GABA (A) receptor subunits in frontal cortical brain region. J Neurosci 24:1478–1485

Mercier G, Lennon AM, Renouf B, Dessouroux A, Ramauge M, Courtin F, Pierre M (2004) MAP kinase activation by fluoxetine and its relation to gene expression in cultured rat astrocytes. J Mol Neurosci 24:207–216

Minguet EG, Vera-Sirera F, Marina A, Carbonell J, Blazquez MA (2008) Evolutionary diversification in polyamine biosynthesis. Mol Biol Evol 25:2119–2128

Moinard C, Cynober L, de Bandt JP (2005) Polyamines: metabolism and implications in human diseases. Clin Nutr 24:184–197

Molnar BE, Berkman LF, Buka SL (2001) Psychopathology, childhood sexual abuse and other childhood adversities: relative links to subsequent suicidal behaviour in the US. Psychol Med 31:965–977

Mullen PE, Martin JL, Anderson JC, Romans SE, Herbison GP (1993) Childhood sexual abuse and mental health in adult life. Br J Psychiatry 163:721–732

Mullen PE, Martin JL, Anderson JC, Romans SE, Herbison GP (1996) The long-term impact of the physical, emotional, and sexual abuse of children: a community study. Child Abuse Negl 20:7–21

Murgatroyd C, Patchev AV, Wu Y, Micale V, Bockmuhl Y, Fischer D, Holsboer F, Wotjak CT, Almeida OF, Spengler D (2009) Dynamic DNA methylation programs persistent adverse effects of early-life stress. Nat Neurosci

Nakatani N, Hattori E, Ohnishi T, Dean B, Iwayama Y, Matsumoto I, Kato T, Osumi N, Higuchi T, Niwa S, Yoshikawa T (2006) Genome-wide expression analysis detects eight genes with robust alterations specific to bipolar I disorder: relevance to neuronal network perturbation. Hum Mol Genet 15:1949–1962

Nelson EC, Heath AC, Madden PA, Cooper ML, Dinwiddie SH, Bucholz KK, Glowinski A, McLaughlin T, Dunne MP, Statham DJ, Martin NG (2002) Association between self-reported childhood sexual abuse and adverse psychosocial outcomes: results from a twin study. Arch Gen Psychiatry 59:139–145

Nemeroff CB, Vale WW (2005) The neurobiology of depression: inroads to treatment and new drug discovery. J Clin Psychiatry 66(Suppl 7):5–13

Pandey GN, Ren X, Rizavi HS, Conley RR, Roberts RC, Dwivedi Y (2008) Brain-derived neurotrophic factor and tyrosine kinase B receptor signalling in post-mortem brain of teenage suicide victims. Int J Neuropsychopharmacol 11:1047–1061

Pariante CM, Lightman SL (2008) The HPA axis in major depression: classical theories and new developments. Trends Neurosci 31:464–468

Pesold C, Impagnatiello F, Pisu MG, Uzunov DP, Costa E, Guidotti A, Caruncho HJ (1998) Reelin is preferentially expressed in neurons synthesizing gamma-aminobutyric acid in cortex and hippocampus of adult rats. Proc Natl Acad Sci USA 95:3221–3226

Polesskaya OO, Sokolov BP (2002) Differential expression of the "C" and "T" alleles of the 5-HT2A receptor gene in the temporal cortex of normal individuals and schizophrenics. J Neurosci Res 67:812–822

Poulter MO, Du L, Weaver IC, Palkovits M, Faludi G, Merali Z, Szyf M, Anisman H (2008) GABAA receptor promoter hypermethylation in suicide brain: implications for the involvement of epigenetic processes. Biol Psychiatry 64:645–652

Rajkowska G, O'Dwyer G, Teleki Z, Stockmeier CA, Miguel-Hidalgo JJ (2007) GABAergic neurons immunoreactive for calcium binding proteins are reduced in the prefrontal cortex in major depression. Neuropsychopharmacology 32:471–482

Regier DA, Hirschfeld RM, Goodwin FK, Burke JD Jr, Lazar JB, Judd LL (1988) The NIMH depression awareness, recognition, and treatment program: structure, aims, and scientific basis. Am J Psychiatry 145:1351–1357

Rhee HJ, Kim EJ, Lee JK (2007) Physiological polyamines: simple primordial stress molecules. J Cell Mol Med 11:685–703

Robins LN, Price RK (1991) Adult disorders predicted by childhood conduct problems: results from the NIMH epidemiologic catchment area project. Psychiatry 54:116–132

Rogoz Z, Skuza G, Legutko B (2005) Repeated treatment with mirtazepine induces brain-derived neurotrophic factor gene expression in rats. J Physiol Pharmacol 56:661–671

Rose CR, Blum R, Pichler B, Lepier A, Kafitz KW, Konnerth A (2003) Truncated TrkB-T1 mediates neurotrophin-evoked calcium signalling in glia cells. Nature 426:74–78

Roth TL, Lubin FD, Funk AJ, Sweatt JD (2009) Lasting epigenetic influence of early-life adversity on the BDNF gene. Biol Psychiatry 65:760–769

Santa Mina EE, Gallop RM (1998) Childhood sexual and physical abuse and adult self-harm and suicidal behaviour: a literature review. Can J Psychiatry 43:793–800

Santoro R, Grummt I (2001) Molecular mechanisms mediating methylation-dependent silencing of ribosomal gene transcription. Mol Cell 8:719–725

Schratt G (2009a) microRNAs at the synapse. Nat Rev Neurosci 10:842–849

Schratt G (2009b) Fine-tuning neural gene expression with microRNAs. Curr Opin Neurobiol 19: 213–219

Sen S, Duman R, Sanacora G (2008) Serum brain-derived neurotrophic factor, depression, and antidepressant medications: meta-analyses and implications. Biol Psychiatry 64:527–532

Sequeira A, Gwadry FG, Ffrench-Mullen JM, Canetti L, Gingras Y, Casero RA Jr, Rouleau G, Benkelfat C, Turecki G (2006) Implication of SSAT by gene expression and genetic variation in suicide and major depression. Arch Gen Psychiatry 63:35–48

Sequeira A, Klempan T, Canetti L, ffrench-Mullen J, Benkelfat C, Rouleau GA, Turecki G (2007) Patterns of gene expression in the limbic system of suicides with and without major depression. Mol Psychiatry 12:640–655

Siomi H, Matunis MJ, Michael WM, Dreyfuss G (1993) The pre-mRNA binding K protein contains a novel evolutionarily conserved motif. Nucleic Acids Res 21:1193–1198

Tamura Y, Kunugi H, Ohashi J, Hohjoh H (2007) Epigenetic aberration of the human REELIN gene in psychiatric disorders. Mol Psychiatry 12(519):593–600

Tsankova NM, Berton O, Renthal W, Kumar A, Neve RL, Nestler EJ (2006) Sustained hippocampal chromatin regulation in a mouse model of depression and antidepressant action. Nat Neurosci 9:519–525

Turecki G, Briere R, Dewar K, Antonetti T, Lesage AD, Seguin M, Chawky N, Vanier C, Alda M, Joober R, Benkelfat C, Rouleau GA (1999) Prediction of level of serotonin 2A receptor binding by serotonin receptor 2A genetic variation in postmortem brain samples from subjects who did or did not commit suicide. Am J Psychiatry 156:1456–1458

Turner JD, Muller CP (2005) Structure of the glucocorticoid receptor (NR3C1) gene 5′ untranslated region: identification, and tissue distribution of multiple new human exon 1. J Mol Endocrinol 35:283–292

Turner JD, Pelascini LP, Macedo JA, Muller CP (2008) Highly individual methylation patterns of alternative glucocorticoid receptor promoters suggest individualized epigenetic regulatory mechanisms. Nucleic Acids Res 36:7207–7218

Vaquero-Lorenzo C, Baca-Garcia E, Diaz-Hernandez M, Perez-Rodriguez MM, Fernandez-Navarro P, Giner L, Carballo JJ, Saiz-Ruiz J, Fernandez-Piqueras J, Baldomero EB, de Leon J, Oquendo MA (2008) Association study of two polymorphisms of the serotonin-2A receptor gene and suicide attempts. Am J Med Genet B Neuropsychiatr Genet 147B: 645–649

Veldic M, Caruncho HJ, Liu WS, Davis J, Satta R, Grayson DR, Guidotti A, Costa E (2004) DNA-methyltransferase 1 mRNA is selectively overexpressed in telencephalic GABAergic interneurons of schizophrenia brains. Proc Natl Acad Sci USA 101:348–353

Weaver IC, Cervoni N, Champagne FA, D'Alessio AC, Sharma S, Seckl JR, Dymov S, Szyf M, Meaney MJ (2004) Epigenetic programming by maternal behavior. Nat Neurosci 7:847–854

Weaver IC, D'Alessio AC, Brown SE, Hellstrom IC, Dymov S, Sharma S, Szyf M, Meaney MJ (2007) The transcription factor nerve growth factor-inducible protein a mediates epigenetic programming: altering epigenetic marks by immediate-early genes. J Neurosci 27:1756–1768

Weeber EJ, Beffert U, Jones C, Christian JM, Forster E, Sweatt JD, Herz J (2002) Reelin and ApoE receptors cooperate to enhance hippocampal synaptic plasticity and learning. J Biol Chem 277:39944–39952

Weissman MM, Kidd KK, Prusoff BA (1982) Variability in rates of affective disorders in relatives of depressed and normal probands. Arch Gen Psychiatry 39:1397–1403

Widom CS, DuMont K, Czaja SJ (2007) A prospective investigation of major depressive disorder and comorbidity in abused and neglected children grown up. Arch Gen Psychiatry 64:49–56

Xu H, Chen Z, He J, Haimanot S, Li X, Dyck L, Li XM (2006) Synergetic effects of quetiapine and venlafaxine in preventing the chronic restraint stress-induced decrease in cell proliferation and BDNF expression in rat hippocampus. Hippocampus 16:551–559

Yen S, Shea MT, Sanislow CA, Skodol AE, Grilo CM, Edelen MO, Stout RL, Morey LC, Zanarini MC, Markowitz JC, McGlashan TH, Daversa MT, Gunderson JG (2009) Personality traits as prospective predictors of suicide attempts. Acta Psychiatr Scand 120:222–229

Ystgaard M, Hestetun I, Loeb M, Mehlum L (2004) Is there a specific relationship between childhood sexual and physical abuse and repeated suicidal behavior? Child Abuse Negl 28: 863–875

Zhao L, Ku L, Chen Y, Xia M, LoPresti P, Feng Y (2006) QKI binds MAP1B mRNA and enhances MAP1B expression during oligodendrocyte development. Mol Biol Cell 17:4179–4186

Zhou Z, Hong EJ, Cohen S, Zhao WN, Ho HY, Schmidt L, Chen WG, Lin Y, Savner E, Griffith EC, Hu L, Steen JA, Weitz CJ, Greenberg ME (2006) Brain-specific phosphorylation of MeCP2 regulates activity-dependent Bdnf transcription, dendritic growth, and spine maturation. Neuron 52:255–269

Zomkowski AD, Hammes L, Lin J, Calixto JB, Santos AR, Rodrigues AL (2002) Agmatine produces antidepressant-like effects in two models of depression in mice. Neuroreport 13: 387–391

Zomkowski AD, Santos AR, Rodrigues AL (2006) Putrescine produces antidepressant-like effects in the forced swimming test and in the tail suspension test in mice. Prog Neuropsychopharmacol Biol Psychiatry 30:1419–1425

Chapter 5
Epidemiology Research and Epigenetics: Translational Epidemiology of Schizophrenia

Mary Perrin, Karine Kleinhaus, Mark Opler, Julie Messinger, and Dolores Malaspina

Abstract Epigenetic processes can explain some of the epidemiological associations between environmental exposure and disease, particularly when the exposure occurs at a critical developmental stage. In this chapter, we present several epigenetic pathways associated with the risk for schizophrenia. We discuss nongenetic factors – such as paternal age, toxin exposure, and psychological stressors – which may influence human development by way of epigenetic mechanisms.

Keywords Environmental toxins · Imprinting · Intrauterine stress · Paternal age · X-chromosome

5.1 Introduction

The science of epigenetics has emerged in the last decade to study and define the molecular mechanisms that control gene expression. This field promises to illuminate some key risk pathways of complex genetic disorders, including schizophrenia. After decades of genetic studies, the risk for common human diseases remains largely unexplained. Before the Human Genome Project, scientists anticipated finding as many as 150,000 human genes. By 2001, the expected number of human genes was revised to less than 40,000, and based on the recent estimates, we now expect to count just 20,000 human genes. A related line of studies has demonstrated that humans are remarkably similar in their genetic codes, sharing 99.9% of nucleotide sequences. Human variability is therefore associated with only a 0.1% variation in nucleotide sequences. How can the great diversity among

M. Perrin (✉), K. Kleinhaus, M. Opler, J. Messinger, and D. Malaspina
New York University Langone Medical Center, Institute for Social and Psychiatric Initiatives:
InSPIRES, 500 First Avenue, NBV 22N-10, New York, NY 10016, USA
e-mail: Mary.Perrin@nyumc.org

A. Petronis and J. Mill (eds.), *Brain, Behavior and Epigenetics*,
Epigenetics and Human Health, DOI 10.1007/978-3-642-17426-1_5,
© Springer-Verlag Berlin Heidelberg 2011

individual people be explained, given so few genes and so much similarity in nucleotide sequences?

Epigenetic mechanisms provide a fresh perspective on human heredity and variation, particularly in the areas of behavior and metabolism. In classic genetic models, alterations of nucleotide sequences are predicted to influence the phenotype and determine disease risk, typically by generating greater or lesser amounts of a protein or somewhat different proteins. This is still the major focus of most genetic research. However, epigenetic mechanisms can initiate, sustain, control, and silence gene expression through DNA methylation, RNA-associated silencing, and histone modifications. Some animal studies have suggested that epigenetic information may be heritable (Roth et al. 2009a, b). Epigenetic processes are critically important for cell functioning and their marks can be altered during development. These epigenetic marks may arise during our life course or possibly through our more immediate ancestors (Mirabello et al. 2010). Most importantly, some epigenetic marks may be biologically determined in response to environmental exposure, which may then be transmitted to descendants. Epigenetic marks are metastable and may be altered through stochastic processes and gained or regained, presumably to enhance the survival of the current organism and possibly of future generations. RNA can direct epigenetic modifications to specific gene promoter regions, usually causing these regions to be silenced. Such RNA-associated silencing arises from the transcription of segments that were previously considered to be junk DNA.

This previously unknown mechanism led to a major paradigm shift, as we have learned more about this formerly obscure layer of complexity in our genome. Contrary to the "central dogma" that "DNA makes RNA and RNA makes protein," we now know that RNA can also epigenetically regulate DNA expression. RNA interference molecules are coded by the antisense strand of small interfering RNAs (siRNAs) (Anway et al. 2005; Gibney and Nolan 2010). New research in epigenetic mechanisms will reveal how and why certain genes are silenced or expressed and whether these epigenetic marks remain stable or fade over generations or disappear within a single lifetime. There are bound to be other surprises in the systems that determine human variation.

Alterations in gene expression likely occur over short periods of time in response to homeostatic and recuperative requirements and environmental stimuli, including interactions with other people (Anway et al. 2005; Morgan et al. 1999; Roth et al. 2009a, b). However, other epigenetic pathways that influence our molecular identity are more stable; there is evidence that these may be established to optimize the fit of each individual human being to his or her expected environment. The establishment of such epigenetic marks may be based on intergenerational influences, such as the exposures and challenges of our parents and grandparents and whether certain genes are maternally or paternally inherited, and on the intrauterine environment. While these events precede our birth, it appears that they may have lasting effects on our physiology by way of epigenetic mechanisms. In essence, the environment of our immediate ancestors and our own life course exposures may transform our identity at the molecular level to enhance our adaptability.

There are now scores of exciting topics in the field of the epigenetic regulation of gene expression. Epigenetic information modulates our growth and metabolism and surely influences the risk for chronic disorders such as diabetes and cardiovascular disease. As this book demonstrates, however, epigenetic processes hold particular interest with respect to the behavior and the risks for neuropsychiatric disorders. Epigenetic mechanisms powerfully explain neuroplasticity and the necessary adaptability of human behavioral repertoires.

This chapter demonstrates that data from epidemiological research can indicate possible epigenetic pathways – including intergenerational effects, prenatal programming, and later paternal age – to schizophrenia.

5.2   Schizophrenia

Schizophrenia is a severe neuropsychiatric syndrome with a prevalence of 0.30–0.66% and an incidence of 10.2–22.0/100,000 person years (reviewed in van Os and Kapur 2009). The symptoms typically begin in late adolescence or early adulthood, whereupon lifelong disability typically ensues. Onset is defined by the emergence of psychosis in the setting of deteriorating function and other symptoms (van Os and Kapur 2009). Before the onset of psychosis, during a prodromal period of several weeks to many years, nonspecific and variable subtle abnormalities worsen and coalesce into the classic disease features. These include alterations in the perception of reality, changes in the form and content of thoughts and speech, and social and emotional deficits including a disturbed sense of self, social dysfunction, apathy, and peculiar behavior (Perkins 2004). The symptoms of schizophrenia are often grouped into positive and negative subtypes, although there may be substantive diversity in the pathophysiology of the symptoms within these groups. Positive symptoms (so named because these phenomena occur in addition to usual experiences) include hallucinations and delusions and disorganized thinking or behavior. Negative symptoms arise from the absence of normal behaviors or experiences, including affective flattening, alogia (impoverished thinking manifested by diminished speech output or content), apathy, avolition (lack of energy and drive), and social withdrawal (van Os and Kapur 2009).

5.2.1   Genetic Etiology of Schizophrenia

Early family, twin, and adoption studies showed that heritable factors were the major components of schizophrenia vulnerability. Indeed, a century of research demonstrated substantially increased morbidity risks for schizophrenia in thousands of the first degree relatives of schizophrenia probands (parents' mean, 5.6%; siblings' mean, 10.1%; and children' mean, 12.8%) compared with the general population (Gottesman and Shields 1982). These early findings remained robust against more modern studies that directly interviewed all relatives and made operationalized diagnoses "blind" to kinship status (Goldstein et al. 1990; Pulver et al. 2004; Wolyniec et al. 1992). Since family studies cannot distinguish between genetic and environmental influences on familial aggregation, twin studies were also employed. Monozygotic (MZ) and dizygotic (DZ) twin pairs differ in their genetic endowment (sharing 100% of genetic variability and an average of 50% of genetic variability, respectively) and are typically exposed to the same familial environment. Accordingly, and in keeping with genetic hypotheses, MZ and DZ co-twins of schizophrenia probands differ in their risk for the disease. Since the initial twin studies of Luxenburger (1928), conducted over 80 years ago, the mean probandwise concordance for MZ twins are consistently threefold higher than for DZ twins (e.g., 59.2 and 15.2% in Kendler 1986). These risks are 40–60 times the risk to the general population, supporting genetic causation. Genetic studies show schizophrenia to be a highly heritable disorder with a heterogeneous clinical presentation. Although dominant, recessive, sex-linked, oligogenic, and polygenic models for schizophrenia transmission have been proposed and variably supported, research has favored the likelihood of a prominent polygenic component involving rare and common alleles, each having a very small effect on the overall population risk (Purcell et al. 2009). Recently, however, it has been suggested that highly penetrant, rare variants of recent origin, affecting neurodevelopmental pathways, may account for some of the population risk (Walsh et al. 2008).

There is an ample room for epigenetic explanations for the risk, onset, and progression of illness. For example, while the significant pairwise concordance for illness in monozygotic twins confirmed the genetic influence for the risk, it did not explain the nonconcordance in identical twins. Viewing the twin study data from the elegant perspective of epigenetics is informative. Petronis et al. (2003) made a leap forward for the field when he showed that monozygotic twins exhibit numerous epigenetic differences, which could explain their discordance. Epigenetic factors can contribute to phenotypic discordance in genetically identical organisms because these factors influence the silencing and expression of genes. They can be determined in development by individual exposures and/or subjected to addition or loss by stochastic processes – an elegant rebuttal to the warring camps of nature vs. nurture!

5.2.2   Nature and Nurture

Over the history of psychiatric discourse, debates have continued as to whether mental outcomes, ranging from intelligence to temperament to schizophrenia, are better explained by "nature" or "nurture." From the new perspective of epigenetics, gene–environment interaction pathways may form or activate molecular modulators that control gene expression, for the purpose of enhancing the adaptability of the organism to an expected environment. If metastable changes in gene expression that arise from exposures (i.e., nurture) are heritable, then the boundary between nature and nurture is obviated. In the setting where epigenetic changes can be inherited and passed on to subsequent generations, the "nurture" of one generation contributes to the "nature" of subsequent generations. Thus, nature and nurture are not distinct, and are certainly not at war.

Human disease may result from failures of epigenetic modifications, as can occur with a mutation in the DNA that precludes methylation, or from the continuance of an epigenetic modification that evolved to enhance survival in our ancestors when food was limited, but which now increases the risk for obesity and diabetes in a setting of food abundance (Gluckman et al. 2008). Likewise, epigenetic changes related to prenatal adversity may have yielded a vigilant and a hyperactive offspring, whose chances for survival were enhanced in an unstable ecosystem, perhaps with new predators. Yet in our society, the same molecular program may be associated with behavioral malfunction or mental illness.

5.3 Epigenetics, Fetal Environment, and Effects on the Offspring

Epidemiological studies show that several environmental factors increase the risk for schizophrenia. These exposures may act alone or in concert with variants in certain genes, or may alter epigenetic mechanisms that control gene expression. The intrauterine environment may be particularly salient for alterations in fetal gene expression. Currently, laboratory evidence is being sought to demonstrate that changes in epigenetic mechanisms are the link between the environmental exposures and the risk for schizophrenia.

5.3.1 Epigenetics and the Intrauterine Environment

DNA methylation can vary due to environmental factors including nutrition, chemical exposures, or psychosocial issues (Bergman et al. 2010; Cooney et al. 2002; Pilsner et al. 2007; Roth et al. 2009a, b). Future laboratory research should continue to investigate epigenetic mechanisms that may underlie the relationship between the environment and the risk for psychosis (Rutten and Mill 2009). While epidemiologic studies do not often prove causality, translational research linking epidemiologic and basic science studies are likely to advance our understanding of both the etiology of schizophrenia and potential therapies (McGrath and Richards 2009).

There is continuing debate about the contribution of the intrauterine environment to the later risk for schizophrenia. While high rates of discordance for schizophrenia in monozygotic twins is often cited as evidence for the role of environmental factors in the etiology of schizophrenia, the discordance could potentially result from changes occurring in DNA methylation from the early embryonal development period onwards (Schaefer et al. 2007). These epigenetic changes could plausibly be stochastic in nature and independent of the environment (Fraga et al. 2005; Petronis et al. 2003).

5.3.2   Epigenetic Processes, Intrauterine Exposures, and Schizophrenia

Because schizophrenia is considered to be a neurodevelopmental disease, current research is focusing on epigenetic processes in the context of the intrauterine environment. The large array of diverse fetal exposures associated with schizophrenia includes maternal infection (Brown 2006), famine (St Clair et al. 2005), preeclampsia (Cannon et al. 2002), diabetes (Cannon et al. 2002), stress (Malaspina et al. 2008), and other adversities. These disparate intrauterine events may cause schizophrenia by way of unique unrelated pathways, such as immune effects on the fetal brain, direct effects of infectious agents, compromised blood flow, decreased caloric intake, and other mechanisms (Koenig et al. 2002).

A more parsimonious expectation is that they may act through a final common pathway that is a nonspecific indicator of prenatal adversity. If so, the mechanism may involve the corticotropin-releasing hormone (CRH) and glucocorticoid hormones, which are thought to induce changes in gene expression (Cottrell and Seckl 2009; Seckl 2004; Seckl and Holmes 2007; Welberg et al. 2000). In animal studies, epigenetic changes in offspring have been linked to intrauterine exposure to endogenously or exogenously administered glucocorticoids, which are known to be associated with stress in pregnancy.

In humans, glucocorticoids from the maternal adrenal glands stimulate placental CRH production and gene expression (King et al. 2001). While CRH is well appreciated for its activity as the central regulator of the stress response in rodents and humans, it plays additional roles in human pregnancy, during which a large amount of CRH is synthesized by the placenta and secreted into the maternal and fetal circulatory systems (Mastorakos and Ilias 2003; Reis et al. 1999). CRH is a primary determinant of gestational length (Buss et al. 2009; Smith and Nicholson 2007; Wadhwa et al. 2004, 1998) and an important mediator of fetal growth and development (Ellman et al. 2008; Wadhwa 2005; Weinstock 2005). In the setting of a threatened pregnancy, either from maternal or fetal complications or from extrinsic factors, the secretion of maternal cortisol and CRH can ramp up the placental CRH production to accelerate parturition and restrict fetal growth independent of other effects of the medical complications (Hobel et al. 1999; Wadhwa et al. 2004). Low birth weight and preterm birth, both of which have been linked to schizophrenia, can result (Wadhwa et al. 2004). These actions of CRH are consistent with the hypothesis that a number of adversities influence the health and viability of the fetus, including the later risk for schizophrenia, via a final common pathway.

It is a challenge to disentangle the impact of CRH on an adverse pregnancy outcome when it arises secondarily to medical complications, which can themselves cause fetal adversity. However, if CRH mediates the risk, then severe stress and stress sensitivity alone should be associated with the risk for schizophrenia in susceptible individuals. Indeed, a number of epidemiologic studies link prenatal stress with schizophrenia risk, particularly when the stress occurs in early pregnancy (Khashan et al. 2008; Malaspina et al. 2008). Epidemiologic studies show that acute psychological trauma and nutritional deprivation in pregnant mothers from war (Malaspina et al. 2008), famine (St Clair et al. 2005), or bereavement (Khashan et al. 2008) is associated with increased risk for schizophrenia in the offspring, as well as for autism, intellectual dysfunction, and decreased language abilities (Beversdorf et al. 2005; Khashan et al. 2008; King and Laplante 2005; Kinney et al. 2008; Laplante et al. 2004, 2008; Malaspina et al. 2008; Susser and Lin 1992). The increased risk for schizophrenia depends, in part, on the timing of the insult during early pregnancy, suggesting that environmental exposures affect risk only during certain critical periods of fetal development (Khashan et al. 2008; Malaspina et al. 2008; Susser and Lin 1992).

We analyzed the effects of fetal exposure to acute maternal stress by month of gestation. The Arab/Israeli Six Day War of June 1967 was a severe psychological stressor that lasted for a month, but with no long-term nutritional deprivation or displacement for Israeli mothers. In May 1967, Egypt closed the Gulf of Aqaba to Israeli shipping, effectively beginning the war and its associated stress. The war was ended by the UN-arranged cease-fire on June 10. Our study found that the risk for schizophrenia in offspring was associated only with a maternal exposure to the stress of war in the second month of pregnancy; exposure during other months showed no effect on the risk for schizophrenia. Furthermore, the effects differed by sex, as illustrated in Fig. 5.1 (Malaspina et al. 2008), with female offspring showing a greater increase in the risk of schizophrenia in the presence of stress in pregnancy.

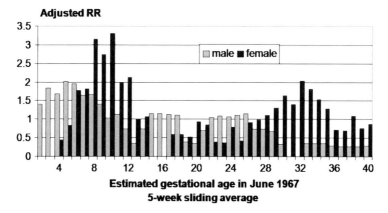

Fig. 5.1 Schizophrenia in males and females, by estimated gestational age on June 1967. Five-week sliding average incidence, adjusted for paternal and maternal age, month of birth, low social class, and duration of marriage (Malaspina et al. 2008)

5.3.3   Longitudinal Epidemiological Research in Birth Cohort Studies Can Identify Possible Epigenetic Pathways

Longitudinal research in a population-based cohort is the optimal method for identifying possible epigenetic factors in epidemiological models. Disorders that are associated with environmental exposures in critical developmental periods suggest that the epigenetic mechanisms have a causal role in the pathway to disease. Our group's work on severe intrauterine stress and paternal age was conducted using data from the Jerusalem Perinatal Study. This is a population-based cohort derived from data on all births from 1964 to 1976 to residents of a defined geographic area in Jerusalem and nearby. The cohort includes core information from the birth certificate supplemented with data from multiple sources, including maternal interviews and pediatric admissions. The Ministry of Health linked the Jerusalem Perinatal Study with Israel's Psychiatric Case Registry, providing information on psychiatric morbidity. Run by the Ministry of Health since 1950 (Lichtenberg et al. 1999), the Psychiatric Case Registry contains a record of all admissions to psychiatric hospitals or psychiatric wards within general hospitals, and admissions to day facilities for psychiatric treatment. It includes dates of admission and discharge and a single discharge diagnosis for each episode, assigned by a board-certified psychiatrist. These diagnoses are coded with the International Classification of Diseases (ICD); codes from earlier years have been updated to the tenth revision and those for psychotic disorders have been validated (Weiser et al. 2005).

In our research, we defined schizophrenia broadly so as to include discharge diagnoses of schizophrenia, schizotypal disorder, delusional disorders, nonaffective psychoses, and schizoaffective disorders, hereafter called "schizophrenia-related disorders" (ICD-10; codes F20-29).

Of the original 92,408 births in the cohort, the identities of 90,079 (97.5%) were verified through Israel's population registry and their vital status ascertained. Approximately, 0.7% were lost to follow-up due to changes in identity number (e.g., adopted, formally emigrated, or in witness protection programs). The remaining 1.8% untraced included 37% who had been born to unmarried mothers (likely to have been adopted) and 12% whose mother had no ID number (likely to have been diplomats or foreign exchange students). There were 861 cases of schizophrenia-related diagnoses in the traced cohort, and 761 individuals with "other" causes of psychiatric hospital admission. The median age at the first hospital admission was 22.8 (range 5–39) for the schizophrenia-related diagnoses and 21.4 (range 5–40) for the other diagnoses. The annual incidence of first hospital admissions in individuals with schizophrenia-related diagnoses was 0.02/1,000 by ages 8–9, increasing to 0.9/1,000 by ages 19–20, 0.5/1,000 by ages 29–30, and during the next decade 0.01/1,000. The life-table estimate of cumulative incidence of schizophrenia was 1.2% by ages 39–40.

This cohort was established by farseeing investigators. It now provides 28–40 years of follow-up from pregnancy and birth through the age of risk for adult diseases including schizophrenia. This rich resource of prospectively collected exposure data permits powerful and precise studies of environmental influences in critical developmental periods. Since the Jerusalem Perinatal Study contains information on the both maternal and paternal grandfathers, parents, and offspring, it allows for an intergenerational view along with intrauterine environment and life course perspectives.

5.3.4   Confirming Stress-in-Pregnancy Effects in Translational Studies

Animal studies have corroborated findings of epidemiologic studies that the intrauterine environment is crucial to adult health, and have also demonstrated that prenatal nutrition (e.g., folate and neural tube defects) (Fleming and Copp 1998) and other environmental factors (Zhong et al. 2010) can affect neurodevelopment. For instance, mice whose mothers received a choline supplemented diet during pregnancy showed significantly improved sensory inhibition (a biomarker for schizophrenia) compared to control mice; they also showed an increase in α-7 receptor numbers in both the CA1 and the dentate gyrus regions of the hippocampus (Stevens et al. 2008). Nutritional supplementation during gestation resulted in permanent improvement in a physiological task that is deficient in animal models of schizophrenia, suggesting that the intrauterine environment might also ameliorate the risk for schizophrenia.

Obstetric complications may also influence the risk for schizophrenia. A study found that certain single nucleotide polymorphisms (SNPs) in four genes regulated by hypoxia are involved in neural vascular functioning interact with serious obstetric complications to influence the risk of schizophrenia. Offspring with "risk" alleles at these SNPs and the history of obstetric complications had a higher risk of schizophrenia than those without the polymorphisms (Nicodemus et al. 2008). These findings correlate well with epidemiologic findings that obstetric complications, including preeclampsia, hemorrhage, maternal sepsis at childbirth, and manual extraction of the baby (Byrne et al. 2007) are associated with increased risk of schizophrenia.

Building on epidemiologic studies that associate stress early in pregnancy with schizophrenia (Brown 2006; Malaspina et al. 2008; St Clair et al. 2005), researchers analyzed the effects of intrauterine exposure to glucocorticoids during early gestation. Pregnant rats that had been injected with synthetic glucocorticoid during early pregnancy delivered offspring that showed decreased juvenile social play, a blunted acoustic startle reflex, increased prepulse inhibition of startle, and reduced amphetamine-induced motor activity, which are animal behaviors considered relevant to schizophrenia. In addition, dams, which were treated, exhibited increased milk ejection bouts during nursing. The frequency of milk ejections significantly interacted with the effects of dexamethasone on play behavior and acoustic startle reflex.

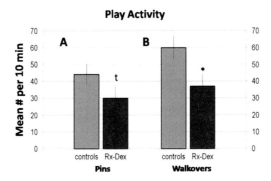

Fig. 5.2 Social play behaviors in juvenile offspring of dams treated with saline (CON; $n = 6$; *gray bars*) or DEX ($n = 5$; *red bars*). *Bars* show litter means ($\pm$SEM) for the number of pins (A) and walkovers (B) per a 10-min period of interaction between two same-sexed littermates. DEX offspring showed decreases in play behavior. *$p < 0.05$, $^t p = 0.16$ (Kleinhaus et al. 2010)

Both intrauterine conditions and postnatal maternal behavior likely contributed to the effects of early environment on an increase in schizophrenia-related behaviors as demonstrated in Fig. 5.2 (Kleinhaus et al. 2010).

Prenatal stress has been shown to influence hippocampal development in a dose-dependent manner. Mild stress of short duration enhances its development, whereas long-lasting and severe stress disturbs its development (Fujioka et al. 2006). Although prenatal stress reduces hippocampal cell proliferation throughout life, as well as cell survival and differentiation (Lemaire et al. 2006), these effects can be completely counteracted by increased infantile stimulation consisting of postnatal handling (Lemaire et al. 2006). Rats that were prenatally stressed also have decreased levels of 5-HT1A immunobinding in the ventral hippocampus as compared with controls (Van den Hove et al. 2006). Rat pups whose dams were stressed during pregnancy have more anxiogenic behavior and impaired spatial learning. Adrenalectomy of the pregnant dams precluded these effects on the pups, suggesting that the high levels of corticosterone secreted by pregnant rats in response to stress mediates the intrauterine stress effects on the developing fetal brain (Zagron and Weinstock 2006).

Epigenetic mechanisms may certainly underlie these environmental effects on the risk for aberrant behavior. A rat model of maltreatment in the first week of life showed increased DNA methylation of the *BDNF* gene in the adult prefrontal cortex. Even the offspring of the females that had experienced the maltreatment regimen showed increased *BDNF* methylation, which suggests that early environment can trigger a heritable epigenetic change (Roth et al. 2009a). The molecular mechanism potentially perpetuates changes in gene expression and behavior throughout the lifespan of the stressed female and into the next generation (Roth et al. 2009a, b). *BDNF* has also been linked to schizophrenia (Weickert et al. 2003). Despite these changes in *BDNF* methylation, it is not yet established whether epigenetic regulation of gene expression is a common underlying mechanism for the link between environmental factors and schizophrenia.

5.4   Genomic Imprinting

The phenomenon of genomic imprinting is ancient, having arisen in a common ancestor to marsupials and eutherian mammals over 150 million years ago (Killian et al. 2000). The evolutionary implications of this mechanism are intriguing. Imprinted genes date back to the branching of the evolutionary tree about 180 million years ago, when live births began for placental mammals. As it is true for most sex differences in mammals, this mechanism may have arisen to account for the differential contribution of resources by the mother and father to the offspring of the next generation. Sex differences are commonly related to sexual reproduction, and the reciprocal silencing and expression of genes from one parent or the other is no exception. The roles of male and female differ with respect to the parturition and nurture of offspring. Likewise, the epigenetic complement of sperm and egg inherited by the young serves the paternal and maternal investments by optimizing the survival and reproduction of the young.

Genomic imprinting of genes runs counter to the usual expectation of biallelic inheritance and expression. Imprinted genes are haploid, as only a single allele is expressed. Such genes are susceptible to environmental mutagens or random mutations, as there is no alternative allele. We have proposed that these mechanisms may be particularly sensitive to later paternal age (Malaspina et al. 2001). Errors in erasure or reestablishment of these imprinting patterns may lead to defective gene expression profiles in the offspring. Human imprinted genes have a critical role in the growth of the placenta, fetus, and central nervous system; in behavioral development; and in adult body size. Imprinted genes are essential for intrauterine development through parturition.

5.4.1   An Imprinting Mechanism

Imprinted genes generally, but not always, reside in clusters, which include both paternally and maternally imprinted genes. The clusters are about 1 Mb and contain a noncoding RNA gene whose product helps to regulate the imprinting of nearby genes. Imprinting control regions, called differentially methylated regions (DMR), coordinate the imprinting of genes in these clusters. During gametogenesis, the methylation marks of the previous generation (the grandparents of the offspring) are erased and subsequently re-established. Though this process is not well understood, there are several proposed mechanisms to explain it [see review in Weaver et al. (2009) for more detail].

In peripheral blood cells, the insulin-like growth factor 2 (*IGF2*) gene is silenced on the maternal allele and expressed from the paternal allele (Feinberg and Tycko 2004). The mechanism involved in this silencing or inactivation is complex, and involves the pattern of methylation at a nearby locus. *IGF2* is found in an imprinted region on chromosome 11 that also includes *H19,* a putative tumor suppressor gene, and several differentially methylated regions (DMR). A DMR 2–4 kb upstream of *H19* contains a *CCCTC*-motif binding site for the CTCF protein (Lewis and Murrell 2004). The maternal DMR is unmethylated and accessible to CTCF, which acts as an insulator, preventing the promoters of *IGF2* from accessing the endodermal enhancers, thus silencing the maternal copy of *IGF2*. Methylation of the DMR on the paternal allele prevents the binding of CTCF, leading to its expression (Murrell et al. 2004).

Imprinting is tissue-specific, maybe even cell-specific, and may differ by the stage of development (Davies et al. 2005). For example, *IGF2* is monoallelically expressed in all tissues except the brain and the liver, where it is biallelically expressed.

Errors in imprinting may occur at any point during erasure, establishment, or maintenance of an imprint. Loss of imprinting occurs when a previously silenced maternal or paternal allele is partially or completely expressed. Loss of imprinting of *IGF2* has been consistently recognized as a risk factor for colon cancer; it is detected in blood and tumor tissue (Cruz-Correa et al. 2004; Cui et al. 2003; Cui et al. 2002). In a percentage of individuals with Angelman and Praeder-Willi (PWS) syndromes, there is a loss of gene expression due to the failure to erase in the parental germline and the imprint established in the grandparental germline (Horsthemke and Buiting 2006). Though both these syndromes are associated with behavioral, cognitive, and neurologic impairment, in the case of PWS, 5–10% of cases experience schizophrenia-like psychotic symptoms (Davies et al. 2001). Epigenetic dysregulation in the parental gametes or in the fetus could therefore influence the gene expression and function of the placenta, which would likely have a substantial impact on fetal development.

5.5   Paternal Age-Related Schizophrenia

While siblings receive similar genetic contributions from their parents, their epigenetic profiles may vary substantially. Changes may occur in sperm and egg cells due to aging or environmental exposures of the parents and differing intrauterine and postnatal environments. It is possible that these differences can alter behavior. We showed that the risk of schizophrenia continues to linearly increase with advancing paternal age, which helps to explain the effect of birth order on schizophrenia within families (Malaspina 2001).

5.5.1   *De Novo Mutations and Later Paternal Age*

We have speculated that the maintenance of schizophrenia in the population, despite the reduced fecundity of affected individuals, might be explained by the replenishment of disease susceptibility genes through new mutations. If so, then the risk for schizophrenia is expected to be related to paternal age, as this is the major source of de novo mutations in humans and other mammals. This fact is explained by the constant cell replication cycles that are ongoing in spermatogenesis. Following puberty, spermatogonia undergo some 23 divisions per year. At ages 20 and 40, a man's germ cell precursors will have undergone about 200 and 660 such divisions, respectively. By contrast, oogonia undergo only a dozen or so cell divisions, predominantly during the mother's fetal life. During a man's lifetime, the constantly dividing spermatogonia are vulnerable to random errors, DNA damage from toxins, and other mutations. These lead to errors in spermatogonia that accumulate in expanding clones as men age (Crow 1999).

5.5.2 Imprinting as a Mechanism Linking Paternal Age to the Risk for Schizophrenia

Advancing paternal age could also plausibly involve epigenetic mechanisms (Brown et al. 2002; Byrne et al. 2003; Dalman and Allebeck 2002; El-Saadi et al. 2004; Malaspina et al. 2001; Sipos et al. 2004; Tsuchiya et al. 2005; Zammit et al. 2003). Paternal age has been shown in repeated studies to be a strong risk factor for schizophrenia, second only to family history of the disorder.

There are several characteristics of imprinted genes that make them reasonable candidates for schizophrenia vulnerability. Paternally and maternally expressed genes are both necessary for embryogenesis (Surani et al. 1990), playing greater roles in placental and embryo development, respectively (Kato et al. 1999). The influence of paternal genes in the placenta may represent a mechanism for the father to ensure that his offspring derives adequate resources from the maternal in utero environment, even if it may be in the best interest of the mother to limit these resources (Iwasa 1998).

Imprinted genes play a key role in brain development, leading to lasting changes in cognition and behavior (Isles and Wilkinson 2000; Keverne et al. 1996). In fact, it has been reported that among males but not females, average DNA methylation of the IGF2, a paternally expressed gene is significantly correlated with brain weight (Pidsley et al. 2010). There appears to be a neuroanatomic localization pattern for the expression of certain imprinted genes in mice: the paternal or maternal allele expression patterns correspond to the limbic and neocortical regions, respectively (Allen et al. 1995; Keverne et al. 1996). The conceptualization of schizophrenia symptoms as deriving from an imbalance or modulatory disturbance between these regions (Weinberger et al. 1992) might be pertinent to these expression differences. In addition, genes for several neurotransmitters implicated in schizophrenia may be imprinted, including those for the serotonin 2A receptor, the dopamine 3 receptor, and several GABA A receptors (see Meguro et al. 1997; Petronis et al. 2000).

5.6   Imprinting and the X-Chromosome

There is strong circumstantial evidence that there are imprinted genes on the X-chromosome. This evidence includes studies in women with Turner's syndrome. Additional support comes by way of epidemiologic studies, which are also discussed below. Further, we will look at the paternal X-chromosome as it may play a role in schizophrenia. We will also discuss skewed X-chromosome inactivation and schizophrenia.

5.6.1   Evidence Supporting the Role of Imprinted Genes on the X-Chromosome

Although several imprinted genes on the X-chromosome have been detected in mice (Kobayashi et al. 2010), as of yet, none have been found on the human X-chromosome. A study by Susan Harlap investigated whether imprinted genes may play a role in schizophrenia (Harlap et al. 2009). In this study, the authors examined the association between schizophrenia in the offspring and birthplace of the maternal and paternal grandfather. The study reported that a *paternal* grandfather from Romania or Hungary increased the risk of schizophrenia in the offspring [RR 1.9; 95% confidence interval (CI) 1.3–2.8 and RR 1.6; 95% CI 1.0–2.6, respectively] whereas a *maternal* grandfather from Romania or Hungary reduced the risk of schizophrenia in the offspring (RR 0.5; 95% CI 0.3–0.8 and RR 0.4; 95% CI 0.2–0.8, respectively). The increased risk associated with having a paternal grandfather from Romania or Hungary was more apparent in female offspring than in male offspring, whereas the decreased risk associated with a maternal grandfather from these countries was similar in males and females. The authors posited that the sex differences reported in this study could be explained by an imprinted locus on the X-chromosome.

5.6.2   Other Research Suggesting the Presence of Imprinted Genes on the X-Chromosome

On the basis of studies in women with Turner's syndrome (45, X), many genes related to neurocognition and social function are thought to lie on the X-chromosome. Women with Turner's syndrome have a constellation of symptoms such as short stature, neurocognitive and social function decrements, and failure to undergo puberty due to ovarian failure. Several studies have suggested that the constellation of symptoms in women with Turner's syndrome may differ between women with a maternal X (Xm) and a paternal X (Xp) chromosome. Some studies have noted that women with an Xp have better social and executive function than Xm women

(Skuse et al. 1997). Others have noted that there is strong correlation with cardio-vascular disease in Xm women but not in Xp women (Chu et al. 1994). Another more recent study reported morphological differences in superior temporal gyrus gray matter between Xm and Xp women (Kesler et al. 2003). The results of these studies strongly suggest the presence of imprinted genes on the X-chromosome.

5.6.3   Skewed X-Chromosome Inactivation and Schizophrenia

Since women receive an X-chromosome from each parent, they have both a maternal (Xm) and a paternal (Xp) X-chromosome. One X-chromosome is silenced in early embryogenesis in each cell line to maintain dosage compensation with males who have only one X-chromosome (46, Xm Y). In women, silencing of one X-chromosome is usually a random process resulting in 50% of cells with an Xm chromosome and 50% of cells with an Xp chromosome actively transcribed. Deviations from the expected 50:50 ratio of paternal to maternal X-chromosome silencing appear to be relatively common in females. More than 30% of women have ratios of 75:25 or more extreme distributions (Kim et al. 2004; Kristiansen et al. 2003; Lanasa et al. 1999; Struewing et al. 2006), though only 1–10% has ratios of 90:10 or more extreme distributions (Kim et al. 2004; Lanasa et al. 1999). Random inactivation is considered protective if one allele has a deleterious muta-tion. However, skewed inactivation can lead to a functional loss of heterozygosity (Buller et al. 1999) resulting in predominant expression of a deleterious mutation or other genetic or epigenetic error (Hedera and Gorski 2003; Kinoshita et al. 2004; Parolini et al. 1998; Pegoraro et al. 1997; Valleix et al. 2002).

   Through the study of X-linked retardation syndromes and Turner's syndrome, it is thought that many loci on the X-chromosome are related to cognition and social functioning. A study by Rosa et al. (2008) reported that differential methylation of the X-chromosome in female monozygotic twin pairs was greater in discordant twin pairs than in concordant twin pairs for bipolar disorder. The results were not significant for schizophrenia. A study is currently being conducted in which it is hypothesized that extreme skewing of 90:10 will be more common in affected sisters than in their nonaffected female siblings. Among those with skewed X-inactivation, it will be determined whether Xp or Xm is preferentially actively transcribed in both affected and nonaffected sisters.

5.6.4   The Paternal X-Chromosome

Sex differences in the age of onset, symptoms, and prognosis are consistently recognized in large groups of patients with schizophrenia. One of the obvious differences between males and females is that only females receive a paternal X-chromosome. It is now becoming well established that important epigenetic changes occur in the paternal X-chromosome through gametogenesis, so later paternal age could conceivably influence the efficiency of the epigenetic processing of the paternal X-chromosome (reviewed in Zamudio et al. 2008). If so, then a greater risk for paternal age-related schizophrenia (PARS) might be observed for females.

We conducted research to determine the influence of advanced paternal age on the risk of schizophrenia in offspring based on the sex of the offspring and their relation to any other first-degree family members who were hospitalized with schizophrenia (Perrin et al. 2010). Among male and female offspring of fathers greater than 35 years of age, mothers diagnosed with schizophrenia conferred the highest overall risk of schizophrenia to their offspring, as has been reported. However, there were marked differences in the risk for schizophrenia in the female and male offspring of older fathers. Sisters of affected females born to older fathers had an almost ninefold increase in their risk of schizophrenia (95% CI 3.9–19.8) compared to the population. By contrast, for the brothers of affected males born to older fathers, the risk of schizophrenia was similar to that of male siblings born to younger fathers.

All female siblings inherit the same paternal X-chromosome. Our results suggest that aberrant epigenetic processes in the paternal X-chromosome and accumulated genetic mutations in the constantly replicating male germline as paternal age advances may increase the risk of schizophrenia in female offspring.

5.7   Environmental Toxins and the Paternal Germline: Epigenetic Effects

Epigenetic changes in sperm from toxic exposures are likely to be of huge public health significance. These effects may be magnified in men of advancing age. Epigenetic changes over the life course in animal studies are consistent with changes in DNA methylation with a trend toward global hypomethylation of repetitive sequences and proto-oncogenes, along with gene-specific hypermethylation increases with age (Ahuja et al. 1998; Wilson and Jones 1983; Wilson et al. 1987). Nonetheless, methylation status fluctuates over the course of development according to cell and tissue type, developmental stage, and experimental conditions. Age-related changes in sperm DNA methylation have not been as carefully studied, although hypermethylation of sequences in sperm ribosomal RNA loci in older animals was reported by Oakes et al. (2003). Both endogenous and exogenous mechanisms have been suggested for age-related changes in methylation.

Exposure to chemicals that inhibit methylation enzymes (e.g., heavy metal exposure such as nickel; Chen et al. 2006) may have long-term consequences, since DNA remethylation processes may be incomplete or prone to error. One study of monozygotic twins reports that epigenetic differences increase over time, providing further support for the theory that the environmental exposures over time alter methylation patterns (Fraga et al. 2005).

While both human and animal studies demonstrate changes in sperm chromatin structure and stability with age, there is a lack of consensus on the nature of the changes and the degree to which these are related to aging. In a rat model, Zubkova et al. (2005) found that sperm chromatin stability was nearly equivalent in young and older rats under normal conditions. However, in the older rats, sperm chromatin was much more susceptible to oxidative stress, causing decreased stability and increases in single- and double-strand breaks. Clinical studies also suggest that stability is decreased in aging men. Using the comet assay to detect single- and double-strand breaks in DNA, Singh et al. (2003) reported a positive correlation between age and DNA fragmentation levels. Measures of reproductive health in male rodents consider pathology and outcome of proximal (pathology of testicular tissue and direct microscopic examination of spermatogenic cells), intermediate (sperm concentration, motility, and morphology), and distal processes (mating behavior and success, litter number, weight, and viability). In studies of lead-induced reproductive toxicity, there are inconsistencies in the extent to which distal vs. proximal and direct vs. indirect effects are reported (Apostoli et al. 1998; Mangelsdorf et al. 2003). Some of these differences may be related to interspecies and interstrain differences in toxicokinetics due to genetic differences.

Despite ongoing controversy regarding the precise level of exposure at which effects may be apparent in a given species or strain, there is consensus that high-level lead exposure negatively affects male reproductive health and may be responsible for reduced male fertility. Stowe and Goyer (1971) were among the first to report that mating behavior may be altered in lead exposed rats, as well as the likelihood of fertilization. Silbergeld et al (2003) found that male rats exposed to lead through their drinking water (average BPb levels of 60 μg/dL) were less likely to successfully fertilize unexposed females. In contrast, Nelson et al. (1997; see later) report no effects on fertility in rabbits (at levels of 80 μg/dL), although the viability of offspring at very high levels (110 μg/dL) was reduced.

The importance of fertility in the context of neurodevelopmental disorders has been demonstrated in work by our own group on time-to-pregnancy and risk of schizophrenia in offspring (Opler et al. 2010).

Using data from the Jerusalem Perinatal Study, postpartum interview data on the number of months required for a couple to conceive were analyzed. Compared with offspring conceived in less than 3 months, the unadjusted relative risks (RR) of schizophrenia associated with conception times of 3–5, 6–11, and 12+ months were 1.10 (95% CI 0.62–1.94), 1.41 (95% CI 0.79–2.52), and 1.88 (95% CI 1.05–3.37) with p for trend = 0.035. It should be noted that in such studies, it is difficult to attribute time-to-pregnancy changes to either male- or female-related factors. However, these findings suggest that factors associated with fecundability, either male or female, may contribute to the risk of schizophrenia.

In vitro studies have shown that lead and other heavy metals may interfere with DNA binding to protamines, small proteins critical both to sperm chromatin stability, and for condensation/decondensation events during fertilization. Foster et al. (1996)

studied the effect of lead on sperm chromatin in cynomolgus monkeys and found changes in chromatin structure at exposure levels below the limit generally thought to have fertility effects in humans. Results from both in vitro and in vivo studies (Hernandez-Ochoa et al. 2006) have suggested that lead has differential effects on chromatin condensation depending on timing and dose, i.e., chromatin of immature spermatocytes that have not completed postmeiotic processing appears to be *less* condensed in lead-exposed animals. By contrast, chromatin from more mature spermatocytes that have undergone late-stage processing including incorporation of protamines appears to be *more* condensed in lead-exposed animals. The authors postulate that the negative effects on fertility are primarily due to "overstabilization" of disulfide bonds in protamines.

5.7.1 Heavy Metals, Solvents, Epigenetics, and Outcomes in Offspring

Many DNA methyltransferases are zinc-dependent, making them potential targets for toxicity following exposure to lead and other heavy metals. Shiao et al. (2005) demonstrated that the specific gene coding for the promoter for 45s ribosomal RNA in mice is altered in the sperm of mice that were exposed to Chromium(III) [Cr(III)], which is known to be a transgenerational carcinogen. Key events in DNA methylation, including methioninesynthase activity have been shown to be affected by chemical exposures such as lead, ethanol, mercury, and aluminum (Waly et al. 2004).

There is some evidence to suggest that epigenetic mechanisms might mediate behavioral and other outcomes in offspring from heavy metal-exposed males. Nelson et al. (1997) demonstrated abnormalities in exploratory behavior, novelty seeking, and the rates of physical activity in the offspring of male rabbits exposed to high lead levels of 40 μg/dL or more. Statistically significant reductions in activity were seen at postnatal day 25 in offspring with paternal exposures of lead at 40 and 80 μg/dL. Both maternal and paternal lead exposure may influence offspring behavior (Brady et al. 1975), including spatial learning measured by increased swimming times in water maze tests. Offspring groups that had both parents exposed to lead demonstrated the highest level of impairment, with significantly longer swim times than either maternal or paternal exposure separately.

Researchers have also examined the growth and development of hippocampal neurons in the brains of animals paternally exposed to lead (Silbergeld et al. 2003). Hippocampal cells were removed from neonatal brains of the offspring of lead-exposed sires (postnatal day 1), and cultured; after 7 days, surviving cells (largely pyramidal) were subjected to morphological analysis. Cultures from paternally exposed animals showed two principal differences from controls: larger cell bodies and increases in the total number of cells with "higher order" branching (i.e., increased numbers of dendrites per axon). The authors suggest changes in timing and regulation of pruning may be responsible for observed behavioral findings.

From a public health perspective, exposure to epigenetically active compounds should be of concern in men of reproductive age (Sharpe 2010). Studies by Opler et al. (2004, 2008) have suggested a link between second and third trimester lead exposure and risk of schizophrenia in adulthood. While certain airborne pollutant levels, for example, lead levels, have fallen in the US since the 1970s, occupational settings still offer the opportunity for exposure. Although no longer sold commercially to the public, tetraethyl lead is used as a gasoline additive in military engines (particularly aircraft) and has only been recently removed from gasoline at NASCAR sporting events. Concern regarding exposure levels for individuals working in these settings is justifiable, particularly since there is an overrepresentation of men entering their peak reproductive years. A study of blood lead levels among a sample of NASCAR employees shows that up to 40% may have elevated blood lead levels (O'Neil et al. 2006).

Our group previously reported that paternal occupation as dry cleaner was associated with a threefold (95% CI 1.0–9.3) increased risk of schizophrenia in the offspring (Perrin et al. 2007). Tetrachloroethylene, a volatile aromatic halogenated hydrocarbon, has been used as a dry cleaning solvent for several decades. It is absorbed readily in adipose tissue and the brain is a target organ. It is primarily excreted through exhalation exposing others to contamination and it is also excreted in breast milk. In animal studies, intrauterine exposure to tetrachloroethylene has been reported to reduce postnatal levels of dopamine and acetylcholine (Nelson et al. 1979), whereas postnatal exposure caused disruption of habituation behaviors at 60 days (Fredrickson and Richelson 1979). Exposure to tetrachloroethylene in humans was found to disturb neuronal processing and alter perception of contrast (Altmann et al. 1990). Reproductive effects of tetrachloroethylene exposure have been reported to include spontaneous abortions in female workers (Ahlborg 1990; Doyle et al. 1997; Kyyronen et al. 1989; Windham et al. 1991), reduced sperm quality in male workers (Eskenazi et al. 1991b), and infertility or prolonged conception time in their wives (Eskenazi et al. 1991a). As men and women in occupational settings are likely to be of reproductive age, these types of exposures become increasingly relevant to the health of their future offspring.

5.8 Conclusion

Breakthrough research in epigenetics has offered new insight into the ways in which disposition to mental illness is transmitted, the biological nature of the inherited factors, and the mechanisms by which these genetic factors interact with environmental determinants. Recent advances in epidemiology have created a new and more promising context for epigenetic discovery. Prenatal and life course environmental exposures associated with schizophrenia risk, including later paternal age and prenatal adversity, could act by altering epigenetic information. Epigenetic influences on behavior may extend from the exposures of earlier generations, to those in the womb and perhaps throughout the life course.

Acknowledgments We would like to thank Dr. Susan Harlap and Benjamin Barasch for reviewing this manuscript and providing many insightful comments.

References

Ahlborg G Jr (1990) Pregnancy outcome among women working in laundries and dry-cleaning shops using tetrachloroethylene. Am J Ind Med 17(5):567–575

Ahuja N, Li Q, Mohan AL, Baylin SB, Issa JP (1998) Aging and DNA methylation in colorectal mucosa and cancer. Cancer Res 58(23):5489–5494

Allen ND, Logan K, Lally G, Drage DJ, Norris ML, Keverne EB (1995) Distribution of parthenogenetic cells in the mouse brain and their influence on brain development and behavior. Proc Natl Acad Sci USA 92(23):10782–10786

Altmann L, Bottger A, Wiegand H (1990) Neurophysiological and psychophysical measurements reveal effects of acute low-level organic solvent exposure in humans. Int Arch Occup Environ Health 62(7):493–499

Anway MD, Cupp AS, Uzumcu M, Skinner MK (2005) Epigenetic transgenerational actions of endocrine disruptors and male fertility. Science 308(5727):1466–1469

Apostoli P, Kiss P, Porru S, Bonde JP, Vanhoorne M (1998) Male reproductive toxicity of lead in animals and humans. ASCLEPIOS Study Group. Occup Environ Med 55(6):364–374

Bergman K, Sarkar P, Glover V, O'Connor TG (2010) Maternal prenatal cortisol and infant cognitive development: moderation by infant-mother attachment. Biol Psychiatry 67:1026–1032

Beversdorf DQ, Manning SE, Hillier A, Anderson SL, Nordgren RE, Walters SE, Nagaraja HN, Cooley WC, Gaelic SE, Bauman ML (2005) Timing of prenatal stressors and autism. J Autism Dev Disord 35(4):471–478

Brady K, Herrera Y, Zenick H (1975) Influence of parental lead exposure on subsequent learning ability of offspring. Pharmacol Biochem Behav 3(4):561–565

Brown AS (2006) Prenatal infection as a risk factor for schizophrenia. Schizophr Bull 32 (2):200–202

Brown AS, Schaefer CA, Wyatt RJ, Begg MD, Goetz R, Bresnahan MA, Harkavy-Friedman J, Gorman JM, Malaspina D, Susser ES (2002) Paternal age and risk of schizophrenia in adult offspring. Am J Psychiatry 159(9):1528–1533

Buller RE, Sood AK, Lallas T, Buekers T, Skilling JS (1999) Association between nonrandom X-chromosome inactivation and BRCA1 mutation in germline DNA of patients with ovarian cancer. J Natl Cancer Inst 91(4):339–346

Buss C, Entringer S, Reyes JF, Chicz-DeMet A, Sandman CA, Waffarn F, Wadhwa PD (2009) The maternal cortisol awakening response in human pregnancy is associated with the length of gestation. Am J Obstet Gynecol 201(4):398, e391–398

Byrne M, Agerbo E, Ewald H, Eaton WW, Mortensen PB (2003) Parental age and risk of schizophrenia: a case-control study. Arch Gen Psychiatry 60(7):673–678

Byrne M, Agerbo E, Bennedsen B, Eaton WW, Mortensen PB (2007) Obstetric conditions and risk of first admission with schizophrenia: a Danish national register based study. Schizophr Res 97 (1–3):51–59

Cannon M, Jones PB, Murray RM (2002) Obstetric complications and schizophrenia: historical and meta-analytic review. Am J Psychiatry 159(7):1080–1092

Chen H, Ke Q, Kluz T, Yan Y, Costa M (2006) Nickel ions increase histone H3 lysine 9 dimethylation and induce transgene silencing. Mol Cell Biol 26(10):3728–3737

Chu CE, Donaldson MD, Kelnar CJ, Smail PJ, Greene SA, Paterson WF, Connor JM (1994) Possible role of imprinting in the Turner phenotype. J Med Genet 31(11):840–842

Cooney CA, Dave AA, Wolff GL (2002) Maternal methyl supplements in mice affect epigenetic variation and DNA methylation of offspring. J Nutr 132(8 Suppl):2393S–2400S

Cottrell EC, Seckl JR (2009) Prenatal stress, glucocorticoids and the programming of adult disease. Front Behav Neurosci 3:19

Crow JF (1999) Spontaneous mutation in man. Mutat Res 437(1):5–9

Cruz-Correa M, Cui H, Giardiello FM, Powe NR, Hylind L, Robinson A, Hutcheon DF, Kafonek DR, Brandenburg S, Wu Y, He X, Feinberg AP (2004) Loss of imprinting of insulin growth factor II gene: a potential heritable biomarker for colon neoplasia predisposition. Gastroenterology 126(4):964–970

Cui H, Onyango P, Brandenburg S, Wu Y, Hsieh CL, Feinberg AP (2002) Loss of imprinting in colorectal cancer linked to hypomethylation of H19 and IGF2. Cancer Res 62(22):6442–6446

Cui H, Cruz-Correa M, Giardiello FM, Hutcheon DF, Kafonek DR, Brandenburg S, Wu Y, He X, Powe NR, Feinberg AP (2003) Loss of IGF2 imprinting: a potential marker of colorectal cancer risk. Science 299(5613):1753–1755

Dalman C, Allebeck P (2002) Paternal age and schizophrenia: further support for an association. Am J Psychiatry 159(9):1591–1592

Davies W, Isles AR, Wilkinson LS (2001) Imprinted genes and mental dysfunction. Ann Med 33 (6):428–436

Davies W, Isles AR, Wilkinson LS (2005) Imprinted gene expression in the brain. Neurosci Biobehav Rev 29(3):421–430

Doyle P, Roman E, Beral V, Brookes M (1997) Spontaneous abortion in dry cleaning workers potentially exposed to perchloroethylene. Occup Environ Med 54(12):848–853

Ellman LM, Schetter CD, Hobel CJ, Chicz-Demet A, Glynn LM, Sandman CA (2008) Timing of fetal exposure to stress hormones: effects on newborn physical and neuromuscular maturation. Dev Psychobiol 50(3):232–241

El-Saadi O, Pedersen CB, McNeil TF, Saha S, Welham J, O'Callaghan E, Cantor-Graae E, Chant D, Mortensen PB, McGrath J (2004) Paternal and maternal age as risk factors for psychosis: findings from Denmark, Sweden and Australia. Schizophr Res 67(2–3):227–236

Eskenazi B, Fenster L, Hudes M, Wyrobek AJ, Katz DF, Gerson J, Rempel DM (1991a) A study of the effect of perchloroethylene exposure on the reproductive outcomes of wives of dry-cleaning workers. Am J Ind Med 20(5):593–600

Eskenazi B, Wyrobek AJ, Fenster L, Katz DF, Sadler M, Lee J, Hudes M, Rempel DM (1991b) A study of the effect of perchloroethylene exposure on semen quality in dry cleaning workers. Am J Ind Med 20(5):575–591

Feinberg AP, Tycko B (2004) The history of cancer epigenetics. Nat Rev Cancer 4(2):143–153

Fleming A, Copp AJ (1998) Embryonic folate metabolism and mouse neural tube defects. Science 280(5372):2107–2109

Foster WG, McMahon A, Rice DC (1996) Sperm chromatin structure is altered in cynomolgus monkeys with environmentally relevant blood lead levels. Toxicol Ind Health 12(5):723–735

Fraga MF, Ballestar E, Paz MF, Ropero S, Setien F, Ballestar ML, Heine-Suner D, Cigudosa JC, Urioste M, Benitez J, Boix-Chornet M, Sanchez-Aguilera A, Ling C, Carlsson E, Poulsen P, Vaag A, Stephan Z, Spector TD, Wu YZ, Plass C, Esteller M (2005) Epigenetic differences arise during the lifetime of monozygotic twins. Proc Natl Acad Sci USA 102(30):10604–10609

Fredrickson P, Richelson E (1979) Mayo seminars in psychiatry: dopamine and schizophrenia–a review. J Clin Psychiatry 40(9):399–405

Fujioka A, Fujioka T, Ishida Y, Maekawa T, Nakamura S (2006) Differential effects of prenatal stress on the morphological maturation of hippocampal neurons. Neuroscience 141 (2):907–915

Gibney ER, Nolan CM (2010) Epigenetics and gene expression. Heredity 105(1):4–13

Gluckman PD, Hanson MA, Beedle AS, Raubenheimer D (2008) Fetal and neonatal pathways to obesity. Front Horm Res 36:61–72

Goldstein JM, Faraone SV, Chen WJ, Tolomiczencko GS, Tsuang MT (1990) Sex differences in the familial transmission of schizophrenia. Br J Psychiatry 156:819–826

Gottesman II, Shields J (1982) Schizophrenia: the epigenetic puzzle. Cambridge University Press, New York, NY

Harlap S, Perrin MC, Deutsch L, Kleinhaus K, Fennig S, Nahon D, Teitelbaum A, Friedlander Y, Malaspina D (2009) Schizophrenia and birthplace of paternal and maternal grandfather in the Jerusalem perinatal cohort prospective study. Schizophr Res 111(1–3):23–31

Hedera P, Gorski JL (2003) Oculo-facio-cardio-dental syndrome: skewed X chromosome inactivation in mother and daughter suggest X-linked dominant Inheritance. Am J Med Genet A 123A(3):261–266

Hernandez-Ochoa I, Sanchez-Gutierrez M, Solis-Heredia MJ, Quintanilla-Vega B (2006) Spermatozoa nucleus takes up lead during the epididymal maturation altering chromatin condensation. Reprod Toxicol 21(2):171–178

Hobel CJ, Dunkel-Schetter C, Roesch SC, Castro LC, Arora CP (1999) Maternal plasma corticotropin-releasing hormone associated with stress at 20 weeks' gestation in pregnancies ending in preterm delivery. Am J Obstet Gynecol 180(1 Pt 3):S257–263

Horsthemke B, Buiting K (2006) Imprinting defects on human chromosome 15. Cytogenet Genome Res 113(1–4):292–299

Isles AR, Wilkinson LS (2000) Imprinted genes, cognition and behaviour. Trends Cogn Sci 4 (8):309–318

Iwasa Y (1998) The conflict theory of genomic imprinting: how much can be explained? Curr Top Dev Biol 40:255–293

Kato Y, Rideout WM 3rd, Hilton K, Barton SC, Tsunoda Y, Surani MA (1999) Developmental potential of mouse primordial germ cells. Development 126(9):1823–1832

Kendler KS (1986) A twin study of mortality in schizophrenia and neurosis. Arch Gen Psychiatry 43(7):643–649

Kesler SR, Blasey CM, Brown WE, Yankowitz J, Zeng SM, Bender BG, Reiss AL (2003) Effects of X-monosomy and X-linked imprinting on superior temporal gyrus morphology in Turner syndrome. Biol Psychiatry 54(6):636–646

Keverne EB, Fundele R, Narasimha M, Barton SC, Surani MA (1996) Genomic imprinting and the differential roles of parental genomes in brain development. Brain Res Dev Brain Res 92 (1):91–100

Khashan AS, Abel KM, McNamee R, Pedersen MG, Webb RT, Baker PN, Kenny LC, Mortensen PB (2008) Higher risk of offspring schizophrenia following antenatal maternal exposure to severe adverse life events. Arch Gen Psychiatry 65(2):146–152

Killian JK, Byrd JC, Jirtle JV, Munday BL, Stoskopf MK, MacDonald RG, Jirtle RL (2000) M6P/IGF2R imprinting evolution in mammals. Mol Cell 5(4):707–716

Kim JW, Park SY, Kim YM, Kim JM, Han JY, Ryu HM (2004) X-chromosome inactivation patterns in Korean women with idiopathic recurrent spontaneous abortion. J Korean Med Sci 19(2):258–262

King S, Laplante DP (2005) The effects of prenatal maternal stress on children's cognitive development: Project Ice Storm. Stress 8(1):35–45

King BR, Smith R, Nicholson RC (2001) The regulation of human corticotrophin-releasing hormone gene expression in the placenta. Peptides 22(5):795–801

Kinney DK, Miller AM, Crowley DJ, Huang E, Gerber E (2008) Autism prevalence following prenatal exposure to hurricanes and tropical storms in Louisiana. J Autism Dev Disord 38 (3):481–488

Kinoshita K, Miura Y, Nagasaki H, Murase T, Bando Y, Oiso Y (2004) A novel deletion mutation in the arginine vasopressin receptor 2 gene and skewed X chromosome inactivation in a female patient with congenital nephrogenic diabetes insipidus. J Endocrinol Invest 27(2):167–170

Kleinhaus K, Steinfeld S, Balaban J, Goodman L, Craft TS, Malaspina D, Myers MM, Moore H (2010) Effects of excessive glucocorticoid receptor stimulation during early gestation on psychomotor and social behavior in the rat. Dev Psychobiol 52(2):121–132

Kobayashi S, Fujihara Y, Mise N, Kaseda K, Abe K, Ishino F, Okabe M (2010) The X-linked imprinted gene family Fthl17 shows predominantly female expression following the two-cell stage in mouse embryos. Nucleic Acids Res 38:3672–3681

Koenig JI, Kirkpatrick B, Lee P (2002) Glucocorticoid hormones and early brain development in schizophrenia. Neuropsychopharmacology 27(2):309–318

Kristiansen M, Knudsen GP, Tanner SM, McEntagart M, Jungbluth H, Muntoni F, Sewry C, Gallati S, Orstavik KH, Wallgren-Pettersson C (2003) X-inactivation patterns in carriers of X-linked myotubular myopathy. Neuromuscul Disord 13(6):468–471

Kyyronen P, Taskinen H, Lindbohm ML, Hemminki K, Heinonen OP (1989) Spontaneous abortions and congenital malformations among women exposed to tetrachloroethylene in dry cleaning. J Epidemiol Community Health 43(4):346–351

Lanasa MC, Hogge WA, Kubik C, Blancato J, Hoffman EP (1999) Highly skewed X-chromosome inactivation is associated with idiopathic recurrent spontaneous abortion. Am J Hum Genet 65 (1):252–254

Laplante DP, Barr RG, Brunet A, Galbaud du Fort G, Meaney ML, Saucier JF, Zelazo PR, King S (2004) Stress during pregnancy affects general intellectual and language functioning in human toddlers. Pediatr Res 56(3):400–410

Laplante DP, Brunet A, Schmitz N, Ciampi A, King S (2008) Project Ice Storm: prenatal maternal stress affects cognitive and linguistic functioning in 5 1/2-year-old children. J Am Acad Child Adolesc Psychiatry 47(9):1063–1072

Lemaire V, Lamarque S, Le Moal M, Piazza PV, Abrous DN (2006) Postnatal stimulation of the pups counteracts prenatal stress-induced deficits in hippocampal neurogenesis. Biol Psychiatry 59(9):786–792

Lewis A, Murrell A (2004) Genomic imprinting: CTCF protects the boundaries. Curr Biol 14(7): R284–286

Lichtenberg P, Kaplan Z, Grinshpoon A, Feldman D, Nahon D (1999) The goals and limitations of Israel's psychiatric case register. Psychiatr Serv 50(8):1043–1048

Luxenburger H (1928) Vorlaufiger Bericht über psychiatrische Serienuntersuchungen und Zwillingen. Zeiischrift gesamte Neurol Psychiatr 116:297–326

Malaspina D (2001) Paternal factors and schizophrenia risk: de novo mutations and imprinting. Schizophr Bull 27(3):379–393

Malaspina D, Harlap S, Fennig S, Heiman D, Nahon D, Feldman D, Susser ES (2001) Advancing paternal age and the risk of schizophrenia. Arch Gen Psychiatry 58(4):361–367

Malaspina D, Corcoran C, Kleinhaus KR, Perrin MC, Fennig S, Nahon D, Friedlander Y, Harlap S (2008) Acute maternal stress in pregnancy and schizophrenia in offspring: a cohort prospective study. BMC Psychiatry 8:71

Mangelsdorf I, Buschmann J, Orthen B (2003) Some aspects relating to the evaluation of the effects of chemicals on male fertility. Regul Toxicol Pharmacol 37(3):356–369

Mastorakos G, Ilias I (2003) Maternal and fetal hypothalamic-pituitary-adrenal axes during pregnancy and postpartum. Ann NY Acad Sci 997:136–149

McGrath JJ, Richards LJ (2009) Why schizophrenia epidemiology needs neurobiology – and vice versa. Schizophr Bull 35(3):577–581

Meguro M, Mitsuya K, Sui H, Shigenami K, Kugoh H, Nakao M, Oshimura M (1997) Evidence for uniparental, paternal expression of the human GABAA receptor subunit genes, using microcell-mediated chromosome transfer. Hum Mol Genet 6(12):2127–2133

Mirabello L, Savage SA, Korde L, Gadalla SM, Greene MH (2010) LINE-1 methylation is inherited in familial testicular cancer kindreds. BMC Med Genet 11:77

Morgan HD, Sutherland HG, Martin DI, Whitelaw E (1999) Epigenetic inheritance at the agouti locus in the mouse. Nat Genet 23(3):314–318

Murrell A, Heeson S, Reik W (2004) Interaction between differentially methylated regions partitions the imprinted genes IGF2 and H19 into parent-specific chromatin loops. Nat Genet 36(8):889–893

Nelson BK, Taylor BJ, Setzer JV, Hornung RW (1979) Behavioral teratology of perchloroethylene in rats. J Environ Pathol Toxicol 3(1–2):233–250

Nelson BK, Moorman WJ, Schrader SM, Shaw PB, Krieg EF Jr (1997) Paternal exposure of rabbits to lead: behavioral deficits in offspring. Neurotoxicol Teratol 19(3):191–198

Nicodemus KK, Marenco S, Batten AJ, Vakkalanka R, Egan MF, Straub RE, Weinberger DR (2008) Serious obstetric complications interact with hypoxia-regulated/vascular-expression genes to influence schizophrenia risk. Mol Psychiatry 13(9):873–877

O'Neil J, Steele G, McNair CS, Matusiak MM, Madlem J (2006) Blood lead levels in NASCAR Nextel Cup teams. J Occup Environ Hyg 3(2):67–71

Oakes CC, Smiraglia DJ, Plass C, Trasler JM, Robaire B (2003) Aging results in hypermethylation of ribosomal DNA in sperm and liver of male rats. Proc Natl Acad Sci USA 100(4):1775–1780

Opler MG, Brown AS, Graziano J, Desai M, Zheng W, Schaefer C, Factor-Litvak P, Susser ES (2004) Prenatal lead exposure, delta-aminolevulinic acid, and schizophrenia. Environ Health Perspect 112(5):548–552

Opler MG, Buka SL, Groeger J, McKeague I, Wei C, Factor-Litvak P, Bresnahan M, Graziano J, Goldstein JM, Seidman LJ, Brown AS, Susser ES (2008) Prenatal exposure to lead, delta-aminolevulinic acid, and schizophrenia: further evidence. Environ Health Perspect 116 (11):1586–1590

Opler MG, Harlap S, Ornstein K, Kleinhaus K, Perrin M, Gangwisch JE, Lichtenberg P, Draiman B, Malaspina D (2010) Time-to-pregnancy and risk of schizophrenia. Schizophr Res 118:76–80

Parolini O, Ressmann G, Haas OA, Pawlowsky J, Gadner H, Knapp W, Holter W (1998) X-linked Wiskott-Aldrich syndrome in a girl. N Engl J Med 338(5):291–295

Pegoraro E, Whitaker J, Mowery-Rushton P, Surti U, Lanasa M, Hoffman EP (1997) Familial skewed X inactivation: a molecular trait associated with high spontaneous-abortion rate maps to Xq28. Am J Hum Genet 61(1):160–170

Perkins DO (2004) Evaluating and treating the prodromal stage of schizophrenia. Curr Psychiatry Rep 6(4):289–295

Perrin MC, Opler MG, Harlap S, Harkavy-Friedman J, Kleinhaus K, Nahon D, Fennig S, Susser ES, Malaspina D (2007) Tetrachloroethylene exposure and risk of schizophrenia: offspring of dry cleaners in a population birth cohort, preliminary findings. Schizophr Res 90(1–3):251–254

Perrin M, Harlap S, Kleinhaus K, Lichtenberg P, Manor O, Draiman B, Fennig S, Malaspina D (2010) Older paternal age strongly increases the morbidity for schizophrenia in sisters of affected females. Am J Med Genet B Neuropsychiatr Genet 153B:1329–1335

Petronis A, Gottesman II, Crow TJ, DeLisi LE, Klar AJ, Macciardi F, McInnis MG, McMahon FJ, Paterson AD, Skuse D, Sutherland GR (2000) Psychiatric epigenetics: a new focus for the new century. Mol Psychiatry 5(4):342–346

Petronis A, Gottesman II, Kan P, Kennedy JL, Basile VS, Paterson AD, Popendikyte V (2003) Monozygotic twins exhibit numerous epigenetic differences: clues to twin discordance? Schizophr Bull 29(1):169–178

Pidsley R, Dempster EL, Mill J (2010) Brain weight in males is correlated with DNA methylation at IGF2. Mol Psychiatry 15:880–881

Pilsner JR, Liu X, Ahsan H, Ilievski V, Slavkovich V, Levy D, Factor-Litvak P, Graziano JH, Gamble MV (2007) Genomic methylation of peripheral blood leukocyte DNA: influences of arsenic and folate in Bangladeshi adults. Am J Clin Nutr 86(4):1179–1186

Pulver AE, McGrath JA, Liang KY, Lasseter VK, Nestadt G, Wolyniec PS (2004) An indirect test of the new mutation hypothesis associating advanced paternal age with the etiology of schizophrenia. Am J Med Genet B Neuropsychiatr Genet 124B(1):6–9

Purcell SM, Wray NR, Stone JL, Visscher PM, O'Donovan MC, Sullivan PF, Sklar P (2009) Common polygenic variation contributes to risk of schizophrenia and bipolar disorder. Nature 460(7256):748–752

Reis FM, Fadalti M, Florio P, Petraglia F (1999) Putative role of placental corticotropin-releasing factor in the mechanisms of human parturition. J Soc Gynecol Investig 6(3):109–119

Rosa A, Picchioni MM, Kalidindi S, Loat CS, Knight J, Toulopoulou T, Vonk R, van der Schot AC, Nolen W, Kahn RS, McGuffin P, Murray RM, Craig IW (2008) Differential methylation of the X-chromosome is a possible source of discordance for bipolar disorder female monozygotic twins. Am J Med Genet B Neuropsychiatr Genet 147B(4):459–462

Roth TL, Lubin FD, Funk AJ, Sweatt JD (2009a) Lasting epigenetic influence of early-life adversity on the BDNF gene. Biol Psychiatry 65(9):760–769

Roth TL, Lubin FD, Sodhi M, Kleinman JE (2009b) Epigenetic mechanisms in schizophrenia. Biochim Biophys Acta 1790(9):869–877

Rutten BP, Mill J (2009) Epigenetic mediation of environmental influences in major psychotic disorders. Schizophr Bull 35(6):1045–1056

Schaefer CB, Ooi SK, Bestor TH, Bourc'his D (2007) Epigenetic decisions in mammalian germ cells. Science 316(5823):398–399

Seckl JR (2004) Prenatal glucocorticoids and long-term programming. Eur J Endocrinol 151 (Suppl 3):U49–62

Seckl JR, Holmes MC (2007) Mechanisms of disease: glucocorticoids, their placental metabolism and fetal 'programming' of adult pathophysiology. Nat Clin Pract Endocrinol Metab 3 (6):479–488

Sharpe RM (2010) Environmental/lifestyle effects on spermatogenesis. Philos Trans R Soc Lond B Biol Sci 365(1546):1697–1712

Shiao YH, Crawford EB, Anderson LM, Patel P, Ko K (2005) Allele-specific germ cell epimutation in the spacer promoter of the 45S ribosomal RNA gene after Cr(III) exposure. Toxicol Appl Pharmacol 205(3):290–296

Silbergeld EK, Quintanilla-Vega B, Gandley RE (2003) Mechanisms of male mediated developmental toxicity induced by lead. Adv Exp Med Biol 518:37–48

Singh NP, Muller CH, Berger RE (2003) Effects of age on DNA double-strand breaks and apoptosis in human sperm. Fertil Steril 80(6):1420–1430

Sipos A, Rasmussen F, Harrison G, Tynelius P, Lewis G, Leon DA, Gunnell D (2004) Paternal age and schizophrenia: a population based cohort study. BMJ 329(7474):1070

Skuse DH, James RS, Bishop DV, Coppin B, Dalton P, Aamodt-Leeper G, Bacarese-Hamilton M, Creswell C, McGurk R, Jacobs PA (1997) Evidence from Turner's syndrome of an imprinted X-linked locus affecting cognitive function. Nature 387(6634):705–708

Smith R, Nicholson RC (2007) Corticotrophin releasing hormone and the timing of birth. Front Biosci 12:912–918

St Clair D, Xu M, Wang P, Yu Y, Fang Y, Zhang F, Zheng X, Gu N, Feng G, Sham P, He L (2005) Rates of adult schizophrenia following prenatal exposure to the Chinese famine of 1959–1961. JAMA 294(5):557–562

Stevens KE, Adams CE, Yonchek J, Hickel C, Danielson J, Kisley MA (2008) Permanent improvement in deficient sensory inhibition in DBA/2 mice with increased perinatal choline. Psychopharmacology (Berl) 198(3):413–420

Stowe HD, Goyer RA (1971) Reproductive ability and progeny of F1 lead-toxic rats. Fertil Steril 22(11):755–760

Struewing JP, Pineda MA, Sherman ME, Lissowska J, Brinton LA, Peplonska B, Bardin-Mikolajczak A, Garcia-Closas M (2006) Skewed X chromosome inactivation and early-onset breast cancer. J Med Genet 43(1):48–53

Surani MA, Allen ND, Barton SC, Fundele R, Howlett SK, Norris ML, Reik W (1990) Developmental consequences of imprinting of parental chromosomes by DNA methylation. Philos Trans R Soc Lond B Biol Sci 326(1235):313–327

Susser ES, Lin SP (1992) Schizophrenia after prenatal exposure to the Dutch Hunger Winter of 1944–1945. Arch Gen Psychiatry 49(12):983–988

Tsuchiya KJ, Takagai S, Kawai M, Matsumoto H, Nakamura K, Minabe Y, Mori N, Takei N (2005) Advanced paternal age associated with an elevated risk for schizophrenia in offspring in a Japanese population. Schizophr Res 76(2–3):337–342

Valleix S, Vinciguerra C, Lavergne JM, Leuer M, Delpech M, Negrier C (2002) Skewed X-chromosome inactivation in monochorionic diamniotic twin sisters results in severe and mild hemophilia A. Blood 100(8):3034–3036

Van den Hove DL, Lauder JM, Scheepens A, Prickaerts J, Blanco CE, Steinbusch HW (2006) Prenatal stress in the rat alters 5-HT1A receptor binding in the ventral hippocampus. Brain Res 1090(1):29–34

van Os J, Kapur S (2009) Schizophrenia. Lancet 374(9690):635–645

Wadhwa PD (2005) Psychoneuroendocrine processes in human pregnancy influence fetal development and health. Psychoneuroendocrinology 30(8):724–743

Wadhwa PD, Porto M, Garite TJ, Chicz-DeMet A, Sandman CA (1998) Maternal corticotropin-releasing hormone levels in the early third trimester predict length of gestation in human pregnancy. Am J Obstet Gynecol 179(4):1079–1085

Wadhwa PD, Garite TJ, Porto M, Glynn L, Chicz-DeMet A, Dunkel-Schetter C, Sandman CA (2004) Placental corticotropin-releasing hormone (CRH), spontaneous preterm birth, and fetal growth restriction: a prospective investigation. Am J Obstet Gynecol 191(4):1063–1069

Walsh T, McClellan JM, McCarthy SE, Addington AM, Pierce SB, Cooper GM, Nord AS, Kusenda M, Malhotra D, Bhandari A, Stray SM, Rippey CF, Roccanova P, Makarov V, Lakshmi B, Findling RL, Sikich L, Stromberg T, Merriman B, Gogtay N, Butler P, Eckstrand K, Noory L, Gochman P, Long R, Chen Z, Davis S, Baker C, Eichler EE, Meltzer PS, Nelson SF, Singleton AB, Lee MK, Rapoport JL, King MC, Sebat J (2008) Rare structural variants disrupt multiple genes in neurodevelopmental pathways in schizophrenia. Science 320(5875):539–543

Waly M, Olteanu H, Banerjee R, Choi SW, Mason JB, Parker BS, Sukumar S, Shim S, Sharma A, Benzecry JM, Power-Charnitsky VA, Deth RC (2004) Activation of methionine synthase by insulin-like growth factor-1 and dopamine: a target for neurodevelopmental toxins and thimerosal. Mol Psychiatry 9(4):358–370

Weaver JR, Susiarjo M, Bartolomei MS (2009) Imprinting and epigenetic changes in the early embryo. Mamm Genome 20(9–10):532–543

Weickert CS, Hyde TM, Lipska BK, Herman MM, Weinberger DR, Kleinman JE (2003) Reduced brain-derived neurotrophic factor in prefrontal cortex of patients with schizophrenia. Mol Psychiatry 8(6):592–610

Weinberger DR, Berman KF, Suddath R, Torrey EF (1992) Evidence of dysfunction of a prefrontal-limbic network in schizophrenia: a magnetic resonance imaging and regional cerebral blood flow study of discordant monozygotic twins. Am J Psychiatry 149(7):890–897

Weinstock M (2005) The potential influence of maternal stress hormones on development and mental health of the offspring. Brain Behav Immun 19(4):296–308

Weiser M, Kanyas K, Malaspina D, Harvey PD, Glick I, Goetz D, Karni O, Yakir A, Turetsky N, Fennig S, Nahon D, Lerer B, Davidson M (2005) Sensitivity of ICD-10 diagnosis of psychotic disorders in the Israeli National Hospitalization Registry compared with RDC diagnoses based on SADS-L. Compr Psychiatry 46(1):38–42

Welberg LA, Seckl JR, Holmes MC (2000) Inhibition of 11beta-hydroxysteroid dehydrogenase, the foeto-placental barrier to maternal glucocorticoids, permanently programs amygdala GR mRNA expression and anxiety-like behaviour in the offspring. Eur J Neurosci 12(3):1047–1054

Wilson VL, Jones PA (1983) DNA methylation decreases in aging but not in immortal cells. Science 220(4601):1055–1057

Wilson VL, Smith RA, Ma S, Cutler RG (1987) Genomic 5-methyldeoxycytidine decreases with age. J Biol Chem 262(21):9948–9951

Windham GC, Shusterman D, Swan SH, Fenster L, Eskenazi B (1991) Exposure to organic solvents and adverse pregnancy outcome. Am J Ind Med 20(2):241–259

Wolyniec PS, Pulver AE, McGrath JA, Tam D (1992) Schizophrenia: gender and familial risk. J Psychiatr Res 26(1):17–27

Zagron G, Weinstock M (2006) Maternal adrenal hormone secretion mediates behavioural alterations induced by prenatal stress in male and female rats. Behav Brain Res 175(2):323–328

Zammit S, Allebeck P, Dalman C, Lundberg I, Hemmingson T, Owen MJ, Lewis G (2003) Paternal age and risk for schizophrenia. Br J Psychiatry 183:405–408

Zamudio NM, Chong S, O'Bryan MK (2008) Epigenetic regulation in male germ cells. Reproduction 136(2):131–146

Zhong Z, Zhang C, Rizak JD, Cui Y, Xu S, Che Y (2010) Chronic prenatal lead exposure impairs long-term memory in day old chicks. Neurosci Lett 476(1):23–26

Zubkova EV, Wade M, Robaire B (2005) Changes in spermatozoal chromatin packaging and susceptibility to oxidative challenge during aging. Fertil Steril 84(Suppl 2):1191–1198

Chapter 6
Environmental Studies as a Tool for Detecting Epigenetic Mechanisms in Schizophrenia

Wim Veling, L.H. Lumey, Bas Heijmans, and Ezra Susser

Abstract Epigenetic mechanisms may play an important role in the etiological pathways of schizophrenia. Since the epigenetic status of the genome partly depends on environmental factors in pre- and postnatal environments, exposure to such factors should be taken into account in epigenetic studies of schizophrenia. Prenatal famine and childhood ethnic minority status have been identified as environmental risk factors for schizophrenia. These exposures can be used to investigate epigenetic effects on schizophrenia, since environmental exposure can be measured with sufficient precision, homogeneously exposed populations are available for study, and plausible biological pathways have been suggested (albeit less specific for migration). This chapter shows that epidemiological studies of famine and migration can help to detect epigenetic mechanisms in schizophrenia, by comparing the epigenome of exposed and unexposed schizophrenia cases and controls. The results of the comparisons will be different depending on the mechanism involved in the interplay between environment and epigenome. If these epidemiological designs are not applied, the overall result of epigenetic schizophrenia studies may well continue to be inconclusive.

Keywords Environmental risk factors · Epidemiology · Epigenetics · Famine · Migration · Schizophrenia

---

W. Veling
Parnassia Center for Early Psychosis, Lijnbaan 4 2512 VA, The Hague, The Netherlands
e-mail: w.veling@parnassia.nl

L.H. Lumey and E. Susser (✉)
Department of Epidemiology, Columbia University, Mailman School of Public Health, 722 West 168 Street, New York, NY 10032, USA
e-mail: lumey@columbia.edu; ess8@columbia.edu

B. Heijmans
Department of Molecular Epidemiology, Leiden University Medical Center, Albinusdreef 2, 2333 ZA, Leiden, The Netherlands
e-mail: b.t.heijmans@lumc.nl

A. Petronis and J. Mill (eds.), *Brain, Behavior and Epigenetics*,
Epigenetics and Human Health, DOI 10.1007/978-3-642-17426-1_6,
© Springer-Verlag Berlin Heidelberg 2011

6.1   Introduction

There is no doubt that schizophrenia has a strong genetic basis (Sullivan et al. 2003). In the 1990s, hopes that traditional linkage studies could identify major genes for schizophrenia were ignited by some exceptional findings for other complex disorders. Perhaps, most notable was the strong association between APOE genetic alleles and Alzheimer's disease, which was originally identified via traditional linkage studies (Kehoe et al. 1999). In the last decade, we have witnessed enormous progress in the creation of novel methods for associating variation in genes to risk for complex disorders. The advent of genome-wide association studies (GWAS), in particular, was a significant development that fueled new expectations. However, the results obtained from GWAS of schizophrenia have been quite disappointing, as they have been inconsistent and difficult to interpret (Manolio et al. 2009). A continuously updated online database of genetic association studies currently lists over 900 different genes and more than 8,000 different polymorphisms that have all been studied in relation to schizophrenia (Allen et al. 2008). Associations with common alleles generally have small effect sizes, are difficult to replicate and, thus far, rare genetic variants with larger effects only explain a small proportion of the heritability of schizophrenia (Manolio et al. 2009). Other research strategies, extending beyond the current GWAS approach, may therefore be needed. Next generation sequencing-based studies, which include whole genome sequencing among other approaches, may provide the field of schizophrenia research with a much-needed advance. Recent reviews have raised hopes that the "missing heritability" will be revealed by these sophisticated methods (Manolio et al. 2009) – this may be true, to some extent, given the enormous power they will confer in gene discovery, although the vast number of variants will make it immensely difficult to identify those which are causal. Another strategy could involve a reappraisal of (pedigree-based) linkage studies that have sufficient power to detect the effects of rare variants, that is, the situation of genetic heterogeneity where different mutations in different individuals at the same locus (gene) contribute to disease. Similar methods have failed in the past, not due to inherently flawed design, but because the studies were too small and underpowered.

Another development that may advance our understanding of the genetic architecture of schizophrenia has been in the field of epigenetics, which refers to mitotically heritable modifications of DNA that do not involve a change in DNA sequence. One advantage of epigenetics is its potential to integrate studies of the genetic and environmental causes of schizophrenia, thereby achieving more powerful designs. The substantially lower discordance rate of schizophrenia in monozygotic (MZ) twins compared with dizygotic ones argues for a strong genetic component, and also allows for a significant role of environmental factors in the development of this complex disease (Oh and Petronis 2008). In this regard, several risk factors that implicate preconceptional, prenatal, or early childhood exposures have been consistently related to schizophrenia, including paternal age at conception, early prenatal famine, urban birth, and migration (especially in early childhood, see later) (Van Os and Kapur 2009). While some of these associations are likely to be causal, the mechanisms by which they are linked to schizophrenia are still largely unknown. Epigenetic mechanisms may mediate the effects of such risk factors, as the epigenetic status of the genome can be modified in response to the environment during embryonic growth, and probably also in the early years of life (Heijmans et al. 2009). Preliminary evidence suggests that epigenetic differences may be related to schizophrenia (Abdolmaleky et al. 2006; Mill et al. 2008), but these epigenetic studies have not yet included environmental exposures.

To determine the contribution of epigenetic components in the interplay between genes and environment, we must study populations that have been homogeneously exposed to well-defined and meticulously measured environmental exposures (Manolio et al. 2009). In this chapter, we discuss two environmental risk factors for schizophrenia in the light of epigenetics. We present epidemiological evidence of a relationship between schizophrenia and prenatal famine and migration. We then argue that the epidemiological findings are consistent with epigenetic mechanisms, and explore evidence of pathways linking these environmental exposures to schizophrenia via epigenetic effects. Finally, we propose ways to further test these hypotheses and argue that this may advance knowledge of both genetic and environmental causes of schizophrenia.

6.2 Prenatal Famine and Schizophrenia

6.2.1 Epidemiological Findings

Tragic historical events in the Netherlands and China set the stage for investigation of the effects of famine on schizophrenia and other health outcomes. Three studies have reported a link between periconceptional or early gestational exposure to starvation and a risk of schizophrenia in offspring (St Clair et al. 2005; Susser et al. 1996; Xu et al. 2009). The first of these studies was based on the Dutch Hunger Winter during World War II. In October 1944, the Nazis blocked food supplies to the Western part of the country in response to the activities of Dutch resistance groups. The famine ended abruptly with the liberation of the Netherlands in early May 1945. Early studies found an increased risk of neural tube defects among individuals who had been conceived at the height of the famine (Brown and Susser 2008), suggesting that the early gestational period is an important risk window for neurodevelopmental insults. This finding supported the plausibility of prenatal famine as a cause of schizophrenia, since a disturbance in early neurodevelopment has also been implicated in the etiology of this disorder. When the risks for schizophrenia were compared between the birth cohort that had been exposed to prenatal famine and unexposed cohorts born in surrounding years, it was found that periconceptional or early gestational, but not later exposure to famine was associated with a relative risk for schizophrenia of 2.0 (95% confidence interval [CI] 1.2–3.4) (Susser et al. 1996).

Recently, these findings have been replicated in two large studies in China. After the initiation of the Great Leap Forward in the late 1950s, a massive famine affected most parts of China. Causes include collectivization of agriculture and reduction of cultivated land. Estimates of famine-related deaths vary between 15 and 40 million people, making this one of the deadliest tragedies of the twentieth century. The height of the famine differed by region, but in Anhui Province, it was most severe from 1959 to 1960, as indicated by extremely high mortality rates and a reduction in birth rates to one-third of the pre-famine average. A recent study analyzed all in-patient and out-patient psychiatric referrals from 1971 to 2001 to the only psychiatric hospital in the region. The birth cohorts conceived or in early gestation in 1959 and 1960 had a twofold increase in risk for schizophrenia in later life, compared to those who were born before or after the famine (between 1956 and 1958 or between 1963 and 1965) (St Clair et al. 2005). Similarly, in a third study examining the Guanxi autonomous region, another part of China, there was a twofold increase in risk for schizophrenia among those conceived or in early gestation at the height of famine (Xu et al. 2009). The increased risk was found exclusively in rural areas, where famine conditions were most severe. This was due to the provision of food from state grain stores to those living in cities, whereas the rural population was only allowed to retain the grain that remained after they had delivered the imposed quotas.

6.2.2 The Folate Pathway

The biological pathways linking prenatal famine to schizophrenia are currently unknown, but there are many potential mechanisms, including micronutrient deficiencies, maternal stress effects on the neuroendocrine system, toxic effects of maternal ingestion of food substitutes, genetic selection (e.g., genetic differences between women who can and cannot ovulate and conceive during famine conditions), and preconceptional damage to paternal spermatogonia (Brown and Susser 2008).

To illustrate how an environmental exposure may have epigenetic effects in schizophrenia, we introduce the potential mechanism of folate deficiency. It is important to note that the metabolism and functions of folate are complicated (Lucock 2000), and that we use only a simplified example of a pathway in which folate plays a role (Fig. 6.1).

Folate is an important factor in the synthesis and maintenance of DNA, via synthesis of purines and pyrimidines (Lucock 2000). Folate deficiency can lead to chromosomal instability and aberrations of DNA repair, thereby increasing rates of mutation; de novo mutations in multiple genes have been related to schizophrenia (Stefansson et al. 2008). A second potential pathway through which folate deficiency may be related to schizophrenia is by disruption of epigenetic programming; folate is involved in the pathway of DNA methylation (Lucock 2000), which represents one of the major epigenetic processes. Another level of epigenetic information is the methylation of histones, which may similarly affect this process (Feinberg 2007). DNA methylation, meaning the addition of a methyl group to the

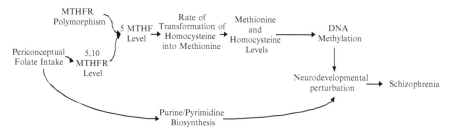

Fig. 6.1 Pathways that could link prenatal folate deficiency to schizophrenia

nucleotide cytosine, occurs at dinucleotide sites in the DNA where a phosphate molecule links cytosine (C) and guanine (G). The CpG dinucleotides can be found throughout the genome, but are highly concentrated in control regions of genes (CpG islands). Methylation modifies transcriptional access to the DNA and, thus, may alter gene expression (Feinberg 2007). The main source of methyl groups in this reaction is methionine, an essential amino acid that is converted from homocysteine to a biologically active methyl donor state. Folate promotes the conversion to methionine by increasing the level of 5,10-methylenetetrahydrofolate reductase (MTHFR) that in turn catalyzes the conversion of 5,10-MTHF to 5-MTHF, a cosubstrate for the homocysteine remethylation to methionine (Lucock 2000). Theoretically, folate deficiency will lead to a lower level of methionine and, therefore, to a lower rate of DNA methylation (Duthie et al. 2000).

Again, it should be realized that these pathways might be far more complicated than described here. This complexity is illustrated by human studies (including one examining the Dutch famine cohort), which also found associations between low folate status and higher level of DNA methylation in some genes (Tobi et al. 2009; Van Engeland et al. 2003). Also, the putative folate-effect may not only represent damage to the epigenome due to the harsh prenatal environment. It is possible that epigenetic changes in metabolic pathways following exposure to prenatal famine are adaptive, occurring either immediately to survive the malnutrition as an embryo/fetus, or in anticipation of the postnatal environment (Heijmans et al. 2009).

6.2.3   Evidence for Influence of Diet on DNA Methylation

Over the last decade, evidence has accumulated in support of the hypothesis that differences in availability of folate are associated with lasting differences in DNA methylation. There may be changes in epigenetic marks throughout an individual's lifetime (e.g., aging appears to be related to changes in DNA methylation; Rakyan et al. 2010), but the epigenome is the most dynamic in early development. Animal studies have suggested that genome-wide demethylation occurs early in gestation, a process in which most parental epigenetic marks are erased (Reik et al. 2001), with remethylation taking place shortly afterwards. The gestational period in which epigenetic reprogramming is thought to occur in humans matches the period in which exposure to famine (and thus folate deficiency) was related to an increased risk for neural tube defects and schizophrenia in the Dutch study. Epigenetic effects as a result of folate deficiency may, therefore, be a mechanism that contributes to the increased risk.

Epigenetic marks are determined by genetic and stochastic factors, but as it turns out, they are also under the influence of environmental factors, such as diet, during early development. A series of experiments with agouti viable yellow (A^{vy}) mice showed that dietary methyl supplements, including folate, in the early gestational period can produce persistent changes in DNA methylation (Waterland and Jirtle 2003; Wolff et al. 1998). A^{vy} mice have a mutation in the regulatory region of the agouti allele. Ectopic agouti transcription is initiated from a promoter in the proximal end of the inserted transposable element. Methylation in this region varies considerably among individual mice and is correlated inversely with ectopic agouti expression. This epigenetic variability causes a wide variation in individual coat color (Wolff et al. 1998). In the offspring of A^{vy} mice that were assigned to a methyl-rich diet, the agouti gene was methylated to a higher level. This resulted in silencing of the gene and downregulated the ectopic agouti expression, which in turn produced a shift in coat color from yellow to brown (Waterland and Jirtle 2003). Since the color differences persisted into adulthood, these findings demonstrated that early life dietary conditions could cause epigenetic changes that are stable into adulthood.

The Dutch famine study provided a unique opportunity to investigate whether prenatal exposure to the prevailing famine conditions is associated with persistent epigenetic differences in humans. Six decades after World War II, individuals who had been exposed prenatally to famine had less methylation of the imprinted insulin-like growth factor II gene (*IGF2*) than their unexposed same-sex siblings (Heijmans et al. 2008). This association was specific for exposure in early gestation: the group that was exposed in late pregnancy did not have lower *IGF2* methylation than their unexposed siblings, although they did have a lower mean birth weight. A subsequent analysis of 15 genes implicated in growth and metabolic diseases, in the same cohort, found that DNA methylation differences were not restricted to only the IGF2 gene, or to early gestational exposure to famine; some genes had less methylation, other genes had a higher degree of methylation in exposed individuals (Tobi et al. 2009). Methylation differences were sex-specific and some associations were found only in those exposed during late gestation, thus persistent changes in DNA methylation may be a common consequence of prenatal exposure to famine.

6.2.4 Epigenetic Effects on Health and the Role of Folate

Persistent alterations in DNA methylation can have a significant influence on health in animals. This is illustrated by the A^{vy} mice, which not only have a more yellow coat than mice without ectopic agouti expression, but also have increases in obesity, diabetes, and susceptibility to tumors (Miltenberger et al. 1997; Wolff et al. 1998). However, it should be noted that this is a very specific genetic transposon model and it cannot be generalized to every DNA sequence or genomic element. Most evidence of epigenetic effects on disease in humans comes from cancer research. Tumor development is regulated by the activation of growth-promoting genes through both global and gene-specific hypomethylation or hypermethylation (Feinberg 2007). The methylation differences may be an indication of genomic instability, and also of altered functioning of specific genes that are relevant to specific diseases, for example, silencing of tumor suppression genes through hypermethylation (Feinberg 2007). Other examples include rare epigenetic diseases, such as Beckwith–Wiedemann syndrome, which is characterized by loss of normal imprinted gene regulation (DeBaun et al. 2002), resulting in affected children typically having macrosomia, abdominal birth defects, and an increased risk of childhood cancer.

The finding that early prenatal exposure to famine was related to neural tube defects, combined with nonrandomized trials, small randomized trials, and observational epidemiological studies of maternal vitamin supplements and neural tube defects (Smithells et al. 1980), provided a strong body of evidence that folate vitamin supplements could reduce the risk of neural tube defects, and prompted initiation of large-scale randomized trials. Definitive randomized trials in the 1990s showed that folate supplementation reduced about 80% of the risk for neural tube defects (Czeizel and Dudás 1992; Group MVSR 1991). These studies also suggested that the critical period for the preventive effect of folate supplementation actually begins shortly prior to conception and ends at 28 days of gestation, when the neural tube closes. As a result, from the 1990s onwards, all women who considered pregnancy were advised to take folate supplementation. Some countries even introduced mandatory folic acid fortification of flour, since the benefits of folate supplementation were large, the costs were low and the intervention had no apparent side effects. With increasing knowledge of the folate pathway and of the involvement of folate in epigenetic programming, however, concerns were raised about other potential long-term consequences for child health and development. A recent study found higher methylation of *IGF2* among children whose mother used folic acid during periconception, indicating that this may indeed lead to epigenetic changes in humans (Steegers-Theunissen et al. 2009). The children of the mothers participating in the original randomized trials of folate supplementation have yet to be investigated, however, some observational studies have found associations between maternal use of folate supplements and an increased risk of asthma and atopy in young children (Haberg et al. 2009; Whitrow et al. 2009), while another study has found an association with decreased risk of childhood behavioral problems and hyperactivity (Schlotz et al. 2009). Conversely, one study did not find a relationship between periconceptional folate supplements and mental or psychomotor development (Tamura et al. 2005). Most recently, data from a large prospective Norwegian birth cohort study (Magnus et al. 2006) suggest that folate supplementation is associated with better neurodevelopmental outcomes (results under review). The studies on folate supplementation should all be regarded as preliminary; nevertheless, they do suggest that periconceptional folate supplements may have consequences for health and neurodevelopment in childhood and later on.

6.2.5 Epigenetic Changes in Schizophrenia

As previously mentioned, epigenetic factors may be related to schizophrenia. Briefly, studies examining postmortem brain tissue reported several potentially important associations. Reelin is a protein involved in neuronal migration in the developing brain, and increased DNA methylation has been found at several positions in the promoter region of the reelin gene in the occipital and prefrontal cortex of schizophrenia patients compared with nonpsychiatric controls (Grayson et al. 2005). A second study, however, showed no detectable DNA methylation at these sites (Tochigi et al. 2008). Another study reported hypomethylation of the membrane-bound catechol-*O*-methyltransferase gene (*MB-COMT*) promoter in the frontal lobe of patients with schizophrenia and bipolar disorder (Abdolmaleky et al. 2006). This may be relevant to the pathophysiology of schizophrenia, since COMT regulates the homeostatic levels of the neurotransmitter dopamine in the synapses, and dopamine plays a central role in schizophrenia (Laruelle 2003). Hypomethylation was related to upregulation of *MB-COMT* (Abdolmaleky et al. 2006), which in turn increases the dopamine degradation in the frontal cortex. *COMT* hypomethylation may be causally related to the cognitive and negative symptoms of schizophrenia, which have been associated with prefrontal hypodopaminergic functioning (Laruelle 2003). Again, a replication study found no evidence of altered *COMT* steady state mRNA or methylation in brains of schizophrenia patients, albeit that this second study used cerebellum rather than frontal lobe tissue (Dempster et al. 2006). In the first genome-wide epigenomic study, Mill et al. (2008) found a number of genes exhibiting differences in DNA methylation in the prefrontal cortex of schizophrenia and bipolar patients vs. healthy controls. The differences included loci involved in glutamatergic and GABAergic neurotransmission and brain development.

There are many caveats in interpreting these findings (see Box 6.1), but even when methodological and conceptual problems are solved, epigenetic studies may continue to yield mixed results when environmental exposures are not taken into account. Given the substantial environmental influence on the epigenome, the epigenetic effects in the pathways leading to schizophrenia may depend on environmental exposures in early life. There are at least two possibilities: (a) environmental exposures may shift the epigenetic status in the exposed population, which results in a higher rate of schizophrenia in that population (Fig. 6.2a) – an example of this principle is that a shift in distribution of high blood pressure in a population can lead to an increase of the occurrence of cardiovascular disease in those individuals (Rose 1985); or (b) epigenetic effects of environmental exposure operate selectively on individuals with genetic predisposition to schizophrenia, i.e., nonadditive gene–environment interaction (Fig. 6.2b).

> **Box 6.1. Methodological and Technical Difficulties in Epigenetic Epidemiology**
> - Epigenetic marks are cell- and tissue-specific – since the brain cannot be accessed in live individuals, other tissues must be used for epigenetic studies of schizophrenia. Epigenetic marks in tissues such as peripheral blood may not correspond to the epigenome of brain regions.
> - The stability of epigenetic marks over the life course is unknown – in cross-sectional studies, it is not possible to test whether epigenetic differences are cause or consequence of illness.
> - Interindividual variation in DNA methylation, and the relationships among methylation, gene expression, and functional consequences are not completely clear for most genes.

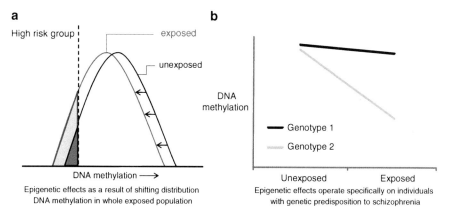

Fig. 6.2 Possible environmental influences on epigenetic effects and schizophrenia risk

Epidemiological studies can help to detect epigenetic mechanisms of disease, with the conditions that measurement of the environmental exposure is precise, timing of exposure is known, and that a homogeneously exposed population is available for study (Foley et al. 2009; Oh and Petronis 2008). In addition, it only makes sense to study causal epigenetic effects mediated by environmental factors if the correlation between the environmental exposure and genetic predisposition to schizophrenia is low (Oh and Petronis 2008).

6.2.6 Famine Studies as a Tool for Detecting Epigenetic Mechanisms in Schizophrenia

The above conditions can be fulfilled in famine studies. We will use the Dutch famine study for illustration purposes here (Box 6.2). Although the sample size of

Box 6.2. Is Prenatal Famine a Useful Environmental Exposure for Epigenetic Studies of Schizophrenia?
The example of the 1944–1945 Dutch famine:
– *Precise measure*: Daily distributed food rations during famine are known. Although some families had more access to food for economic or other reasons, the measures are precise enough to describe changes in average food intake over time.
– *Homogeneous exposure*: The total population of a well-circumscribed geographic area has been exposed to famine, during a well-specified period. While there was substantial individual variation in food intake, the large majority of the population suffered from severe food shortage.
– *Timing of exposure*: Date of birth is an easy measure. It can be used to estimate timing of conception, though with some imprecision.
– *Gene–environment correlation*: War-related famine, it is unlikely that prenatal exposure was strongly influenced by (parental) schizophrenia genes.
– *Plausible biological/genetic pathways*: These are identified; folate-related one-carbon pathway, MTHFR gene, IGF2 gene.

the actual study is too small to investigate epigenetic effects in schizophrenia, there is a great potential for follow-up studies of famine exposure in China, where several hundreds of prenatally exposed schizophrenia cases have been identified (St Clair et al. 2005).

During the World War II famine in the Netherlands, the total population of the larger cities in the western part of the country was exposed to severe food shortages. We know exactly that the height of the famine was from January through April 1945, and that it ended immediately after liberation on 5th May 1945. We know that the daily distributed food ration was less than 500 calories/day at the height of the famine, and we have detailed population data, in addition to detailed information of adult health outcomes, including schizophrenia (Brown and Susser 2008). It is unlikely that a strong correlation exists between (parental) schizophrenia genes and prenatal exposure to famine, because the famine was war-related, unpredicted, and largely inescapable.

In this context, a powerful study design would be to combine the environmental information with epigenetic measures. In a case-control study, DNA methylation should be measured in at least four groups (a) exposed cases – individuals with schizophrenia from the birth cohort conceived during the height of the famine, (b) unexposed cases – individuals with schizophrenia from surrounding birth cohorts, (c) exposed random controls, and (d) unexposed random controls.

Global DNA methylation may be used as an indicator of genomic stability, but hypotheses of gene-specific methylation differences can be tested as well. Methylation loss of the imprinted IGF2 gene is an interesting candidate, because this epigenetic effect has already been found in individuals exposed to the Dutch famine in early gestation (Heijmans et al. 2008), and the gene is involved in (brain) growth and development. We have to keep in mind that epigenetic marks are tissue-specific, and therefore, the best option would be to study brain tissue, but this cannot be sampled during life. There is some evidence, however, that DNA methylation measured in blood may be a marker for less accessible tissues that are directly involved in disease (Talens et al. 2010). Epigenetic changes in brain tissue are also often found in peripheral cells, but this issue has yet to be resolved.

If epigenetic effects of famine on schizophrenia operate through a shift in distribution of DNA methylation profiles in the total exposed population (Fig. 6.2a), we may find differences in DNA methylation between exposed and unexposed controls (reflecting the shift in distribution), but no differences between exposed and unexposed cases (there will be more exposed than unexposed cases, but in both groups, most cases are found in the high risk end of the distribution).

On the other hand, if epigenetic effects of famine on schizophrenia depend on a specific pre-existing genetic vulnerability to schizophrenia (Fig. 6.2b), we would find a different pattern of results. For example, we may find no differences in DNA methylation between exposed and unexposed controls, but instead find differences between exposed and unexposed cases.

These are two basic illustrations of how epidemiological models can be used and how different models may predict different results. We want to emphasize that many other models can be envisioned, such as a model that accounts for the interplay between the postnatal environment and the epigenome. An example of the latter is discussed in the next section. Nevertheless, the prenatal famine example clearly demonstrates that adding environmental exposure to an epigenetic study may increase the chances of detecting epigenetic effects and understanding the epigenetic mechanisms in schizophrenia. If information about famine exposure status is not considered, the overall result may be inconclusive or not confirmed in replication studies.

6.3 Migration/Childhood Ethnic Minority Status

6.3.1 Epidemiological Findings

Associations between the incidence of schizophrenia and international migration have been reported for nearly 80 years. In the early 1930s, Ødegaard (1932) found that Norwegian immigrants in the USA were admitted to a psychiatric hospital for schizophrenia twice as often as native-born Americans or Norwegians in Norway. Observations of higher schizophrenia rates among immigrants were also reported in the 1950s and 1960s in the USA and the UK (Hemsi 1967; Malzberg 1955). These studies had considerable methodological limitations, but later investigations in the UK, using prospective case finding within defined catchment areas, standardized assessments and diagnostic criteria of psychopathology, and more accurate census data, replicated the findings of an increased risk for schizophrenia in immigrant populations (Harrison et al. 1997; King et al. 1994). In the last decade, the large AESOP incidence study, conducted in London, Nottingham, and Bristol, found strikingly increased rates of schizophrenia in African Caribbeans (Incidence Rate Ratio [IRR] = 9.1; 95% CI 6.6–12.6) and Black Africans (IRR = 5.8; 95% CI 3.9–8.4) compared with the white British population, and modestly increased rates in Asian and other immigrants (Fearon et al. 2006). The rates of schizophrenia were significantly increased in second-generation immigrants in London as well (Coid et al. 2008).

The association between migration and schizophrenia has also been studied extensively in the Netherlands. Selten reported significantly higher first-admission rates for schizophrenia in immigrants from Surinam, the Netherlands Antilles, and Morocco in the 1990s (Selten and Sijben 1994; Selten et al. 1997). Subsequently, a prospective first-contact incidence study of psychotic disorders found an increased risk for schizophrenia in Surinamese and Moroccan immigrants, both in the first and second generation (Selten et al. 2001; Veling et al. 2006). The risk was particularly high for Moroccan males (first generation: IRR = 4.0; 95% CI 2.5–6.3 and second generation: IRR = 5.8; 95% CI 2.9–11.4) and was not significantly increased for Turkish immigrants or immigrants from Western countries (Veling et al. 2006).

Taken together, the incidence of schizophrenia is increased in different immigrant groups in several countries around the world. The degree to which rates are increased varies considerably with ethnic group and country, but the increased risk pertains to second-generation immigrants. A meta-analysis of all migrant incidence studies of schizophrenia up to 2003 estimated the mean relative risks of 2.7 and 4.5 for first- and second-generation immigrants, respectively, compared with native populations (Cantor-Graae and Selten 2005). Several potential explanations have been proposed for the migrant findings. We cannot review these here due to space restrictions (see Cantor-Graae and Selten 2005 for a full discussion), but it is necessary to discuss whether migration can be treated as an environmental risk factor in epigenetic studies of schizophrenia (Box 6.3).

Gene–environment correlation is conceivable, as individuals with genetic predisposition to schizophrenia may be more likely to migrate. No studies in the UK directly addressed selective migration. A population register study in Denmark, however, found an increased risk among immigrants who migrated as a child and, thus, did not make the decision to migrate themselves (Cantor-Graae et al. 2003). In the Netherlands, we recently completed an analysis of age at migration in The Hague incidence study. The results are still under review, but show that the risk for schizophrenia among immigrants is still increased when only those immigrants who migrated before the age of 15 were included.

When age at migration data are available, the relevant timing of exposure can be determined precisely. Our age at migration analyses show that the risk for schizophrenia is particularly high for immigrants who migrated in early childhood (between age 0 and 4) and decreases with older age at migration. In combination with the replicated finding of an increased risk among second-generation immigrants (Coid

Box 6.3. Is Migration a Useful Environmental Exposure for Epigenetic Studies of Schizophrenia?
- *Precise measure*: History of international migration.
- *Homogeneous exposure*: First-generation immigrants have all been exposed to migration; the exposure can be considered homogeneous when one country of origin and one country of arrival are studied.
- *Timing of exposure*: Age at migration, easy, and reliable measure.
- *Gene–environment correlation*: Selective migration is unlikely, because the risk for schizophrenia is also increased among immigrants who migrated in childhood.
- *Biological/genetic pathways*: These have not yet been established; hypotheses include sensitization of the mesolimbic dopamine system, and increased inflammatory set-point as a result of stress in early life.

et al. 2008; Veling et al. 2006), the results strongly suggest that not the event of migration itself, but the context of living in an ethnic minority position in early childhood may be the actual environmental exposure influencing risk for psychosis in adulthood.

Several studies in the UK and the Netherlands have found that a disadvantaged ethnic minority position, characterized by low social status, high degree of discrimination against the group, and low proportion of others from one's own ethnic group in the neighborhood (low ethnic density), may lead to an increased risk of psychotic disorders (Veling 2008). This is particularly the case when social resources are insufficient to buffer the impact of the adverse social experiences (compromised family structures, restricted social networks, low access to social capital, and low social cohesion of ethnic group) (Veling 2008). It should be noted that most of these studies investigated the social context at illness onset; however, unpublished data from a US birth cohort study also suggests that low ethnic density at birth increases the risk for adult schizophrenia among ethnic minorities (Dana March, personal communication).

6.3.2   Epigenetic Changes in Postnatal Life

Prenatal folate deficiency can influence epigenetic marks in DNA, such changes may persist into adulthood and may influence health, including neurodevelopmental outcomes. One further step could be to test the association between exposure to famine- and folate-related epigenetic changes in schizophrenia. In the case of migration, however, there are fewer hypotheses of potential pathways and less evidence supporting biological mechanisms. Can we make an argument that epigenetic factors may be involved?

There are two apparent differences, in this respect, between exposure to migration and to famine. First, the epidemiological evidence of migration suggests that early childhood is an important etiological period and, if the effect of migration on schizophrenia is mediated by epigenetic effects, persistent changes in the epigenome should be possible in childhood. This is at least conceivable, as gestation in rats does not equal gestation in humans; brain development in humans takes longer and is still very rapid in the early years of life. Also, the timing of epigenetic programming may be related to tissue differentiation and development, and may occur at a later stage in some tissues (Heijmans et al. 2009). Second, it appears that social context shapes the increased risk among ethnic minorities, rather than dietary conditions. Social experiences should therefore be translated into epigenetic consequences.

Recently, a series of experiments with maternal behavior in rats have suggested that both requirements may be met. Offspring of "high care" mothers are less fearful and show a more modest physiological stress response than offspring of "low care" mothers (Caldji et al. 1998), but biological offspring of "low care" mothers reared by "high care" mothers (cross-fostering) resemble the normal offspring of the "high care" mothers (Francis et al. 1999). These findings suggest a persistent effect of maternal behavior on stress reactivity in offspring that is not associated with DNA sequence. The glucocorticoid receptor (GR) may be involved, because GR gene expression is related to stress reactivity and was increased in the offspring of "high care" mothers (Francis et al. 1999). As gene expression is controlled by the epigenome, Meaney and colleagues investigated whether maternal care alters the methylation of the promoter region of the GR gene in rats (Weaver et al. 2004). They found de novo differences in methylation of the NGFI-A consensus sequence on the exon 1_7 promoter in hippocampal cells between offspring of low care and high care mothers (Weaver et al. 2004). These differences were absent at birth, but emerged over the first week of life and persisted into adulthood. The impact of maternal care on DNA methylation was reversible in adult postmitotic brain cells, as differences in DNA methylation were removed after central infusion of a histone deacetylase (HDAC) inhibitor (Weaver et al. 2004). In another experiment, both methylation pattern and behavioral response to stress normalized after methionine treatment in adult offspring of "low care" mothers (Weaver et al. 2005).

Animal studies also suggest that epigenetic mechanisms are involved in the formation of long-term memory in the hippocampus. Neurons of rats subjected to a conditioned fear paradigm (in which they learn to associate a novel context with an aversive stimulus) showed increased acetylation of histone H3 (Levenson et al. 2004). DNA methylation was also found to regulate synaptic plasticity and memory in adult animals, while fear conditioning was associated with rapid methylation of the memory suppressor gene protein, phosphatase 1, and demethylation of the reelin gene (Miller et al. 2008; Sweatt 2009).

These results suggest that epigenetic regulation of genes may be a much more dynamic process than previously believed. Environmental influences on the epigenome might not be restricted to prenatal life – early social experiences, such as maternal care, may cause epigenetic differences with adult phenotypic consequences. Also, despite the inherent stability of epigenomic marks established in early life, they may be potentially reversible in the adult brain. Moreover, epigenetic processes may be involved in normal brain responses to environmental stimuli.

It should be noted, however, that it is uncertain how these rat models apply to human physiology and psychology. We do not know whether social experiences affect epigenetic programming in humans. It is also unclear whether significant epigenetic changes due to environmental exposures occur throughout life or are limited to critical points perinatally and perhaps in early life (Szyf et al. 2008). Still, there is some evidence of changes in epigenetic patterns over the life course: one report suggests that monozygotic twins may show increasingly different global DNA methylation profiles at older ages (Fraga et al. 2005), and a recent study of normal human aging identified aging-associated differentially methylated regions in different tissues (Rakyan et al. 2010). These changes may reflect not only the genetic control, but also the influence of environmental exposures over the life course. One recent study examining epigenetic regulation of the glucocorticoid receptor gene (*GR*) in the human brain suggests that the maternal care results in rats may be relevant to humans. Suicide victims with a history of childhood abuse were found to have decreased levels of *GR* mRNA, as well as mRNA transcripts bearing the *GR 1F* splice variant and an increase in cytosine methylation of the *NR3C1* promoter, compared to either suicide victims with no childhood abuse or controls (McGowan et al. 2009).

These issues have not been resolved as of yet, and epidemiological studies are needed to clarify the role of epigenetics over the life course. Migration studies can help to test whether social experiences of early life adversity can have long-term effects on epigenetic processes in humans, and whether and how these may increase the risk of schizophrenia.

6.3.3 Ethnic Minority Status and Potential Epigenetic Effects

As previously discussed, the high rates of schizophrenia among ethnic minorities are difficult to explain outside of the context of social factors. More specifically, having an ethnic minority status in early childhood is related to an increased risk. Few biological hypotheses have been proposed to explain these findings, and none have been tested in humans. We use two examples to illustrate potential epigenetic pathways.

Social defeat has been used as a paradigm to relate epidemiological findings to potential neurobiological mechanisms. Selten and Cantor-Graae (2007) proposed that childhood ethnic minority status represents the long-term experience of social defeat, defined as a subordinate position or as "outsider status." In rodents, chronic exposure to social defeat (carried out by placing an experimental mouse in the home cage of a different aggressive mouse repeatedly for several days) has been associated with dopaminergic hyperactivity in the mesocorticolimbic system (Tidey and Miczek 1996), in particular, when the experimental animals were socially isolated after defeat (Isovich et al. 2001). Heightened dopaminergic transmission is likely to play a central role in schizophrenia. Several studies demonstrated that drug naïve schizophrenia patients have an increase in mesolimbic dopamine release after acute amphetamine challenge (Laruelle 2003), suggesting an abnormal responsiveness of dopaminergic neurons. Among other factors, the neurotrophic factor brain-derived neurotrophic factor (BDNF) may be a key regulator of the mesolimbic dopamine pathway (Berton et al. 2006). In an animal study, knockdown of *Bdnf* in the nucleus accumbens (NAc) removed most of the effects of repeated social defeat on gene expression within this circuit (Berton et al. 2006). Another study reported that chronic social defeat stress significantly downregulated mRNA levels of HDAC 5 in the NAc (Renthal et al. 2007). This suggests epigenetic control of the response to social defeat, as this HDAC enzyme is capable of repressing *BDNF*, as well as the expression of many other genes (Tsankova et al. 2006).

The second example involves immunological pathways. The hypothesis that chronic inflammation may be a basic biological mechanism of schizophrenia has a long history (Smith 1992). Recent studies of the proinflammatory state of circulating monocytes in patients with bipolar disorder and schizophrenia have reported increased mRNA levels of inflammatory genes (Drexhage et al. 2010; Padmos et al. 2008). The aberrant gene-expression profile was also found in children of bipolar patients (Padmos et al. 2008), and a subsequent twin study suggested that nearly all the variation in proinflammatory gene expression was due to environmental factors (Padmos et al. 2009). There are a multitude of factors that can influence proinflammatory monocyte activation, one of which is exposure to stress in early life (Padmos et al. 2009). Growing up in a low ethnic density context, which is related to increased risk for schizophrenia among ethnic minorities (Veling et al. 2008), is likely to be associated with disturbing experiences and social stress – stress is often implicated in etiological models of schizophrenia (Walker and Diforio 1997). Consistent with this hypothesis, human studies have found that individuals who are genetically vulnerable to psychosis are also more sensitive to daily life stress than healthy controls (Myin-Germeys et al. 2001, 2005). In addition, early childhood trauma has been linked to an increased risk for adult psychosis (Read et al. 2005), and there is preliminary evidence that early trauma may have persistent epigenetic effects on stress reactivity (McGowan et al. 2009). Overall, the maternal care experiments in rats discussed earlier suggest the possibility of epigenetic regulation of stress reactivity (Weaver et al. 2004), and evidence in humans supports that there is an inherent plausibility that different, disturbing experiences in early childhood could have epigenetic effects. In summation, the epigenetic modifications induced by early life stress exposure may mediate the effect of childhood ethnic minority status on schizophrenia.

6.3.4 Migration Studies as a Tool for Detecting Epigenetic Mechanisms in Schizophrenia

Migration studies provide opportunities to investigate potential epigenetic mechanisms in schizophrenia. To enhance the power of the study design and to increase the homogeneity of the exposure, we should study a single ethnic minority group, preferably the group with the highest effect of migration on risk for schizophrenia, i.e., African Caribbeans in the UK or Moroccans in the Netherlands.

The first question to address is whether early postnatal social experiences can influence the epigenome in humans. That is are persistent epigenetic changes associated with early postnatal exposure to the social experience of ethnic minority status? To test this concept, we could assess peripheral blood samples and compare the epigenome of exposed ethnic minority individuals (who arrived in the Netherlands before age 5 or were born in the Netherlands as second generation) with that of unexposed individuals (ethnic minorities who arrived as adults or are native Dutch). Again, an important caveat is that it is uncertain how epigenetic marks in peripheral blood correspond to the epigenome of the brain tissues relevant to schizophrenia. Epigenetic changes occurring later in life in one tissue will not necessarily be visible in another tissue, whereas epigenetic changes induced early in development may be more likely to be propagated throughout the body because the epigenetic marks are partially stable in somatic cells (Heijmans et al. 2009).

The second question is whether: epigenetic changes mediate the effect of ethnic minority status on the risk for schizophrenia. As explained in the famine example, epigenetic effects of childhood ethnic minority status may shift the whole distribution of epigenetic changes in the ethnic minority population (Fig. 6.2a), or they may operate selectively on individuals with a genetic predisposition to schizophrenia (Fig. 6.2b). If epigenetic effects operate through a shift in distribution of DNA methylation, we would find differences in DNA methylation between exposed and unexposed controls (reflecting the shift in distribution), but no differences between exposed and unexposed cases (there will be more exposed than unexposed cases, but in both groups, most cases are found in the high risk end of the distribution). However, if epigenetic effects of childhood ethnic minority status depend on specific pre-existing genetic vulnerability to schizophrenia (Fig. 6.2a), we may find differences in DNA methylation between exposed cases and exposed controls, but no significant epigenetic differences between unexposed cases and unexposed controls.

6.4 Conclusion

Epigenetic mechanisms may play an important role in the etiological pathways of schizophrenia. Since the epigenetic status of the genome partly depends on environmental factors in pre- and postnatal environments, exposure to such factors should be taken into account in epigenetic studies of schizophrenia. Prenatal famine and childhood ethnic minority status have been identified as environmental risk factors for schizophrenia. These exposures can be used to investigate epigenetic effects on schizophrenia, since environmental exposure can be measured with sufficient precision, homogeneously exposed populations are available for study, and plausible biological pathways have been suggested (albeit less specific for migration). We have shown that epidemiological studies of famine and migration can help to detect epigenetic mechanisms in schizophrenia, by comparing the epigenome of exposed and unexposed schizophrenia cases and controls. Since epigenetic marks are tissue-specific, especially when they occur later in life, experimenters should carefully consider the choice of tissues to be used in these studies. The results of the comparisons will be different depending on the mechanism involved in the interplay between environment and epigenome. If these epidemiological designs are not applied, the overall result of epigenetic schizophrenia studies may well continue to be inconclusive. Thus, the examples of prenatal famine and childhood ethnic minority status clearly demonstrate that it is important to add an environmental exposure aspect to epigenetic studies of schizophrenia.

References

Abdolmaleky HM, Cheng KH, Faraone SV, Wilcox M, Glatt SJ, Gao F, Smith CL, Shafa R, Aeali B, Carnevale J, Pan H, Papageorgis P, Ponte JF, Sivaraman V, Tsuang MT, Thiagalingam S (2006) Hypomethylation of MB-COMT promoter is a major risk factor for schizophrenia and bipolar disorder. Hum Mol Genet 15:3132–3145

Allen NC, Bagade S, McQueen MB, Ioannidis JP, Kawoura FK, Khoury MJ, Tanzi RE, Bertram L (2008) Systematic meta-analyses and field synopsis of the genetic association studies in schizophrenia: the SzGene database. Nat Genet 40:827–834

Berton O, McClung CA, DiLeone RJ, Krishnan V, Renthal W, Russo SJ, Graham D, Tsankova NM, Bolanos CA, Rios M, Monteggia LM, Self DW, Nestler EJ (2006) Essential role of BDNF in the mesolimbic pathway in social defeat stress. Science 311:864–868

Brown AS, Susser ES (2008) Prenatal nutritional deficiency and risk of adult schizophrenia. Schizophr Bull 34:1054–1063

Caldji C, Tannenbaum B, Sharma S, Francis D, Plotsky PM, Meany MJ (1998) Maternal care during infancy regulates the development of neural systems mediating the expression of fearfulness in the rat. Proc Natl Acad Sci 28:5335–5340

Cantor-Graae E, Selten JP (2005) Schizophrenia and migration: a meta-analysis and review. Am J Psychiatry 162:12–24

Cantor-Graae E, Pedersen CB, McNeil TF, Mortensen PB (2003) Migration as a risk factor for schizophrenia: a Danish population-based cohort study. Br J Psychiatry 182:117–122

Coid JW, Kirkbride JB, Barker D, Cowden F, Stamps R, Yang M, Jones PB (2008) Raised incidence rates of all psychoses among migrant groups. Arch Gen Psychiatry 65:1250–1258

Czeizel AE, Dudás I (1992) Prevention of the first occurrence of neural-tube defects by periconceptual vitamin suppletion. New Eng J Med 327:1832–1835

DeBaun MR, Niemitz EL, McNeil DE, Brandenburg SA, Lee MP, Feinberg AP (2002) Epigenetic alterations of H19 and LIT1 distinguish patients with Beckwith-Wiedemann syndrome with cancer and birth defects. Am J Hum Genet 70:604–611

Dempster EL, Mill J, Craig IW, Collier DA (2006) The quantification of COMT mRNA in post mortem cerebellum tissue: diagnosis, genotype, methylation and expression. BMC Med Genet 7:10

Drexhage RC, Knijff EM, Padmos RC, Heul-Nieuwenhuijzen L, Beumer W, Versnel MA, Drexhage HA (2010) The mononuclear phagocyte system and its cytokine inflammatory networks in schizophrenia and bipolar disorder. Expert Rev Neurother 10:59–76

Duthie SJ, Narayanan S, Blum S, Pirie L, Brand GM (2000) Folate deficiency in vitro induces uracil misincorporation and DNA hypomethylation and inhibits DNA excision repair in immortalized normal human colon epithelial cells. Nutr Cancer 37:245–251

Fearon P, Kirkbride JB, Morgan C, Dazzan P, Morgan K, Lloyd T, Hutchinson G, Tarrant J, Fung WLA, Holloway J, Mallett R, Harrison G, Leff J, Jones PB, Murray RM (2006) Incidence of schizophrenia and other psychoses in ethnic minority groups: results from the MRC AESOP study. Psychol Med 36:1541–1550

Feinberg AP (2007) Phenotypic plasticity and the epigenetics of human disease. Nature 447:433–440

Foley DL, Craig JM, Morley R, Olsson CA, Dwyer T, Smith K, Saffery R (2009) Prospects for epigenetic epidemiology. Am J Epidemiol 169:389–400

Fraga MF, Ballestar E, Paz MF, Ropero S, Setien F, Ballestar ML, Heine-Suner D, Cigudosa JC, Urioste M, Benitez J, Boix-Chornet M, Sanchez-Aguilera A, Ling C, Carlsson E, Poulsen P, Vaag A, Stephan Z, Spector TD, Wu YZ, Plass C, Esteller M (2005) Epigenetic differences arise during the lifetime of monozygotic twins. Proc Natl Acad Sci 102:10604–10609

Francis D, Diorio J, Liu D, Meany MJ (1999) Nongenomic transmission across generations of maternal behavior and stress responses in the rat. Science 286:1155–1158

Grayson DR, Jia X, Chen Y, Sharma RP, Mitchell CP, Guidotti A, Costa E (2005) Reelin promoter hypermethylation in schizophrenia. Proc Natl Acad Sci 102:9341–9346

Group MVSR (1991) Prevention of neural tube defects: results of the Medical Research Council Vitamin Study. Lancet 338:131–137

Haberg S, London SJ, Stigum H, Nafstad P, Nystad W (2009) Folic acid supplements in pregnancy and early childhood respiratory health. Arch Dis Child 94:180–184

Harrison G, Glazebrook C, Brewin J, Cantwell R, Dalkin T, Fox R, Jones P, Medley I (1997) Increased incidence of psychotic disorders in migrants from the Caribbean to the United Kingdom. Psychol Med 27:799–806

Heijmans BT, Tobi EW, Stein AD, Putter H, Blauw GJ, Susser ES, Slagboom PE, Lumey LH (2008) Persistent epigenetic differences associated with prenatal exposure to famine in humans. Proc Natl Acad Sci 105:17046–17049

Heijmans BT, Tobi EW, Lumey LH, Slagboom PE (2009) The epigenome; archive of the prenatal environment. Epigenetics 4:526–531

Hemsi LK (1967) Psychotic morbidity of West Indian immigrants. Soc Psychiatry 2:95–100

Isovich E, Engelmann M, Landgraf R, Fuchs E (2001) Social isolation after a single defeat reduces striatal dopamine transporter binding in rats. Eur J Neurosci 13:1254–1256

Kehoe PG, Russ C, McIlory S, Williams H, Holmans P, Holmes C, Liolitsa D, Vahidassr D, Powell J, McGleenon B, Liddell M, Plomin R, Dynan K, Williams N, Neal J, Cairns NJ, Wilcock G, Passmore P, Lovestone S, Williams J, Owen MJ (1999) Variation in DCP1, encoding ACE, is associated with susceptibility to Alzheimer disease. Nat Genet 21:71–72

King M, Coker E, Leavy G, Hoare A, Johnson-Sabine E (1994) Incidence of psychotic illness in London: comparison of ethnic groups. Br Med J 309:1115–1119

Laruelle M (2003) Dopamine transmission in the schizophrenic brain. In: Hirsch SR, Weinberger D (eds) Schizophrenia. Blackwell, Oxford, pp 365–387

Levenson JM, O'Riordan KJ, Brown KD, Trinh MA, Molfese DL, Sweatt JD (2004) Regulation of histone acetylation during memory formation in the hippocampus. J Biol Chem 279:40545–40549

Lucock M (2000) Folic acid: nutritional biochemistry, molecular biology, and role in disease processes. Mol Genet Metab 71:121–138

Magnus P, Irgens LM, Haug K, Nystad W, Skjaerven R, Stoltenberg C, Group TMS (2006) Cohort profile: the Norwegian mother and child cohort study. Int J Epidemiol 35:1146–1150

Malzberg B (1955) Mental disease among the native and foreign-born white populations of New York State, 1939–41. Ment Hyg 39:545–563

Manolio TA, Collins FS, Cox NJ, Goldstein DB, Hindorff LA, Hunter DJ, McCarthy MI, Ramos EM, Cardon LR, Chakravarti A, Cho JH, Guttmacher AE, Kong A, Kruglyak L, Mardis E, Rotimi CN, Slatkin M, Valle D, Whittemore AS, Boehnke M, Clark AG, Eichler EE, Gibson G, Haines JL, Mackay TF, McCarroll SA, Visscher PM (2009) Finding the missing heritability of complex disorders. Nature 461:747–753

McGowan PO, Sasaki A, D'Alessio AC, Dymov S, Labonté B, Szyf M, Turecki G, Meany MJ (2009) Epigenetic regulation of the glucocorticoid receptor in human brain associates with childhood abuse. Nat Neurosci 12:342–348

Mill J, Tang T, Kaminsky Z, Khare T, Yazdanpanah S, Bouchard L, Jia P, Assadzadeh A, Flanagan J, Schumacher A, Wang SC, Petronis A (2008) Epigenomic profiling reveals DNA-methylation changes associated with major psychosis. Am J Hum Genet 82:696–711

Miller CA, Campbell SL, Sweatt JD (2008) DNA methylation and histone acetylation work in concert to regulate memory formation and synaptic plasticity. Neurobiol Learn Mem 89:599–603

Miltenberger RJ, Mynatt RL, Wilkinson JE, Woychik RP (1997) The role of the agouti gene in the yellow obese syndrome. J Nutr 127:1902S–1907S

Myin-Germeys I, van Os J, Schwartz JE, Stone AA, Delespaul PA (2001) Emotional reactivity to daily life stress in psychosis. Arch Gen Psychiatry 58:1137–1144

Myin-Germeys I, Delespaul P, Van Os J (2005) Behavioural sensitization to daily life stress in psychosis. Psychol Med 35:733–741

Ødegaard O (1932) Emigration and insanity: a study of mental disease among Norwegian-born population in Minnesota. Acta Psychiatrica et Neurologica Scandinavica 7:1–206

Oh G, Petronis A (2008) Environmental studies of schizophrenia through the prism of epigenetics. Schizophr Bull 34:1122–1129

Padmos RC, Hillegers MH, Knijff EM, Vonk R, Bouvy A, Staal FJ, de Ridder D, Kupka RW, Nolen WA, Drexhage HA (2008) A discriminating messenger RNA signature for bipolar disorder formed by an aberrant expression of inflammatory genes in monocytes. Arch Gen Psychiatr 65:395–407

Padmos RC, Van Baal GC, Vonk R, Wijkhuijs AJ, Kahn RS, Nolen WA, Drexhage HA (2009) Genetic and environmental influences on pro-inflammatory monocytes in bipolar disorder: a twin study. Arch Gen Psychiatr 66:957–965

Rakyan VK, Down TA, Maslau S, Andrew T, Yang TP, Beyan H, Whittaker P, McCann OT, Finer S, Valdes AM, Leslie RD, Deloukas P, Spector TD (2010) Human aging-associated DNA hyper-methylation occurs preferentially at bivalent chromatin domains. Genome Res 20:434–439

Read J, Van Os J, Morrison AP, Ross CA (2005) Childhood trauma, psychosis and schizophrenia: a literature review with theoretical and clinical implications. Acta Psychiatrica Scandinavica 112:330–350

Reik W, Dean W, Walter J (2001) Epigenetic reprogramming in mammalian development. Science 293:1089–1092

Renthal W, Maze I, Krishnan V, HEr C, Xiao G, Kumar A, Russo SJ, Graham A, Tsankova N, Kippin TE, Kerstetter KA, Neve RL, Haggarty SJ, McKinsey TA, Bassel-Duby R, Olson EN, Nestler EJ (2007) Histone deacetylase 5 epigenetically controls behavioral adaptations to chronic emotional stimuli. Neuron 56:517–529

Rose G (1985) Sick individuals and sick populations. Int J Epidemiol 14:32–38

Schlotz W, Jones A, Phillips DI, Gale CR, Robinson SM, Godfrey KM (2009) Lower maternal folate status in early pregnancy is associated with childhood hyperactivity and peer problems in offspring. J Child Psychol Psychiatry Published online, 28 October 2009

Selten JP, Cantor-Graae E (2007) Hypothesis: social defeat is a risk factor for schizophrenia? Br J Psychiatry 191:s9–s12

Selten JP, Sijben N (1994) First admission rates for schizophrenia in immigrants to The Netherlands. The Dutch National Register. Soc Psychiatry Psychiatr Epidemiol 29:71–77

Selten JP, Slaets JPJ, Kahn RS (1997) Schizophrenia in Surinamese and Dutch Antillean immigrants to The Netherlands: evidence of an increased incidence. Psychol Med 27:807–811

Selten JP, Veen N, Feller W, Blom JD, Schols D, Camoenie W, Oolders J, van der Velden M, Hoek HW, Rivero VM, van der Graaf Y, Kahn R (2001) Incidence of psychotic disorders in immigrant groups to The Netherlands. Br J Psychiatry 178:367–372

Smith RS (1992) A comprehensive macrophage-T-lymphocyte theory of schizophrenia. Med Hypotheses 39:248–257

Smithells RW, Sheppard S, Schorah CJ, Seller MJ, Nevin NC, Harris R, Read AP, Fielding DW (1980) Possible prevention of neural-tube defects by periconceptional vitamin supplementation. Lancet 315:339–340

St Clair D, Xu M, Wang P, Yu Y, Fang Y, Zhang F, Zheng X, Gu N, Feng G, Sham P, He L (2005) Rates of adult schizophrenia following prenatal exposure to the Chinese famine of 1959–1961. J Am Med Assoc 294:557–562

Steegers-Theunissen RP, Obermann-Borst SA, Kremer D, Lindemans J, Siebel C, Steegers EA, Slagboom PE, Heijmans BT (2009) Periconceptual maternal folic acid use of 400 ug per day is related to increased methylation of the IGF2 gene in the very young child. PLoS One 4:e7845. doi:10.1371/journal.pone.0007845

Stefansson H, Rujescu D, Cichon S, Pietilainen OP, Ingason A, Steinberg S, Fossdal R, Sigurdsson E, Sigmundsson T, Buizer-Voskamp JE, Hansen T, Jakobsen KD, Muglia P, Francks C, Matthews PM, Gylfason A, Halldorsson BV, Gudbjartsson D, Thorgeirsson TE, Sigurdsson A, Jonasdottir A, Bjornsson A, Mattiasdottir S, Blondal T, Haraldsson M, Magnusdottir BB, Giegling I, Moller HJ, Hartmann A, Shianna KV, Ge D, Need AC, Crombie C, Fraser G, Walker N, Lonnqvist J, Suvisaari J, Tuulio-Henriksson A, Paunio T, Toulopoulou T, Bramon E, Di Forti M, Murray R, Ruggeri M, Vassos E, Tosato S, Walshe M, Li T, Vasilescu C, Muhleisen TW, Wang AG, Ullum H, Djurovic S, Melle I, Olesen J, Kiemeney LA, Franke B, Sabatti C, Freimer NB, Gulcher JR, Thorsteinsdottir U, Kong A, Andreassen OA, Ophoff RA, Georgi A, Rietschel M, Werge T, Petursson H, Goldstein DB, Nothen MM, Peltonen L, Collier DA, St Clair D, Stefansson K (2008) Large recurrent microdeletions associated with schizophrenia. Nature 455:232–236

Sullivan PF, Kendler KS, Neale MC (2003) Schizophrenia as a complex trait: evidence from a meta-analysis of twin studies. Arch Gen Psychiatry 60:1187–1192

Susser E, Neugebauer R, Hoek HW, Brown AS, Lin S, Labovitz D, Gorman JM (1996) Schizophrenia after prenatal famine. Further evidence. Arch Gen Psychiatry 53:25–31

Sweatt JD (2009) Experience-dependent epigenetic modifications in the central nervous system. Biol Psychiatry 65:191–197

Szyf M, McGowan PO, Meany MJ (2008) The social environment and the epigenome. Environ Mol Mutagen 49:46–60

Talens RP, Boomsma DI, Tobi EW, Kremer D, Jukema JW, Willemsen G, Putter H, Slagboom PE, Heijmans BT (2010) Variation, patterns, and temporal stability of DNA methylation: considerations for epigenetic epidemiology. FASEB J: doi:10.1096/fj.09-150490

Tamura T, Goldenberg RL, Chapman VR, Johnston KE, Ramey SL, Nelson KG (2005) Folate status of mothers during pregnancy and mental and psychomotor development of their children at five years of age. Pediatrics 116:703–708

Tidey JW, Miczek KA (1996) Social defeat stress selectively alters mesocorticolimbic dopamine release: an in vivo microdialysis study. Brain Res 721:140–149

Tobi EW, Lumey LH, Talens RP, Kremer D, Putter H, Stein AD, Slagboom PE, Heijmans BT (2009) DNA methylation differences after exposure to prenatal famine are common and timing- and sex-specific. Hum Mol Genet 18:4046–4053

Tochigi M, Iwamoto K, Bundo M, Komori A, Sasaki T, Kato N, Kato T (2008) Methylation status of the reelin promoter region in the brain of schizophrenic patients. Biol Psychiatry 63:530–533

Tsankova NM, Berton O, Renthal W, Kumar A, Neve RL, Nestler EJ (2006) Sustained hippocampal chromatin regulation in a mouse model of depression and antidepressant action. Nat Neurosci 9:519–525

Van Engeland M, Weijenberg MP, Roemen GMJM, Brink M, De Bruine AP, Goldbohm RA, Van den Brandt PA, Baylin SB, De Goeij AFPM, Herman JG (2003) Effects of dietary folate and alcohol intake on promoter methylation in sporadic colorectal cancer: The Netherlands cohort study on diet and cancer. Cancer Res 63:3133–3137

Van Os J, Kapur S (2009) Schizophrenia. Lancet 374:635–645

Veling W (2008) Schizophrenia among ethnic minorities. Erasmus University, Rotterdam

Veling W, Selten JP, Veen N, Laan W, Blom JD, Hoek HW (2006) Incidence of schizophrenia among ethnic minorities in the Netherlands: a four-year first-contact study. Schizophr Res 86:189–193

Veling W, Susser E, Van Os J, Mackenbach JP, Selten JP, Hoek HW (2008) Ethnic density of neighborhoods and incidence of psychotic disorders among immigrants. Am J Psychiatry 165:66–73

Walker EF, Diforio D (1997) Schizophrenia: a neural diathesis-stress model. Psychol Rev 104:667–685

Waterland RA, Jirtle RL (2003) Transposable elements: targets for early nutritional effects on epigenetic gene regulation. Mol Cell Biol 23:5293–5300

Weaver IC, Cervoni N, Champagne FA, D'Alessio AC, Sharma S, Seckl JR, Dymov S, Szyf M, Meany MJ (2004) Epigenetic programming by maternal behavior. Nat Neurosci 7:847–854

Weaver IC, Champagne FA, Brown SE, Dymov S, Sharma S, Meany MJ, Szyf M (2005) Reversal of maternal programming of stress responses in adult offspring through methyl supplementation: altering epigenetic marking later in life. J Neurosci 25:11045–11054

Whitrow MJ, Moore VM, Rumbold AR, Davies MJ (2009) Effect of supplemental folic acid in pregnancy on childhood asthma: a prospective birth cohort study. Am J Epidemiol 170:1486–1493

Wolff GL, Kodell RL, Moore SR, Cooney CA (1998) Maternal epigenetics and methyl supplements affect *agouti* gene expression in A^{vy}/a mice. FASEB J 12:949–957

Xu MQ, Sun WS, Liu BQ, Feng BY, Yu L, Yang L, He G, Sham P, Susser E, St Clair D, He L (2009) Prenatal malnutrition and adult schizophrenia: further evidence from the 1959–1961 Chinese famine. Schizophr Bull 35:568–576

Chapter 7
Imprinting, Inactivation and the Behavioural Genetics of the X Chromosome

Ian W. Craig

Abstract The X chromosome presents some unique features in the context of DNA modifications including methylation and histone deposition. In some ways, the patterns of epigenetic changes during the life cycle of the X chromosome resemble those affecting autosomal loci in parent-of-origin effects. Similarly, chromatin changes to the X chromosome of somatic cells may occur in response to the impact of external environmental factors. In addition to any imprinting, the X chromosome of placental mammals has the distinction of random inactivation in diploid females. The focus of this chapter is to examine what consequences these X-chromosomal modifications may have for human phenotypes and in particular that of behaviour. It is of particular interest in this context that, of the few loci escaping inactivation and expressed at higher levels in females, several are notable for their involvement in chromatin remodelling.

Keywords Behaviour · Chromatin remodelling · Histone modification · Twin studies · X-inactivation

7.1 X Chromosome Imprinting and Inactivation Cycle

As reviewed elsewhere in this volume, one of the most easily studied aspects of epigenetic modification is that of methylation of the cytosine residue at CpG dinucleotides. Studies in mice indicate that, at fertilisation, about 20% of CpG sites are methylated. At the blastocyst stage, there is a dramatic removal of most of these (although it is supposed that a number of key methylated cytosine marks may be maintained) to be later followed by waves of de novo methylation at the trophoblast stage – with somatic and germ cell lineages subsequently achieving different overall levels of about 60 and 30%, respectively (Reik et al. 2001;

I.W. Craig
SGDP Centre, Institute of Psychiatry, King's College London, PO Box 82, Denmark Hill, London SE5 8AF, UK
e-mail: ian.craig@kcl.ac.uk

A. Petronis and J. Mill (eds.), *Brain, Behavior and Epigenetics*,
Epigenetics and Human Health, DOI 10.1007/978-3-642-17426-1_7,
© Springer-Verlag Berlin Heidelberg 2011

Jaenisch and Bird 2003). Following fertilisation, there are significant differences in the mechanisms involved in the demethylation of maternal and paternal genomes. Whereas the chromatin of paternal chromosomes is reprogrammed before replication by an active process, which involves the replacement of protamines by acetylated histones and extensive demethylation, loss of methylation from the maternal genome is replication dependent (Reik et al. 2001).

Against this genomic background, subsequent epigenetic modification of the X chromosome also follows different pathways depending on the parent of origin. The paternal X (X^P) arrives in the zygote in a pre-inactivated state because, during the meiotic process in spermatogenesis, its regions that do not pair with homologous regions on the Y undergo inactivation in a process that appears to differ mechanistically from that seen in the differentiating embryo and which does not involve the *Xist* locus (see below). Furthermore, it seems that following meiotic inactivation in males, some regions of the X are reactivated in spermatids enabling many multi-copy genes, including some encoding testes-specific transcripts, to be expressed. Following fertilisation, preferential inactivation of X^P is followed by its reactivation and the subsequent random inactivation of maternally and paternally inherited X chromosomes. Unlike spermatogenic meiotic inactivation, the pathway of preferential paternal X-inactivation that follows fertilisation appears to require de novo *Xist* expression (Mueller et al. 2008).

7.1.1 The Role of XIST in X Chromosome Epigenetic Modification

Initiation of random X-inactivation, which is the norm for somatic tissues of eutherian mammals, requires both that the number of X chromosomes relative to autosomes be counted and that a random choice made as to which of two Xs in a diploid chromosome set is inactivated (Heard and Disteche 2006). The locus controlling this process is referred to as the inactivation centre (*XIC*). This region (located at Xp13.2 in humans) contains several elements and regulatory sequences. Much of what is known concerning X-inactivation in eutherian mammals is based on studies in mice with some support from parallel investigations in humans. Although there are some differences in precise mechanism, it is recognised that one common aspect of epigenetic modification is the role of the product of the *XIST* locus (referred to as *Xist* in mice) located within the X-inactivation centre (*XIC* – *Xic* in mice). *XIST* is responsible for the production of the non-translated RNA that coats and interacts with the chromosome and which signals the first stage of inactivation (Ng et al. 2007). This precedes histone modifications and the extensive methylation of CpG dinucleotides that together are responsible for the relatively stable subsequent silencing of a majority of the X chromosome's transcriptional activity.

In mice, at the first examinable stages following fertilisation, both paternal and maternal X chromosomes appear to be active and both *Xic* sites switched off

(Okamoto and Heard 2006); however, there persists some epigenetic mark on the paternal X predisposing subsequent preferential *Xist*-linked inactivation. Such imprinting-linked inactivation of the paternal X persists in all tissues of marsupials and in the extra-embryonic membranes of some eutherians including mice and to a limited degree in human trophoblasts. The paternal X-inactivation is well established by the blastocyst stage and some studies suggest its onset as early as the eight-cell stage (Heard and Disteche 2006). This X^P-specific inactivation is generally accompanied by similar chromatin changes to those seen in regular inactivation observed in cellular differentiation, although CpG methylation of gene promoters does not feature. Murine paternal X-inactivation is consolidated in trophoectoderm; however, in the embryo proper (inner cell mass), the inactive X^P become reactivated during blastocyst differentiation, coincident with a general erasure of epigenetic marks throughout the genome at this point. This, thereby, sets the stage for the process of random inactivation of paternal and maternal chromosomes – mediated by a counting process that results in the inactivation of $N - 1$ X chromosomes, where N is the total number of Xs. Hence in XXX individuals only a single one remains active. The condensed (and hence inactive X) chromosome in females was first described by Barr and Bertram (1949) and as a result has subsequently been referred to as a Barr body. Although some details differ, specifically with respect to a key role in mice for an antisense transcript to *Xist* (*Tsix*), overall murine and human patterns appear to be similar.

7.2 Skewing of X Chromosome Inactivation

Broadly speaking, X-inactivation enables males and females to achieve parity in gene expression; however, as a result of the contribution of genes that escape inactivation, potentially important consequences arise for sex differences in behaviour. Additional complications may arise as a result of skewing in the inactivation process. It is of interest that, although it might be anticipated that random inactivation in somatic tissues should result in a 50:50 distribution between cells having an active paternal X ($X_p{}^a$) and those having an active maternal X ($X_m{}^a$), quite significant differences in inactivation ratios are observed in practice. These can result from a variety of genetic and stochastic processes. For example, although inactivation in differentiating cells is generally independent of parental origin, in mice, different strains carry X-inactivation centres of differing "strengths" so that in inter-strain crosses the X from one strain may preferentially remain active. This is thought to be controlled by a locus-controlling variation and which is coincident with a regulator of *Tsix*, the locus encoding an antisense transcript to *Xist* (Ogawa and Lee 2003; Boumil et al. 2006). There is also evidence in humans that, in a possibly analogous manner, skewed X-chromosome inactivation segregates in some pedigrees in a manner consistent with mutations affecting the *XIST* locus (Plenge et al. 1997). In other cases, extremely skewed inactivation patterns may arise from X-chromosomal mutations that may result in

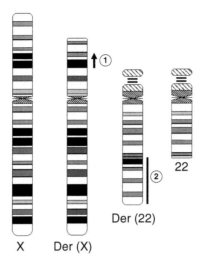

X   Der (X)

Fig. 7.1 Chromosome ideograms illustrating an X:autosome translocation (in this case X;22) and the consequences arising from inactivation. If the normal (non-rearranged) X is inactivated, any gene that would normally be expressed, but which crosses the breakpoint, will be rendered non-functional and consequently, the cell will lack any product from either X-locus. If the rearranged (der X) is inactivated, two consequences arise. Firstly, the inactivation spread from the *XIST* locus may penetrate into the portion of chromosome 22 attached. Secondly, the distal part of the X short arm will fail to be inactivated. The latter result particularly is likely to have cell-lethal consequences leaving only the cells with an inactive normal X to survive and hence the female translocation carrier will manifest any pathological symptoms associated with the lack of product from any gene situated across the breakpoint. In the case illustrated, the translocation carrier would exhibit Duchenne muscular dystrophy, as the DMD gene is located at Xp21.2. Ideograms drawn using http://www.cydas.org/OnlineAnalysis/ (Hiller B, Bradtke J, Balz H and Rieder H, 2004)

selection against cells carrying the defective X (Heard et al. 1997). X chromosome translocations also often result in selective cell death as a result of isolation of X-chromosomal regions from the inactivation centre, which can result in diploid expression of normally inactivated X-linked genes, as is the case in girls with X autosomal translocations. Surviving cells will have an inactive normal X and will lack expression of any gene crossing the breakpoint on the derived X chromosome with potentially pathological consequences (Fig. 7.1). Finally, skewing may simply result from stochastic processes, particularly if tissues develop from relatively few cells and the number of stem cells existing at the various stages will affect any skewing observed. This process is generally thought to underpin most of the deviations from a 50:50 distribution of inactive X^p and X^m observed. Indeed, skewing in favour of the activity of one or other of the X chromosomes is relatively common in adults, with about 35% of individuals showing > 70:30 skewed in either direction and with severe skewing (ratios > 90:1) seen in 7% of women under 25 and in 16% of women over 60 (Sharp et al. 2000; Amos-Landgraf et al. 2006), probably as a result of random events occurring on a small number of progenitor cells.

The X chromosome skewing resulting from X mutations and translocations can have very significant phenotypic consequences. Skewed inactivation in the absence of obvious chromosomal aberrations can also cause profound phenotypic differences even between otherwise genetically identical individuals, most convincingly evidenced by monozygous (MZ) girl twin pairs discordant for the expression of haemophilia, fragile X mental retardation and Duchenne muscular dystrophy (Tiberio 1994; Brown and Robinson 2000). The significance of skewed inactivation leading to the identification of X-linked quantitative trait loci (QTLs) affecting behaviour through twin studies is discussed later.

7.3   Chromatin Modifications Associated with the Inactive X Chromosome

In general, active regions of chromosomes are packed in a loose structure (euchromatin) that contains a high proportion of histone H3 and H4 molecules with acetylated lysine residues at their N-terminal tails and, where present, active genes are characterised by unmethylated CpG islands; furthermore, the promoter regions of active genes are frequently marked by methylation of lysine-4 of histone H3 (H3-K4). In contrast, heterochromatic regions reflect an inactive status and, in addition to the methylation of CpG islands, are typically enriched in methylated lysine residue 9 at the terminus of histone 3 (H3K9me), a modification that is observed from early stages of X-inactivation (Heard et al. 2001). The categorisation into either euchromatic or heterochromatic state, however, does not depend solely on a particular epigenetic mark, but on the collective influence of many different modifications. The inactivation of the X chromosome in differentiating cells can be separated into two distinct stages. The first involves the initiation and primary steps in which *XIST* RNA plays a key role, although this may be dependent on the particular cellular context (Sengupta et al. 2008). The complete manifestation of inactivation requires a regulated multi-layering of chromatin modifications. Transition from initiation to maintenance phase appears to involve the polycomb group proteins – known for their activity in repression of the *Hox* genes and which are implicated in the control of body patterns and cell differentiation. Other chromatin and nuclear architectural proteins are recruited to enforce the inactivation status; these include scaffold attachment factors, the trithorax group protein Ash2l and the histone variant macro-H2A2.1 (Pullirsch et al. 2010). As in other chromatin silencing, X-inactivation is typically characterised by additional changes in histone methylation, histone deacetylation and DNA methylation. Once stable inactivation is established, the X chromatin can be divorced from its *cis*-acting inactivation centre and its epigenetic downregulation will persist in its complete absence.

7.4   The Spread of X-Inactivation and the Role
of LINE Elements

It has long been recognised that the spread of inactivation and the epigenetic marks
that accompany it do not penetrate far into the autosomal sequences adjacent to the
X chromosome in X/A translocations and it has been therefore surmised that
changes in the pattern of genomic features may be responsible for the lack of
transmission. Mary Lyon (1998) suggested that LINE-1 motifs may be the key
elements forming the way-stations that had been proposed to exist along the
spreading inactivation path (Gartler and Riggs 1983). The LINE-1 hypothesis is
circumstantially supported by their approximately twofold higher density on the
X chromosome sequence (29%) compared to only 17% for autosomes and their
relative dearth around loci for which evidence exists that they escape the inactivation process. LINE-1 motifs are particularly enriched around the inactivation centre
as predicted for agents instrumental in propagating the inactivation process (Ross
et al. 2005). Further support for the model comes from studies on an X/4 translocation in a female mouse embryonic stem cell line, T37H. Popova et al. (2006)
demonstrated that the ingress of inactivation into chromosome 4 material, as
evidenced from the spreading of *Xist* RNA and histone hypoacetylation, from the
Xic locus was correlated with its encounter with an extensive 20 Mb region depleted
in Line-1 sequences located close to the translocation breakpoint. Other features
may also control the spread of inactivation; for example, studies on genes believed
to escape inactivation revealed that their 5′ ends were protected by CTCF insulator
elements (Filippova et al. 2005).

7.5   Patterns of Inactivation and Loci Which Escape

In the foregoing account, it has been assumed that genes on the inactive X are not
expressed, apart from regions of X/Y homology that include both pseudoautosomal
regions and some scattered isolated regions mostly found on the X short arm in
humans. Obviously, transcripts from any loci that escape inactivation and which do
not have expressed Y homologues may be expected to be found at relatively higher
concentration in females than males and potentially contribute to sex differences in
phenotypes including behaviour (Craig et al. 2004a). Because of this, there has been
considerable interest in establishing the number and nature of any such escapee
genes.

   A variety of strategies have been employed to track the potential expression and
hence the inactivation status of specific loci on paternal and maternal X chromosomes and resulted in widely differing conclusions. Early studies were based
on animals and human individuals heterozygous for the X-linked enzyme glu-
cose-6-phosphate dehydrogenase (G6PD), which was taken as a representative
marker for the inactivation status of the entire X. Heterozygotes were chosen to

have electrophoretically distinguishable allelic variants. If both alleles are active in cells or tissues, an intermediate hybrid dimeric band appears following electrophoresis of the enzyme resulting in a three-banded pattern. In contrast, single cells or clonal cell lines with X^p or X^m exclusively active exhibit a single band, and tissues with a mixture of both cell types will exhibit two bands with no intermediate form. The presence of a hybrid-band pattern in post-meiotic germ cells in both humans and mice constituted evidence for X-chromosome reactivation during female germ-line development (Gartler and Riggs 1983). This inactivation assay was later employed in studies leading to the first strong evidence that at least one human X-linked gene (steroid sulphatase, STS) escapes partially from inactivation (Gartler and Riggs 1983). Since this time, a variety of other approaches has been employed to monitor the inactivation status of X-linked genes and to assess the degree of skewing, thereby enabling an investigation of the relationship between CpG island methylation, transcription and mono-allelic expression. Many methods employed to monitor inactivation patterns have been based on the epigenetic methylation of CpG islands associated with genes on the inactive X. This results in resistance to digestion by one of the isoschizomer pairs of restriction enzymes, for example *Msp*I and *Hpa*II, both of which cleave at CCGG sites; however, digestion with *Hpa*II but not *Msp*I is inhibited by methylation of the internal cytosine. The size of products from PCR amplification across the non-digested template of heterozygous females can then be distinguished by the selection of target regions that contain both the CCGG site(s) and appropriate variable tandem repeat polymorphisms allowing the products to be distinguished. Systems based on tandem repeats at the androgen receptor, AR (Allen et al. 1992), and the DXS255 loci have been commonly employed (Boyd and Fraser 1990).

More recently, the focus has shifted to studies scanning the entire chromosome for loci and regions that remain active on an otherwise inactive X chromosome. One of the first preliminary chromosome-wide studies was based on the application of non-quantitative PCR detection of human transcripts from somatic cell hybrids carrying an inactive human X chromosome in an essentially otherwise rodent cell-line background. It was concluded that about 20% of genes tested escaped inactivation and that a significant proportion of these were located on the short arm (Carrel et al. 1999). This study was followed up with more detailed investigations employing a similar strategy supplemented with a quantitative allele-specific assay on a subset of loci examined. Broadly similar general conclusions were reached with about 15% of loci escaping to some degree with an additional 10% of X-linked genes showing variable patterns and extents of inactivation (Carrel and Willard 2005). The somatic cell hybrid approach, however, will detect even low levels of expression from an inactive X and furthermore relates specifically to the situation in a transformed rodent cell background, which may not represent the environment of a more typical somatic cell. Other techniques such as quantitative evaluation of data from expression microarrays are better suited to assess whether, or not, escapees contribute overall to differences in gene dosage between males and females. Comparisons between cell lines with supernumerary X chromosomes, and on lymphocytes, lymphoblastoid lines and tissues from males and females have been reported (Sudbrak et al. 2001; Craig et al. 2004b; Talebizadeh et al. 2006; McRae et al. 2007). In a comprehensive survey, Johnston et al. (2008) established that male and female expression levels were generally similar and, in an important extension to the observations of Nugyen and Disteche (2006), noted that expression from the single X in male cell lines is upregulated twofold relative to autosomes, thereby achieving dosage parity between the X and autosomes. In addition, they provided compelling data that relatively few loci consistently escape inactivation in females.

Confidence in the potentially significant implications of the microarray expression approach is the coincident identification of some key regulatory and protein-modifying loci in several of the studies. These are highlighted in bold in Table 7.1. Of particular relevance in the present context of epigenetics and disease is the identification as escapees of *SMC1L1* (HGNC Symbol: *SMC1A* – structural maintenance of chromosomes 1A) and of its close distal neighbour *SMCX*. SMC1L1 is a component of the cohesion complex, which, in turn, interacts with PDS5, a protein implicated in chromosome cohesion, condensation and recombination in yeast. *SMCX* encodes one of the families of histone H3 lysine-4 demethylases and reverses the trimethylated H3K4me3 to di- and mono-methylated status and presumptively results in transcriptional repression at target sites. *SMCX* is also one of the more frequently mutated targets in X-linked mental retardation (XLMR) and there is evidence that it both escapes inactivation and has a distinct function from its Y-linked counterpart (*SMCY*). In a manner similar to some of the other confirmed loci that escape inactivation, its Y homologue differs in amino acid sequence and in its levels and patterns of expression. Both *SMCX* and *SMCY* are expressed in mouse brain in a sex-specific fashion with *SMCX* being expressed at a significantly higher level in the adult mouse brain of females compared with males, and expression of the Y homologue in males being insufficient to compensate for the female bias in X-gene expression (Xu et al. 2002). Moreover, *SMCX* has been implicated in neuronal survival and dendritic survival and its mutation in several XLMR patients is associated with reduced demethylase activity (Iwase et al. 2007).

UTX (ubiquitously transcribed TPR gene on the X chromosome) is another gene escaping inactivation and which is involved in epigenetic modification. It catalyses the demethylation of tri/di-methylated H3 lysine-27 (H5K27me3/2) and has been implicated in HOX gene regulation. A further escapee with potentially important significance in epigenetic regulation is *MSL3L1* (male-specific lethal 3-like 1) – given that *Drosophila* male-specific lethal (msl) genes regulate transcription from the male X chromosome in a dosage compensation pathway (see http://www.ncbi. nlm.nih.gov/omim/ for details).

It is, therefore, of considerable interest to discover that, of the relatively few genes that escape inactivation, several have roles in epigenetic modification and consequently have considerable potential for gene regulation. Overall, it is reasonable to suppose that such loci have the potential to contribute to sex differences in a range of phenotypes including behaviour.

Table 7.1 Loci escaping inactivation based on over-expression in females detected by microarray analyses

Gene name	Escapees Johnston et al. (2008)	Escapees Craig et al. (2004b)	Escapees Talebizadeh et al. (2006)	Escapees McRae et al. (2007)	Escapees based on somatic cell hybrids Carrel and Willard (2005)	Position Kb from pter
ACSL4			Yes		0 of 5	108,884,564–108,976,621 reverse strand
ALG13	Yes					110,909,043–111,003,877 forward strand
AP1S2			Yes		9 of 9	15,843,929–15,873,100 reverse strand
DDX3		Yes		Yes	9 of 9	41,192,651–41,223,725 forward strand
CA5B/CA5BL	Yes			Yes		15,706,953–15,805,747 forward strand
CDR1			Yes		2 of 9	139,865,425–139,866,723 reverse strand
CLCN4		Yes			5 of 9	10,125,024–10,205,700 forward strand
EIF1A	Yes			Yes		20,142,636–20,159,962 reverse strand
EIF2S	Yes	Yes		Yes	9 of 9	24,072,833–24,096,088 forward strand
EIF2S3						
FUNDC1	Yes					44,382,885–44,402,247 reverse strand
HDHD1A	Yes		Yes	Yes	8 of 9	6,966,961–7,066,231 reverse strand
MSL3L1/MSL3	Yes			Yes		11,776,278–11,793,870 forward strand
PCTK1	Yes	Yes			9 of 9	47,077,528–47,089,396 forward strand
RBBP7				Yes		16,857,406–16,888,537 reverse strand
PNPLA4	Yes		Yes		9 of 9	7,866,288–7,895,780 reverse strand
PRKX	Yes			Yes		3,522,411–3,631,649 reverse strand

(continued)

Table 7.1 (continued)

Gene name	Escapees Johnston et al. (2008)	Escapees Craig et al. (2004b)	Escapees Talebizadeh et al. (2006)	Escapees McRae et al. (2007)	Escapees based on somatic cell hybrids Carrel and Willard (2005)	Position Kb from pter
RPGR			Yes		0 of 9	38,128,424–38,186,817 reverse strand
RPS4X	Yes		Yes			71,475,529–71,497,150 reverse strand
SEDL/TRAPPC2		Yes			9 of 9	13,730,363–13,752,742 reverse strand
SMC1L1/SMC1A	Yes	Yes		Yes	7 of 9	53,401,070–53,449,677 reverse strand
SMCX/JARID1C	Yes			Yes		53,221,334–53,254,604 reverse strand
SRSP2/SMS		Yes			9 of 9	21,958,691–22,025,318 forward strand
STK3		Yes			9 of 9	131,157,245–131,209,971 forward strand
STS	Yes	Yes			9 of 9	7,137,497–7,272,851 forward strand
SYP		Yes			2 of 9	49,044,269–49,056,718 reverse strand
TBL1		Yes			7 of 9	9,431,335–9,687,780 forward strand
U2AF1L2 *ZRSR*	Yes			Yes		15,808,595–15,841,383 forward strand
UBE1/UBA1	Yes	Yes[a]				47,050,260–47,074,527 forward strand
USP9X	Yes					40,944,888–41,092,185 forward strand
UTX/KDM6A	Yes	Yes	Yes	Yes		44,732,423–44,971,847 forward strand
ZFX	Yes	Yes	Yes	Yes	9 of 9	24,167,290–24,234,206 forward strand

[a]Weak signal and very partial escape

7.6   Somatic Imprinting of X-Linked Genes and Potential Impact on Behaviour

The chromosome constitution of individuals with Turner's syndrome (TS), who have a single X and no other sex chromosome (45, X0), provides an opportunity to examine possible differences in expression from paternally or maternally inherited X chromosomes. In a series of studies on Turner's syndrome females, a range of behavioural phenotypes were observed, which appeared to differ depending on the parent of origin of the single X. Those who retained the maternal X (X^m0) had greater difficulties in socialisation than those with a paternal X (Skuse et al. 1997). The authors speculated that an X-linked gene (or group of genes) existed, which was implicated in social behaviour and which was inactive (imprinted) on the maternally inherited X chromosome. This raised the interesting possibility that the generally accepted relative lack of such skills in boys is a result of their inheritance of their X chromosome from their mothers. Other evidence for X-linked socialisation QTLs has come more recently from twin studies (see below). A variety of subsequent investigations has supported the existence of behavioural differences in X^P0 compared with X^m0 Turner's syndrome individuals; however, the situation is complicated by the existence of mosaicism where some individuals may retain some tissues containing cells with additional sex chromosome fragments (Henn and Zang 1997). Although there is some direct experimental evidence for imprinted loci in mice (Davies et al. 2005; Raefski and O'Neill 2005), none is yet available for humans and the issue requires further clarification.

7.7   Behavioural Impact of Epigenetic Status at Specific X-Linked Genes

7.7.1   Fragile X Mental Retardation Syndrome, FRAXA

Fragile X syndrome is the most common inherited cause of mental retardation, with an incidence of around 1 in 4,000 males (Turner et al. 1996). The mental impairment is often co-morbid with further symptoms including macro-orchidism and, in around 25% cases, epileptic seizures (Hagerman 1995, 1996). The gene implicated is referred to as *FMR1* and in unaffected individuals its 5' untranslated region located in exon 1 contains about 30 copies of a CGG trinucleotide repeat. This repeat has intrinsic instability thought to result from a propensity to form an abnormal hairpin-like secondary structure which predisposes replication slippage; however, the somatic instability is relatively low compared to some other trinucleotide repeats such as the CAG sequence in the myotonic dystrophy gene (*DM1*). Instability can lead to increasing copy number of the repeat, which in the fully mutated state expands to contain more than 200 CGG repeats leading to the formation of a target for extensive DNA methylation within the CGG repeat and in the flanking DNA (e.g. Sutcliffe et al. 1992; Hornstra et al. 1993). This in turn predicates the formation of altered chromatin structure, which can be manifested through specific treatments as a visible fragile site at Xq27.3 in metaphase chromosome preparations. The methylation and chromatin changes result in the cessation of *FMR1* expression and a lack of its protein product FMRP, which is responsible for the mental retardation phenotype in FRAXA. Fragile X mental retardation protein, FMRP, is a selective RNA-binding protein; it forms messenger ribonucleoprotein (mRNP) complexes which associate with polyribosomes in the brain and which can suppress protein translation in vitro (Laggerbauer et al. 2001) and in vivo (Li et al. 2001; Stefani et al. 2004).

Two intermediate stages are recognised before full expansion is reached; these are "intermediate" alleles (~41–55 repeats) and "premutations" (55–200 repeats). Both are now recognised as more than a generational stepping stone between normal allele size and the full mutation (Hagerman and Hagerman 2004). In addition, some studies have found an association between expanded alleles in these size ranges and cognitive/behavioural measures (e.g. Youings et al. 2000). Other studies indicate a significant negative correlation between allele lengths within the generally accepted normal range and a standardised score for IQ and general cognitive ability in young males, suggesting that modest increases in repeat numbers may have a limiting influence on cognitive performance (Loat et al. 2006). Interestingly, epigenetic modification and partial suppression of *FMR1* expression do not seem to be associated with phenotypes determined by such intermediate stages. Paradoxically, the intermediate alleles are associated with increased transcription, but lower levels of FMRP, and it seems that intermediate and premutation alleles manifest effects on the carrier by a distinct mechanism from the full mutation. Hagerman et al. (2001) have proposed an RNA "toxic-gain-of-function" model, whereby it is not an absence of protein, but rather an excess of RNA that causes the phenotypes associated with alleles in this range.

Recent studies have provided an insight into the possible mechanism underlying the hypermethylation of the expanded 5′ untranslated region of the *FMR1* locus. Naumann et al. (2009) have identified a methylation boundary existing at 650 and 800 nucleotides upstream of the CGG repeat, where the boundary separates a hypermethylated area from the normally unmethylated *FMR1* promoter, thereby protecting it from the spread of methylation. This boundary is lost in individuals with the fragile X syndrome and methylation extends into the *FMR1* promoter resulting in inactivation of the *FMR1* gene. It is speculated that the boundary in the *FMR1* 5′-upstream region coincides with a specific chromatin structure that, when destabilised, allows methylation to spread downstream, with concomitant repression of the *FMR1* transcript.

Other epigenetic changes accompany the hypermethylation of the expanded repeat. Use of immunoprecipitation approaches to analyse the histone patterns in the *FMR1* region near the expanded repeat revealed high levels of methylated histone 3 at Lys9 (H3K9me), lower levels of acetylated (Ac)H3 and H4 together with histone H3-K4 demethylation, suggesting that, unlike their normal-length counterparts, expanded CGG repeats at this locus carry epigenetic marks typical of condensed heterochromatin (Oberlé et al. 1991; Coffee et al. 1999, 2002; O'Donnell and Warren 2002). Intermediate expansion may sometimes reflect the partial transition to heterochromatinisation, and some individuals with 60–200 CGG repeats display variable patterns of DNA methylation in different tissues (Saveliev et al. 2003). More recently, an intriguing novel gene, *ASFMR1*, has been identified. The *ASFMR1* transcript overlaps the CGG repeat region of the *FMR1* gene in the antisense orientation and is elevated in peripheral blood leucocytes of individuals with premutation alleles, but not expressed from full mutation alleles, suggesting that the locus may contribute to pathogenesis in premutation individuals (Ladd et al. 2007).

Primary and transformed cell cultures obtained from rare individuals of normal phenotype with an unmethylated full mutation in the *FMR1* gene have been used to show that CGG expansion per se does not block transcription (Smeets et al. 1995; Pietrobono et al. 2005).

There is a well-established parent-of-origin effect on the expansion of the CCG repeat in which asymptomatic mothers carrying permutation alleles produce male offspring with full expansions in all tissues (apart from testes in which contraction may occur). This results from repeat expansion in the maternal germline. Additional evidence indicates that changes in repeat copy number can also occur early in embryogenesis, which is particularly well illustrated by the observation of monozygotic (MZ) twins with different repeat lengths (Dion and Wilson 2009). The somatic instability of CGG repeats is low in patients with extensively methylated full mutations; however, unmethylated large expansions in FRAXA males who express *FMR1* show a high degree of instability (Wöhrle et al. 1998). Eiges et al. (2007) investigated the impact of differentiation on the methylation process in a model system based on embryonic stem cells derived from a male pre-implantation fragile X-affected embryo whose mother was a carrier of a premutation (170 repeats). The undifferentiated male cell line was shown to have expanded repeats in the range 200–> 1,000; however, the 5′ CGG expansion was unmethylated and the FMR1 protein expressed. Methylation and histone modification of the region, however, occurred once the stem cells were manipulated to differentiate. On differentiation, the promoter region, originally enriched in acetylated histone H3 and unmethylated at H3K9, on differentiation, showed loss of acetylated histone H3 together with increased methylation at H3K9. It seems that the critical stages of transcription-downregulation of the expanded repeat at this locus are coincident with the epigenetic changes occurring on cell differentiation.

In recent studies employing matrix-assisted laser desorption/ionisation time of flight mass spectroscopy (MALDI-TOF MS), Godler et al. (2010) have identified a number of novel elements at the FMR1 locus. The methylation of two of these termed FREE1 and FREE2 appeared to be highly correlated with the methylation of the CpG island and repression of gene activity in lymphocytes in blood from partially methylated "high functioning" full mutation males. Methylation of both markers in blood DNA from carrier females appeared to be inversely correlated with the *FMR1* activation ratio.

7.7.2   Monoamine Oxidases A and B

The neurotransmitter metabolising enzymes MAOA and MAOB play an important role in the metabolism of biogenic amines in the central nervous system and in the periphery. They are the products of closely similar and abutting genes arranged in a tail-to-tail configuration on the short arm at Xp11.23. Although both are capable of metabolising neurotransmitter amines, MAOB is also active towards dietary amines. As a consequence, in the context of behaviour, monoamine oxidase A (MAOA) has received detailed attention concerning its expression and inactivation status mainly because of its perceived significant role in aggression. This was first recognised in humans through observations on a family segregating an allele with a nonsense mutation that was associated with extremely disturbed and violent behaviour in affected males. Apart from this very rare deleterious mutation, there are two common alleles in most populations characterised by the presence of either three or four copies of a 30 base pair VNTR found within the promoter region of the gene and which are respectively associated with low vs. high transcriptional activity. This is of particular interest given the observations of gene by environment effects, which indicate that males carrying the low activity variant appear to be more vulnerable to childhood abuse and as a result are more likely to be involved in violent and antisocial behaviour, thereby perpetuating the "cycle of violence" (Caspi et al. 2002). Many subsequent studies have generally supported the interaction between adverse environments and the low activity allele, although different conclusions have been reached by some, depending on the sex, age and behavioural measures employed (Craig 2007; Craig and Halton 2009, 2010). The potential impact of epigenetic modifications to genes encoding members of the HPA axis and monoamine metabolism pathways (including monoamine oxidases), which may result from early exposure to stress are therefore of intense interest. Similarly, the inactivation statuses of the monoamine oxidases have been the object of several investigations. Some preliminary studies suggested that MAOA escaped (at least partly) from inactivation. This, however, was inconsistent with observations on allele differences in methylation of its CpG-rich regions and was also in conflict with studies examining RNA expression in myoblasts. By employing a PCR-based transcription assay on cloned myoblasts, which has the advantage of directly assessing transcription rather than the passive measure of methylation, Benjamin et al. (2000) showed that clonal populations expressed (at the level of detection on agarose gels) only either one or the other allele, which strongly suggests that the locus is regularly inactivated.

Pinsonneault et al. (2006) in a series of detailed investigations have examined the potential roles of inactivation and cis-acting regulatory factors on the expression of MAOA in human brain tissues. By employing two SNPs expressed at the mRNA level, they were able to evaluate relative allelic expression in females heterozygous for the high and low expressing VNTR genotypes (expressed as allelic expression imbalance ratios, AEI). Evidence of significant cis-acting effects was demonstrated by the wide range of AEI observed (0.3–4) in prefrontal cortex. However, although extensive methylation in the promoter region VNTR was observed in females, but not males, this did not correlate with inactivation ratios as determined by an independent assay at the androgen receptor locus (Allen et al. 1992), which the authors took to indicate the existence of an alternative process of dosage compensation in females. Methylation at two CpG sites was examined in detail and showed extensive variation, but also correlated to some extent with allelic expression ratios. Local sequence also contributed to expression differences and it seems that allele-specific expression of MAOA in females depends on both genetic and epigenetic phenomena.

The impact of epigenetic programming coupled with the inactivation status of the MAOA locus may contribute significantly to the variable reports of association of low activity MAOA genotype and aggression in females. Very recently, a detailed bioinformatics study of the upstream region of the MAOA gene has provided valuable insight into the potential epigenetic modulation of expression from the locus and shown that the regulatory region extends up to 2,000 bp upstream of the transcription start site and contains a variety of potential methylation-sensitive regions (Shumay and Fowler 2010). In addition to the well-recognised VNTR, the analysis predicts a second putative promoter region whose activity is supported by the reported detection of a transcript (BC044787) apparently initiated within a CpG island distal to the conventional promoter. These data, taken together with the previous reports, suggest the potential for additional levels of regulation and epigenetic modulation of the control of MAOA expression in addition to those currently recognised.

There has also been some debate regarding the inactivation status of monoamine oxidase B (MAOB), whose levels in platelets provide a readily accessible source for monitoring its enzymic activity in various disorders. MAOB levels are lower in Turner's syndrome (X0) individuals than in control females (Good et al. 2003), providing suggestive evidence that the gene may escape inactivation and consequently that haploinsufficiency in X0 individuals may contribute to the range of symptoms observed in this condition. Subsequent investigations, however, failed to find an association between measured enzyme activity and cognitive skills in normal and X0? individuals (Lawrence et al. 2006). Chip-based expression studies as described above also do not provide any support that the locus escapes from inactivation.

7.7.3 Methyl-CpG-Binding Protein 2, MECP2 and the Chromatin-Modifying Gene, ATRX

The role of *MECP2* in chromatin and genome modifications is of particular interest. This X-linked locus is itself subjected to epigenetic modification as well as having a central role in binding to methylated CpG signatures of other loci. Its significance in context of behaviour is highlighted by its key role in Rett syndrome, RTT, which is one of the most common forms of intellectual disability in young girls. RTT-affected individuals manifest a progressive neurodevelopmental disorder which may include loss of speech, acquired microcephaly, ataxia and growth retardation. The disorder normally results from germline mutations in the gene and the almost exclusive involvement of females is best explained by X-linked dominant inheritance with lethality in the hemizygous males. Because of the normal involvement of MECP2 protein in binding to 7-methyl cytosine residues, it has been speculated that mutations may lead to a failure of binding leading to derepression of otherwise inactive loci; however, the spectrum of loci that it appears to influence is complex (Shahbazian and Zoghbi 2002).

Chahrour et al. (2008) examined gene expression patterns in the hypothalamus of mice that either lack or over-express *Mecp2*. In both conditions, *Mecp2* dysfunction induced changes in the expression levels of thousands of genes, but unexpectedly, the majority of genes (about 85%) appeared to be activated rather than repressed by Mecp2. The authors then selected a subset of six genes (*Sst*, *Oprk1*, *Mef2C Gamt*, *Gprin1* and *A2bp1*) and confirmed that Mecp2 binds to its promoters. In addition, they showed that Mecp2 associates with the transcriptional activator Creb1 at the promoter of an activated target, but not a repressed target. Their studies overall suggested that *Mecp2* regulates the expression of a wide range of genes in the hypothalamus and that it can function as both an activator and a repressor of transcription.

Chromatin immunoprecipitation studies indicated that the regulatory protein encoded by the early growth response 2 gene, *EGR2*, bound to the *MECP2* promoter and that MeCP2 bound to the intron 1 enhancer region of *EGR2* (Swanberg et al. 2009). These authors also noted that post-mortem cortex samples of both RTT and AS disorders showed decreased EGFR2 compared to matched controls and proposed a role for disruption of a pathway embracing these two regulators in both RTT syndrome and AS. Other studies on male mouse embryonic fibroblast cells deleted for *Mecp2* showed reduced levels of the cytoskeletal related gene, neuronal alpha tubulin, *Tuba1a*, and a deteriorated morphology. These defects were reversed by the introduction and expression of the human *MECP2* gene, suggesting that the latter is involved in the regulation of neuronal alpha tubulin, which had been shown to be reduced in brain tissue from both RTT and AS patients (Abuhatzira et al. 2009).

MECP2 is expressed at high levels in post-mitotic neurons and one of its well-characterised and highly significant targets in the context of behaviour is the brain-derived neurotrophic factor gene, BDNF, which is important in regulating neuronal plasticity (Martinowich et al. 2003; Dulac 2010).

The MECP2 protein binds to methylated CpG dinucleotide sites through an 85 amino acid methyl-CpG-binding domain (amino acids 78–162) (Lewis et al. 1992; Nan et al. 1993) and mediates gene silencing by causing changes in chromatin structure through interactions with co-repressor complexes, such as SIN3A, which contains the histone deacetylases HDAC1 and HDAC2 – an interaction that is targeted through a 104 amino acid transcriptional repression domain (amino acids 207–310) (Nan et al. 1993). MECP2 may also interact with other chromatin-modifying enzymes, such as histone methyltransferase and the product of another X-linked gene, *ATRX* (helicase 2, X-linked), mutations in which cause the alpha-thalassaemia/mental retardation syndrome (Nan et al. 2007; Shahbazian and Zoghbi 2002). Interestingly, MECP2 also interacts with the DNA methyltransferase, DNMT1, and consequently could be involved in the regulation of DNA methylation. In addition to its role in interacting with CpG islands, recent studies have shown that MECP2 can bind to intergenic sites and raise the possibility that its role may also include long-range chromatin reconfiguration (Yasui et al. 2007)

7.7.4 MECP2 and Its Association with ATRX Another X-Linked Chromatin Interacting Protein

MECP2 has been implicated in the regulation of parentally imprinted genes – for example, by binding to the paternal allele of *H19* and the maternal alleles of *U2af1-rs1* (e.g. Drewell et al. 2002). Indeed, very recently, it has been observed that MECP2 and ATRX together with cohesin interact and bind to established imprinted domains such as the H19 imprinting control region and the Gtl2/Dlk1 imprinted domain in mouse brain. It is proposed therefore that ATRX, cohesin and MeCP2 cooperate to silence a subset of imprinted genes in the postnatal mouse brain (Kernohan et al. 2010). Furthermore, chromatin immunoprecipitation experiments have indicated that ATRX decorates the single late replicating (inactivated) X chromosome in female somatic cells (trophoblastic stem cells) but only after differentiation onset, as illustrated by its absence from embryonic stem cells. This suggests that the association of the chromatin remodelling protein follows the onset of inactivation and may be significant in the observed skewed X-inactivation observed in patients with ATRX syndrome (Baumann and de la Fuente 2009).

MECP2 mutations have also been observed in a wide variety of other behavioural disorders including autism, bipolar disorder and schizophrenia. Interestingly, milder late-onset versions of Rett syndrome have been attributed to skewed X-inactivation in which the mutant allele is significantly underexpressed (Amir et al. 2000). Mutations in coding and flanking regions of *MECP2* have been observed in autism at low frequency; more frequently, significant increase in promoter methylation associated with decreased expression (detected by immunofluorescence with anti-C-terminal MECP2 antibodies detecting both isoforms) has been observed in the frontal cortex of affected males by bisulphite sequencing. This suggests that the *MECP2* locus is affected by and itself influences the epigenetic programme with potential complex consequences (Nagarajan et al. 2006). The recent demonstration that there may be more common population variants affecting *MECP2*, which contribute to the complex aetiology of autism may be relevant in this context (Loat et al. 2008a).

7.8 Skewing of Inactivation as a Novel Approach to Identifying Behaviours with X-Linked Genetic Input

As noted previously, a variety of mechanisms, both stochastic and directed, may lead to skewed X chromosome inactivation patterns in females, with modest to extreme skewing observed in a significant proportion of women. Extreme bias can additionally occur through cellular selection caused by deletions and translocations on one of the X chromosomes. It is interesting to note that differences in skewing between twin girls can also arise. Indeed, dichorionic MZ twinning, unlike monochorionic MZ twinning, occurs prior to the onset of X-inactivation (Puck 1998) and may lead to a relative increase in skewing of the former. Whatever the mechanism, skewing of X-inactivation should be expected to cause female MZ twins to be, on average, more discordant than their male homozygous twin counterparts for polymorphic X-linked traits. Given that the human X chromosome holds about 880 known protein-coding genes and that an impressive level of genetic heterogeneity exists, such that, on average, each gene may exhibit one or more single nucleotide polymorphisms (SNPs) and a scattering of variable simple sequence repeat motifs, the potential for functional heterozygosity at each locus and the potential for detecting X-linked traits by this process are considerable. In a preliminary study, Loat et al. (2004) examined nine behaviours or composite behavioural traits in 1,000 MZ female and 1,000 MZ male twin pairs taken from the Twins Early Development Study (TEDS) cohort. They found three of the traits (peer problems, prosocial behaviour and verbal ability) had significantly lower correlation coefficients for the female twins compared to males. They also found the same behaviours were significantly less correlated for dizygotic (DZ) male twins, which is to be expected as females share a common paternal X chromosome, so that any variation engendered by the differential inheritance of the two maternal X chromosomes will be moderated by the presence of the common paternal X. In contrast, males will be fully exposed to any functional variation for such traits resulting from the inheritance of one, or other, of the maternal X chromosome. Furthermore, the fact that they are hemizygous for X-linked genes which have no Y homologue means that the male sex as a whole may generally be exposed to extremes of phenotypes that are controlled by alleles on the X chromosome. This may help to explain the commonly recognised, yet infrequently discussed, phenomenon that males exhibit greater variance in the population than females for a large number of traits including intelligence (Hedges and Nowell 1995; Johnson et al. 2008; Craig et al. 2009). Subsequent studies have replicated these findings on older children and the additional data from these studies provided evidence that there are also X-linked QTLs for the social incapacity element of individuals with autism spectrum disorders (Loat et al. 2008b).

References

Abuhatzira L, Shemer R, Razin A (2009) MeCP2 involvement in the regulation of neuronal alpha-tubulin production. Hum Mol Genet 18:1415–1423

Allen RC, Zoghbi HY, Moseley AB, Rosenblatt HM, Belmont JW (1992) Methylation of HpaII and HhaI sites near the polymorphic CAG repeat in the human androgen receptor gene correlates with X chromosome inactivation. Am J Hum Genet 51:1229–1239

Amir RE, Van den Veyver IB, Schultz R, Malicki DM, Tran CQ, Dahle EJ, Philippi A, Timar L, Percy AK, Motil KJ, Lichtarge O, Smith EO, Glaze DG, Zoghbi HY (2000) Influence of mutation type and X chromosome inactivation on Rett syndrome phenotypes. Ann Neurol 47:670–679

Amos-Landgraf JM, Cottle A, Plenge RM, Friez M, Schwartz CE, Longshore J, Willard HF (2006) X chromosome-inactivation patterns of 1, 005 phenotypically unaffected females. Am J Hum Genet 79:493–499

Barr ML, Bertram EG (1949) A morphological distinction between neurones of the male and female, and the behaviour of the nucleolar satellite during accelerated nucleoprotein synthesis. Nature 163:676–677

Baumann C, de la Fuente R (2009) ATRX marks the inactive X chromosome (Xi) in somatic cells and during imprinted X chromosome inactivation in trophoblast stem cells. Chromosoma 118:209–222

Benjamin D, Van Bakel I, Craig I (2000) A novel expression based approach for assessing the inactivation status of human X-linked genes. Eur J Hum Genet 8:103–108

Boumil RM, Ogawa Y, Sun BK, Huynh KD, Lee JT (2006) Differential methylation of Xite and CTCF sites in Tsix mirrors the pattern of X- inactivation choice mice. Mol Cell Biol 26:2109–2117

Boyd Y, Fraser NJ (1990) Methylation patterns at the hypervariable X chromosome locus DXS255 (M27-BETA) correlates with X-inactivation status. Genomics 7:182–187

Brown CJ, Robinson WP (2000) The causes and consequences of random and non-random X-chromosome inactivation in humans. Clin Genet 58:353–563

Carrel L, Willard HF (2005) X-inactivation profile reveals extensive variability in X-linked gene expression in females. Nature 434:400–404

Carrel L, Cottle AA, Goglin KC, Willard HF (1999) A first-generation X inactivation profile of the human X chromosome. Proc Natl Acad Sci USA 96:14440–14444

Caspi A, McClay J, Moffitt TE, Mill J, Martin J, Craig IW, Taylor A, Poulton R (2002) Role of genotype in the cycle of violence in maltreated children. Science 297:851–854

Chahrour M, Jung SY, Shaw C, Zhou X, Wong STC, Qin J, Zoghbi HY (2008) MECP2, a key contributor to neurological disease, activates and represses transcription. Science 320:1224–1229

Coffee B, Zhang F, Warren ST, Reines D (1999) Acetylated histones are associated with FMR1 in normal but not fragile X-syndrome cells. Nat Genet 22:98–101

Coffee B, Zhang F, Ceman S, Warren ST, Reines D (2002) Histone modifications depict an aberrantly heterochromatinized FMR1 gene in fragile x syndrome. Am J Hum Genet 71:923–932

Craig IW (2007) The importance of stress and genetic variation in human aggression. Bioessays 29:227–236

Craig IW, Halton K (2009) Genetics of human aggressive behaviour. Hum Genet 126:101–113

Craig IW, Halton K (2010) The genetics of human aggressive behaviour. In: Encyclopedia of Life Sciences 2010, Wiley, Chichester http://www.els.net/ [DOI: 10.1002/9780470015902.a0022405]

Craig IW, Harper E, Loat C (2004a) The genetic basis for sex differences in human behaviour: role of the sex chromosomes. Ann Hum Genet 68:269–284

Craig IW, Mill J, Craig GM, Loat C, Schalkwyk LC (2004b) Application of micro-arrays to the analysis of the inactivation status of human X-linked genes expressed in lymphocytes. Eur J Hum Gen 12:639–646

Craig IW, Hawarth CMA, Plomin R (2009) Commentary on "A role for the X chromosome in sex differences in variability in general intelligence" (Johnson et al., 2009). Perspect Psychol Sci 4:615–621

Davies W, Isles A, Smith R, Burgoyne P, Wilkinson L (2005) A novel imprinted candidate gene for X-linked parent-of-origin effects on cognitive functioning in mice. Genet Res 86:236–236

Dion V, Wilson JH (2009) Instability and chromatin structure of expanded trinucleotide repeats. Trends Genet 25:288–297

Drewell RA, Goddard CJ, Thomas JO, Surani MA (2002) Methylation-dependent silencing at the H19 imprinting control region by MeCP2. Nucleic Acids Res 30:1139–1144

Dulac C (2010) Brain function and functional plasticity. Nature 425:728–735

Eiges R, Urbach A, Malcov M, Frumkin T, Schwartz T, Amit A, Yaron Y, Eden A, Yanuka O, Benvenisty N, Ben-Yosef N (2007) Developmental study of fragile X syndrome using human embryonic stem cells derived from preimplantation genetically diagnosed embryos. Cell Stem Cell 1:568–577

Filippova GN, Cheng MK, Moore JM, Truong J-P, Hu YJ, Di KN, Tsuchiya KD, Disteche CM (2005) Boundaries between chromosomal domains of X inactivation and escape bind CTCF and lack CpG methylation during early development. Dev Cell 8:31–42

Gartler SM, Riggs AD (1983) Mammalian X-chromosome inactivation. Annu Rev Genet 17:155–190

Godler DE, Tassone F, Loesch ZL, Taylor AK, Gehling F, Hagerman RJ, Burgess T, Ganesamoorthy D, Hennerich D, Gordon L, Evans A, Chool KH, Slater HR (2010) Methylation of novel markers of fragile X alleles is inversely correlated with FMRP expression and FMR1 activation ratio. Hum Mol Genet 19:1618–1632

Good CD, Lawrence K, Thomas NS, Price CJ, Ashburner J, Friston KJ, Frackowiak RSJ, Oreland L, Skuse DH (2003) Dosage sensitive X-linked locus influences the development of the amygdala and orbitofrontal cortex, and fear recognition in humans. Brain 126:1–16

Hagerman RJ (1995) Molecular and clinical correlations in fragile X syndrome. Ment Retard Dev Disabil Res Rev 1:276–280

Hagerman RJ (1996) Biomedical advances in developmental psychology: the case of fragile X syndrome. Dev Psychol 32:416–424

Hagerman PJ, Hagerman RJ (2004) The fragile-X premutation: a maturing perspective. Am J Hum Genet 74:805–816

Hagerman RJ, Leehey M, Heinrichs W, Tassone F, Wilson R, Hills J, Grigsby J, Gage B, Hagerman PJ (2001) Intention tremor, parkinsonism, and generalized brain atrophy in male carriers of fragile X. Neurology 57:127–130

Heard E, Disteche CM (2006) Dosage compensation in mammals: fine-tuning the expression of the X chromosome. Genes Dev 20:1848–1867

Heard E, Clerc P, Avner P (1997) X-chromosome inactivation in mammals. Annu Rev Genet 31:571–610

Heard E, Rougeulle C, Arnaud D, Avner P, Allis CD (2001) Methylation of Histone H3 at Lys-9 Is an early mark on the X chromosome during X inactivation. Cell 107:727–738

Hedges LV, Nowell A (1995) Sex-differences in mental test-scores, variability, and numbers of high-scoring individuals. Science 269:41–45

Henn W, Zang KD (1997) Mosaicism in Turner's syndrome. Nature 390:569

Hornstra IK, Nelson DL, Warren ST, Yang TP (1993) High resolution methylation analysis of the FMR1 gene trinucleotide repeat region in fragile X syndrome. Hum Mol Genet 2:1659–1665

Iwase S, Lan F, Bayliss P, de la Torre-Ubieta L, Huarte M, Qi HH, Whetstine JR, Bonni A, Roberts TM, Shi Y (2007) The X-linked mental retardation gene SMCX/JARID1C defines a family of histone H3 lysine 4 demethylases. Cell 128:1077–1088

Jaenisch R, Bird A (2003) Epigenetic regulation of gene expression: how the genome integrates intrinsic and environmental signals. Nat Genet 33:245–254

Johnson W, Carothers A, Deary IJ (2008) Sex differences in variability in general intelligence: a new look at the old question. Perspect Psychol Sci 3:518–531

Johnston CM, Lovell FL, Leongamornlert DA, Stranger BE, Dermitzakis EY, Ross MT (2008) Large scale population study of human cell lines indicates that dosage compensation is virtually complete. PLoS Genet 4:0088–0098

Kernohan KD, Jiang Y, Tremblay DC, Bonvissuto AC, Eubanks JH, Mann MRW, Bérubé NG (2010) ATRX partners with cohesin and MeCP2 and contributes to developmental silencing of imprinted genes in the brain. Dev Cell 18:191–202

Ladd PD, Smith LE, Rabaia NA, Moore JM, Georges SA, Hansen RS, Hagerman RJ, Tassone F, Tapscot SJ, Filippova GN (2007) An antisense transcript spanning the CGG region of FMR1 is upregulated in permutation carriers but is silenced in full mutation individuals. Hum Mol Genet 16:3174–3187

Laggerbauer B, Ostareck D, Keidel EM, Ostareck-Lederer A, Fischer U (2001) Evidence that fragile X mental retardation protein is a negative regulator of translation. Hum Mol Genet 10:329–338

Lawrence K, Jones A, Oreland L, Spektor D, Mandy W, Campbell R, Skuse D (2006) The development of mental state attributions in women with X- monosomy, and the role of monoamine oxidase B in the socio-cognitive phenotype. Cognition 102:84–100

Lewis JD, Meehan RR, Henzel WJ, Maurer-Fogy I, Jeppesen P, Klein F, Bird A (1992) Purification, sequence, and cellular localization of a novel chromosomal protein that binds to methylated DNA. Cell 69:905–914

Li ZZ, Zhang YY, Ku L, Wilkinson KD, Warren ST, Feng Y (2001) The fragile X mental retardation protein inhibits translation via interacting with mRNA. Nucleic Acids Res 29:2276–2283

Loat CS, Asbury K, Galsworthy MJ, Plomin R, Craig IW (2004) X inactivation as asource of behavioural differences in monozygotic female twins. Twin Res 7:54–61

Loat CS, Craig GM, Plomin R, Craig IW (2006) Investigating the relationship between FMR1 allele length and cognitive ability in children: a subtle effect of the normal allele range on the normal ability range? Ann Hum Genet 70:555–565

Loat CS, Curran S, Lewis CM, Abrahams B, Duvall J, Geschwind D, Bolton P, Craig IW (2008a) Methyl-CpG-binding protein (MECP2) polymorphisms and vulnerability to autism. Genes Brain Behav 7:754–760

Loat CS, Haworth CMA, Plomin R, Craig IW (2008b) A model incorporating potential skewed X-inactivation in MZ girls suggests that X-linked QTLs exist for several social behaviours including Autism Spectrum Disorder. Ann Hum Genet 72:742–751

Lyon MF (1998) X-Chromosome inactivation: a repeat hypothesis. Cytogenet Cell Genet 80:133–137

Martinowich K, Hattori D, Wu H, Fouse S, He F, Hu Y, Fan G, YiE S (2003) DNA methylation-related chromatin remodeling in activity-dependent Bdnf gene regulation. Science 302:890–893

McRae AF, Matigian NA, Vadlamudi L, Mulley JC, Mowry B, Martin NG, Berkovic SF, Hayward NK, Visscher PM (2007) Replicated effects of sex and genotype on gene expression in human lymphoblastoid cell lines. Hum Mol Genet 16:364–373

Mueller JL, Mahadevaiah SK, Park PJ, Warburton PE, Page DC, Turner JM (2008) The mouse X chromosome is enriched for multicopy testis genes showing postmeiotic expression. Nat Genet 40:794–799

Nagarajan RP, Hogart AR, Gwye Y, Martin MR, La Salle JM (2006) Reduced MECP2 expression is frequent in autism frontal cortex and correlates with aberrant MECP2 promoter methylation. Epigenetics 1:e1–e11

Nan X, Meehan RR, Bird A (1993) Dissection of the methyl-CpG binding domain from the chromosomal protein MeCP2. Nucleic Acids Res 21:4886–4892

Nan X, Hou J, Maclean A, Nasir J, Lafuente MJ, Shu X, Kriaucionis S, Bird A (2007) Interaction between chromatin proteins MECP2 and ATRX is disrupted by mutations that cause inherited mental retardation. Proc Nat Acad Sci USA 104:2709–2714

Naumann A, Hochstein N, Weber S, Fanning E, Doerfler W (2009) A distinct DNA-methylation boundary in the 5′ – upstream sequence of the fmr1 promoter binds nuclear proteins and is lost in fragile X syndrome. Am J Hum Genet 85:606–616

140

I.W. Craig

Ng K, Purllirsch D, Loeb M, Wutz A (2007) Xist and the order of silencing. EMBO Rep 8:34–38
Nguyen DK, Disteche CM (2006) Dosage compensation of the active X chromosome in mammals. Nat Genet 38:47–53
O'Donnell WT, Warren ST (2002) A decade of molecular studies of fragile X syndrome. Annu Rev Neurosci 25:315–338
Oberlé I, Rousseau F, Heitz D, Kretz C, Devys D, Hanauer A, Boue J, Bertheas M, Mandel J (1991) Instability of a 550-base pair DNA segment and abnormal methylation in fragile X syndrome. Science 252:1097–1102
Ogawa Y, Lee JT (2003) Xite, X-inactivation intergeneic transcriptional elements that regulate the probability of choice. Mol Cell 11:731–734
Okamoto I, Heard E (2006) The dynamics of imprinted X inactivation during preimplantation development in mice. Cytogenet Genome Res 113:318–324
Pietrobono R, Tabolacci E, Zalfa F, Zito I, Terracciano A, Moscato U, Bagni C, Oostra B, Chiurazzi P, Neri G (2005) Molecular dissection of the events leading to inactivation of the FMR1 gene. Hum Mol Genet 14:267–277
Pinsonneault JK, Papp AC, Sadée W (2006) Allelic mRNA expression of X-linked monoamine oxidase a (MAOA) in human brain: dissection of epigenetic and genetic factors. Hum Mol Genet 15:2636–2649
Plenge RM, Hendrich BD, Schwartz C, Arena JF, Naumova A, Sapienza C, Winter RM, Willard HF (1997) A promoter mutation in the XIST gene in two unrelated families with skewed X-chromosome inactivation. Nat Genet 17:353–356
Popova BC, Takashi T, Takagi N, Brockdorff N, Nesterova TB (2006) Attenuated spread of X-inactivation in an X;autosome translocation. Proc Natl Acad Sci USA 103:7706–7711
Puck JM (1998) The timing of twinning: more insights from x inactivation. Am J Hum Genet 63:327–328
Pullirsch D, Härtel R, Kishimoto H, Leeb M, Steiner G, Wutz A (2010) The Trithorax group protein Ash2l and Saf-A are recruited to the inactive X chromosome at the onset of stable X inactivation. Development 137:935–943
Raefski AS, O'Neill MJ (2005) Identification of a cluster of X-linked imprinted genes in mice. Nat Genet 37:620–624
Reik W, Dean W, Walter J (2001) Epigenetic reprogramming in mammalian development. Science 293:1089–1093
Ross MT, Grafham DV, Coffey AJ, Scherer S, McLay K, Muzny D, Platzer M, Howell GR, Burrows C, Bird CP et al (2005) The DNA sequence of the human X chromosome. Nature 434:325–337
Saveliev A, Everett C, Sharpe T, Webster Z, Festenstein R (2003) DNA triplet repeats mediate heterochromatinprotein-1-sensitive variegated gene silencing. Nature 422:909–913
Sengupta AK, Ohhata T, Wutz A (2008) X chromosome inactivation. In: Tost J (ed) Epigenetics. Caister Academic Press, Norfolk, VA, pp 273–302
Shahbazian MD, Zoghbi HY (2002) Rett syndrome and MeCP2: linking epigenetics and neuronal function. Am J Hum Genet 71:1259–1272
Sharp A, Robinson D, Jacobs P (2000) Age and tissue specific variation of X chromosome inactivation ratios in normal women. Hum Genet 107:343–349
Shumay E, Fowler JS (2010) Identification and characterization of putative methylation targets in the MAOA locus using bioinformatic approaches. Epigenetics 5:325–342
Skuse DH, James RS, Bishop DVM, Coppin B, Dalton P, Aamodt-Leeper G, Bacarese-Hamilton M, Creswell C, McGurk R, Jacobs PA (1997) Evidence from Turner's syndrome of an imprinted X-linked locus affecting cognitive function. Nature 387:705–708
Smeets HJM, Smits APT, Verheij CE, Theelen JPG, Willemsen R, Vandeburgt I, Hoogveen AT, Oosterwijk JC, Oostra BA (1995) Normal phenotype in 2 brothers with a full FMR1 mutation. Hum Mol Genet 4:2103–2108
Stefani G, Fraser CE, Darnell JC, Darnell RB (2004) Fragile X mental retardation protein is associated with translating polyribosomes in neuronal cells. J Neurosci 24:7272–7276

Sudbrak R, Wieczorek G, Nuber UA, Mann W, Kirchner R, Erdogan F, Brown CJ, Wöhrle D, Sterk P, Kalscheuer VM, Berger W, Lehrach H, Ropers HH (2001) X chromosome-specific cDNA arrays: identification of genes that escape from X-inactivation and other applications. Hum Mol Genet 10:77–83

Sutcliffe JS, Nelson DL, Zhang F, Pieretti M, Caskey CT, Saxe D, Warren ST (1992) DNA methylation represses FMR-1 transcription in fragile X syndrome. Hum Mol Genet 1:397–400

Swanberg SE, Nagarajan RP, Peddada S, Yasui DH, LaSalle JM (2009) Reciprocal co-regulation of EGR2 and MECP2 is disrupted in Rett syndrome and autism. Hum Mol Genet 18:525–534

Talebizadeh Z, Simon SD, Butler MG (2006) X chromosome gene expression in human tissues: male and female comparisons. Genomics 88:675–681

Tiberio G (1994) MZ Female twins discordant for X-linked diseases: a review. Acta Genet Med Gemellol 43:207–214

Turner G, Webb T, Wake S, Robinson H (1996) Prevalence of fragile X syndrome. Am J Med Genet 64:196–197

Wöhrle D, Salat U, Gläser D, Mücke J, Meisel-Stosiek M, Schindler D, Vogel W, Steinbach P (1998) Unusual mutations in high functioning fragile X males: apparent instability of expanded unmethylated CGG repeats. J Med Genet 35:103–111

Xu J, Burgoyne PS, Arnold AP (2002) Sex differences in sex chromosome gene expression in mouse brain. Hum Mol Genet 11:1409–1419

Yasui DH, Peddada S, Bieda MC, Vallero RO, Hogart A, Nagarajan RP, Thatcher KN, Farnham PJ, LaSalle JM (2007) Integrated epigenomic analyses of neuronal MeCP2 reveal a role for long-range interaction with active genes. Proc Natl Acad Sci USA 104:19416–19421

Youings SA, Murray A, Dennis N, Ennis S, Lewis C, McKechnie N, Pound M, Sharrock A, Jacobs P (2000) FRAXA and FRAXE: the results of a five year survey. J Med Genet 37:415–421

Chapter 8
The Strategies of the Genes: Genomic Conflicts, Attachment Theory, and Development of the Social Brain

Bernard J. Crespi

Abstract I describe and evaluate the hypothesis that effects of parent–offspring conflict and genomic imprinting on human neurodevelopment and behavior are central to evolved systems of mother–child attachment. The psychological constructs of Bowlby's attachment theory provide phenomenological descriptions of how attachment orchestrates affective-cognitive development, and patterns of imprinted-gene expression and coexpression provide evidence of epigenetic and evolutionary underpinnings to human growth and neurodevelopment. Social-environmental perturbations to the development of normally secure attachment, and alterations to evolved systems of parent–offspring conflict and imprinted-gene effects, are expected to lead to specific forms of maladaptation, manifest in psychiatric conditions affecting social-brain development. In particular, underdevelopment of the social brain in autism may be mediated in part by mechanisms that lead to physically enhanced yet psychologically underdeveloped attachment to the mother, and affective-psychotic conditions, such as schizophrenia and depression, may be mediated in part by forms of insecure attachment and by increased relative effects of the maternal brain, both directly from mothers and via imprinted-gene effects in offspring. These hypotheses are concordant with findings from epidemiology, attachment theory, psychiatry, and genetic and epigenetic analyses of risk factors for autism and affective-psychotic conditions, they make novel predictions for explaining the causes of psychosis in Prader–Willi syndrome and idiopathic schizophrenia, and they suggest avenues for therapeutic interventions based on normalizing alterations to epigenetic networks and targeting public-health interventions toward reduction of perturbations to the development of secure attachment in early childhood and individuation during adolescence.

Keywords Attachment · Autism · Genomic imprinting · Schizophrenia · Social brain

B.J. Crespi
Department of Biosciences, Simon Fraser University, Burnaby, BC V5A 1S6, Canada
e-mail: crespi@sfu.ca

A. Petronis and J. Mill (eds.), *Brain, Behavior and Epigenetics*,
Epigenetics and Human Health, DOI 10.1007/978-3-642-17426-1_8,
© Springer-Verlag Berlin Heidelberg 2011

8.1 Introduction

Conrad Waddington coined the term "epigenetics" to refer to the processes, whereby interactions between genetic and environmental variation lead to the emergence of patterns in phenotypic variation via development (Haig 2004a). In 1957, Waddington explicated in detail his theory of how natural selection and other processes mediate the evolution of ontogenetic trajectories, described by the concept of progressively increasing canalization as depicted in adaptive-developmental landscapes. His "strategy of the genes" thus centers on the evolution of cooperative developmental-genetic networks that can, in part via epigenetic modifications, produce relatively viable phenotypes in response to, and in spite of, genetic and environmental perturbations due to alterations in genes or their patterns of expression.

Epigenetic landscapes represent metaphors for how gene regulation directs pathways of development from the largest to smallest scales – from the first deviation in totipotency of embryonic stem cells, to gene-expression signatures, cell fate determinants and tissue-type differentiation into organs, and to phenotypes that include conditional behavior (Fig. 8.1). Much of modern developmental genetics focuses on elucidating the causal processes that underlie subsections of such landscapes, in the contexts of human ontogenies and disease, yet epigenetics itself, the impetus for Waddington's conception of development, has only recently

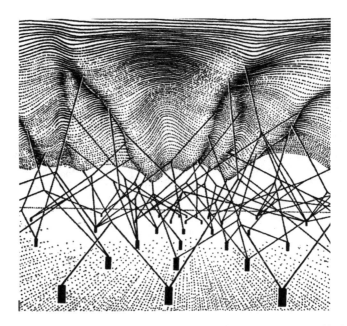

Fig. 8.1 Waddington's (1957) conceptualization of an epigenetic landscape, with the pegs as genes and the strings as developmental effects from gene expression

reemerged as a central focus of research in understanding the orchestration of phenotypic development.

For humans, development proceeds via growth and differentiation of body, brain, and behavior under the joint influences of genes and, for environment, mainly interacting humans. Throughout much of the most formative early years, the mother holds center stage, providing both physiological nurture from uterus, placenta, and breast, and, increasingly, as the infant grows, psychological guidance through interactive processes of bonding, instruction, and other behavior. These developmental processes, perhaps more than many others, are expected to be strongly canalized, yet also sensitive to relatively predictable perturbations, such that epigenetic modifications to gene expression should direct neurodevelopment along conditionally adaptive pathways unless perturbations are too severe. As such, and as Waddington (1957) described, epigenetic landscapes may be considered as structures shaped by long evolutionary histories of selection, representing in their form some more or less long-term integration of past social environments and genomes.

From Waddington's mid-twentieth century perspective, the adaptive strategies of all genes in an individual coincide, and aspects of the environment, such as the agents of other genomes, are not expected to pursue strategies that conflict. Two levels and forms of genetic conflict are now well documented in their effects: conflicts between individuals who are genetically unrelated to some degree, and conflicts within the genomes of individuals, between sets of genes with different patterns of inheritance and genetic relatedness to potential interactants (Hamilton 1964, 1996; Trivers 1974; Haig 1997, 2006a, b; Burt and Trivers 2006; Fox et al. 2010). Both forms of conflict lead to differences in the phenotypic optima toward which they are, and have been, directed by natural selection. Optimal developmental trajectories of a given individual, and thus epigenetic landscapes, may thus vary in systematic ways between mother and child, and between sets of genes, such as imprinted genes that are silenced when inherited from either the mother or the father (Haig 2002). From evolutionary theory, and now-abundant empirical data (e.g., Hrdy 1999; Maestripieri 2002), offspring are expected to solicit more investment from parents, especially mothers as the main caregivers, than parents have been naturally selected to provide, due ultimately to parent–offspring relatedness of only one-half for autosomal genes. Similarly, paternally expressed imprinted genes in the child are expected to exert phenotypic effects that extract more investment from the mother than do maternally expressed imprinted genes, due to a history of paternally inherited genes exhibiting lower genetic relatedness within sibships and matrilines (Haig 2002, 2004b).

Outcomes of conflict between individuals, and between sets of genes, are difficult to predict, but may include stable equilibria, tugs-or-war over resource allocation, one party "winning" due to asymmetries in control over resource allocation, or continued conflict (e.g., Royle et al. 2004; Smiseth et al. 2008). Conflicts such as genomic imprinting also potentiate liability to phenotypes associated with disease (Crespi 2010), due to functional haploidy of imprinted genes, dysregulation of tug-of-war-based systems that evolved in this context, and the expected general higher lability of epigenetic gene-expression control systems (based on DNA methylation and histone modifications) compared to the lability of DNA alterations via mutation. Such disease effects from imprinting have been documented extensively for disorders related to human placentation, overall growth, and neurodevelopment (e.g., Angiolini et al. 2006; McMinn et al. 2006; Wagschal and Feil 2006; Davies et al. 2008a, b).

The main thesis of this chapter is that genomic conflicts and cooperation, especially the epigenetic effects of genomic imprinting, centrally mediate core aspects of mother–child developmental interactions – most notably the processes of attachment – with important consequences for psychological well-being throughout life. I first describe the roles of imprinted genes in development, and recent discoveries of imprinted-gene networks that control growth. Next, I explicate the hypothesis that human early-childhood social development, mainly via interaction with the mother, involves a network of brain-expressed imprinted genes that modulate attachment – the process whereby children, in environments characterized by secure and responsive maternal care, internalize psychological constructs derived from external mother–child interactions to develop a self and psyche centered in their social context (Bowlby 1969; Bretherton 1997). The idea of imprinted genes mediating attachment was originally suggested by Isles and Holland (2005), and I extend and evaluate the hypothesis using information from patterns of imprinted-gene expression and coexpression, phenotypes of imprinting-based disorders, Bowlby's attachment theory, and psychiatric conditions involving the social brain. Finally, I discuss the implications of these ideas and data for pharmacological and behavioral therapies, public-health strategies, and the integration of epigenetic perspectives derived from Waddington into research programs focused on understanding the genetic bases of human development. Most generally, I integrate and synthesize evidence from evolutionary biology, developmental psychology, human genetics and epigenetics, and psychiatry of social-brain disorders to develop and evaluate explicit, testable hypothesis regarding roles of genomic conflicts and epigenetics in human development and evolution.

8.2   Genomic Imprinting in Human Growth

Haig and Graham (1991) developed the kinship theory of imprinting in the context of conflict interactions in fetal mice between paternally expressed *Igf2*, which drives growth, and maternally expressed *Igf2r*, which acts as a "decoy" receptor to reduce *Igf2*'s growth-stimulating effects. Although the predicted pattern of paternally expressed imprinted genes tending to foster overall growth, and maternally expressed imprinted genes constraining it, has been abundantly supported in studies of placentation and body size (e.g., Plagge et al., 2004; Weinstein et al., 2004; Kelsey 2007), the simple, direct tug-of-war system exemplified by *Igf2* and its receptor has proven to be atypical of imprinted-gene effects generally. The first clear evidence for a much more extensive system of imprinted-gene interaction – imprinted-gene networks – emerged from work by Arima et al. (2005), who demonstrated that the imprinted genes *ZAC1*, *LIT1*, and *CDKN1C* jointly mediate growth of human cells. Varrault et al. (2006) used information from experimental mouse knockouts, and microarray databases, to document more directly the existence of a coregulatory imprinted-gene network; thus, gains and losses of *Zac1* altered the expression levels of the imprinted genes *Igf2*, *H19*, *Cdkn1c*, and *Dlk1*, and a broad pattern of imprinted-gene coexpression, involving these five genes as well as *Grb10*, *Gtl2*, *Peg1* (*Mest*), *Sgce*, *Dcn*, *Gatm*, *Gnas*, *Ndn*, and *Peg3*, emerged from analyses of gene coexpression in pooled datasets from mouse muscle and other tissues. Lui et al. (2008) subsequently identified a set of 11 imprinted genes in this network, all of which influence aspects of cell proliferation, whose expression levels across multiple tissues paralleled trajectories of overall body growth, and Gabory et al. (2009) showed that *H19* acts as an important transregulator of this imprinted-gene network that may also "fine-tune" gene coexpression patterns to moderate effects from perturbations; network interactions among unrelated genes are indeed postulated as a major cause of robustness against mutations (Wagner 2000), which should be especially important for functionally haploid, imprinted genes. Gabory et al. (2009) also demonstrated that such regulation via *H19* apparently did not operate in the placenta, which implies a notable degree of tissue and stage specificity of imprinted-gene network dynamics. Most recently, loss of expression of the *ATRX* gene in mice has been shown to cause altered postnatal expression of a suite of imprinted genes including *Igf2, H19, Dlk1, Zac1*, and *Peg1*, as well as the Rett-syndrome gene *MeCP2*, suggesting a role for *ATRX* in transregulation of the imprinted-gene network (Kernohan et al. 2010) and corroborating effects of *MeCP2* expression in the regulation of imprinted genes (Miyano et al. 2008).

Two independent lines of data provide further evidence for fundamental roles of imprinted-gene networks in development. First, two of the best-understood human genetic syndromes, Beckwith–Wiedemann syndrome and Silver–Russell syndrome, are each mediated by alterations to different imprinted genes in the network, which convergently generate similar phenotypes involving, respectively, overgrowth or undergrowth (Eggermann et al. 2008; Eggermann 2009). Similar convergent effects, whereby different epigenetic or genetic alterations produce highly similar phenotypes, have also been described for Prader–Willi syndrome (Crespi 2008a) and Angelman syndrome (Jedele 2007; Crespi 2008a). Convergence from diverse genetic or epigenetic perturbations, to similar phenotypes across multiple traits, represents clear examples of developmental canalization. Such canalization effects can also be generalized to idiopathic conditions, such as autism and schizophrenia, each of which also exhibits diverse genetic, epigenetic, and environmental causes converging to a relatively small set of cognitive, affective, and behavioral phenotypes (Happé 1994; Owen et al. 2007; Abrahams and Geschwind 2008). As imprinted-gene networks have presumably evolved in part due to selection for coordinated, robust control of mammalian growth – yielding specific, syndromic phenotypes when sufficiently perturbed – genomic and epigenetic networks orchestrating human neurodevelopment and behavior may likewise be expected to yield predictable patterns from different forms of alteration.

A second line of evidence pertinent to gene-expression networks in general, and imprinted genes in particular, is the recent discovery of mechanisms, whereby imprinted domains interact across different chromosomes, via allele-specific physical juxtaposition of long-range chromatin loops in interphase nuclei (Smits and Kelsey 2006; Zhao et al. 2006). Such interactions occur genome-wide (Ling and Hoffman 2007), but are strongly enriched to imprinted regions (Zhao et al. 2006), with an apparent central role for the imprinted RNA gene *H19* as a hub for transvection of parent-of-origin specific effects to both imprinted and non-imprinted loci on other chromosomes (Sandhu et al. 2009). Interchromosomal interactions that involve imprinted loci provide a genome-scale mechanism for coordinated expression of imprinted genes (in addition to mechanisms involving, for example, transcription factors such as *Zac1*, and protein–protein interactions such as those between *p57kip2* and *Nurr1*) (Joseph et al. 2003), and for control of non-imprinted genes and loci by specific imprinted genes, that may serve to increase their relative influence on development.

In the context of Haig's kinship theory of imprinting, imprinted-gene networks can be hypothesized as multidimensional generalizations of simple, two-dimensional tugs-of-war, which apparently evolved step by step with the accrual of imprinted domains along the lineages leading to the origins of metatherian and eutherian mammals (Renfree et al. 2009). This conception of imprinted-gene networks shows how cooperation, in a literal sense of the word, can evolve from conflict, when the interests of different mutually dependent parties, here paternally expressed and maternally expressed imprinted genes, overlap partially yet broadly. Thus, paternal and maternal genes, as well as additional genetic "factions" such as genes on the X chromosome (Haig 2006a), share a common interest in successful development via reducing physiological costs of conflict, and (within limits) increasing the robustness of development to perturbations, although natural selection continues to favor paternal-gene variants that solicit marginally more investment from mothers, and maternal and X-linked alleles that reduce such imposition of increased costs.

Consideration of the tissue and stage specifics of imprinted-gene expression, in the context of the kinship theory of imprinting, leads to the inference that more or less different imprinted-gene networks should characterize each of the three main arenas for imprinted-gene effects (1) placentation, (2) overall postnatal growth, and (3) behavioral interactions with the mother, as influenced by imprinted-gene expression in the brain. Indeed, the network presented in Varrault et al. (2006) represents a conglomeration of gene coexpression patterns across multiple tissues and stages, and some central genes in the network, such as *Ndn*, apparently do not exert effects on overall growth (Tsai et al. 1999). Eutherian placentation is known to be orchestrated by imprinted genes in a manner consonant with predictions of the kinship theory (e.g., Bressan et al. 2009), and alterations to imprinted-gene expression underlie a considerable proportion of risk for the major disorders of human pregnancy (e.g., Charalambous et al. 2007); Fauque et al. (2010) describe evidence for imprinted-gene coregulation effects in mouse placentation, which coordinate gene-expression changes in relation to early-embryonic conditions. Postnatal growth effects are similarly mediated by imprinted genes, which appear to predominantly exert their influences through effects on cell proliferation at the tissue level (Reik et al. 2001), and glucose and lipid metabolism at the levels of physiology and metabolism (Sigurdsson et al. 2009). The body growth enhancement effects of Beckwith–Wiedemann syndrome, and growth reduction in Silver–Russell syndrome, indeed represent paradigmatic examples of imprinted-gene disorders with primary effects on both prenatal and postnatal growth. Microarray studies that focus on placental gene expression, and gene expression across the tissues most directly involved in prenatal and postnatal growth, are thus expected to reveal imprinted-gene networks that comprise partially overlapping sets of genes, with imprinted genes exerting effects that are more or less tissue specific. The tissue with the most pervasive effects on growth, development, and behavior – the brain – remains, however, the least well understood.

8.3   Genomic Imprinting in the Brain

The study of imprinted-gene effects in brain development was pioneered by Keverne, whose studies of chimeric mice showed differential contribution of paternally expressed imprinted genes to development of limbic brain regions (especially the hypothalamus), and maternally expressed genes to development of the neocortex (Allen et al. 1995; Keverne et al. 1996; Keverne 2001a, b). Functional and evolutionary hypotheses for the effects of brain-expressed imprinted genes have been described in detail; these include diverse effects on affect, cognition, attention, feeding behavior, and other central brain functions (Isles et al. 2006; Wilkinson et al. 2007; Davies et al. 2008a, b; Champagne et al. 2009), some of which apparently influence resource-related interactions between mothers and offspring. These hypotheses have proved difficult to evaluate critically due to the complexity of the mechanisms involved, and the difficulty of testing alternative hypotheses of neurobehavioral adaptation compared to pleiotropic by-product.

Adaptation is most commonly recognized, at least initially, as convergence or parallelism in causal patterns consistent with theory. For imprinted brain-expressed gene, clear convergent effects of paternally expressed genes on neurodevelopment have been described for the roles of *Peg3, Peg1*, and *Ndn* in promoting development of hypothalamic neurons that secrete oxytocin, the peptide hormone that most strongly mediates social bonding (Davies et al. 2008a, b; Ross and Young 2009; MacDonald and MacDonald 2010). Moreover, in the *Zac1* network (Varrault et al. 2006), these three genes occupy central locations as "hubs", prominently connected, like *Zac1* itself, to relatively large numbers of both imprinted and non-imprinted genes. These findings, from three lines of evidence (mouse knockouts, functional gene-expression data, and gene coexpression networks), suggest a functional and evolutionary role for imprinted genes in fostering bonding and attachment of offspring to mothers, in the context of an imprinted-gene network that affects expression of offspring behaviors that regulate levels of resource accrual from mothers. In mice, bonding of pups to mothers involves olfactory, tactile, and auditory cues, which foster safety and suckling; moreover, suckling behavior is differentially disrupted in mouse knockouts of the paternally expressed genes *Peg3* and *Gnasxl* (Curley et al 2004; Plagge et al. 2004).

In humans, who like mice are highly altricial as neonates, attachment involves the same three categories of sensory cue as in mice, and early suckling and feeding are impaired in the two genomic conditions, Silver–Russell syndrome and Prader–Willi syndrome, that involve strong maternal-gene biases (Blissett et al. 2001; Holland et al., 2003; Dudley and Muscatelli 2007), as well as in humans with paternal deletion of *GNASxl* (Geneviève et al. 2005); in contrast, macroglossia (enlarged tongues, which are expected to facilitate suckling) has been reported in both Beckwith–Wiedemann syndrome and Angelman syndrome (Cohen 2005). But much more extensively than in mice, human cognitive-affective interactions guide early development of the child's "social brain" – the distributed, integrated set of neural systems that control acquisition, processing, and deployment of socially interactive information (Frith 2008). Such interactions have motivated the development of a large body of theory and empirical work in psychology and attachment theory, with direct implications for other fields from genetics, epigenetics, and neurodevelopment to analyses of the etiology of psychiatric conditions that involve alterations to early development and function of the social brain.

8.4 Attachment Theory and Human Social Development

Attachment theory was developed by John Bowlby and Mary Ainsworth to help explain the adaptive significance of physical and psychological interactions between young children and close caregivers (primarily the mother), and how children deprived of care, or subject to dysfunctional forms of caregiver–child interaction, develop along lifelong trajectories characterized by altered emotional and cognitive systems that are explicable in part by the nature of these early perturbations (Bowlby 1969). The majority of children develop "secure" attachment, whereby their intimate interactions with the mother provide for physical safety, nutritional sustenance, and social-emotion-cognitive guidance that generates a "secure base", increasingly explorative behavior with age, and an environmental conducive to development of a social brain – internalized schema – with robust sense of self, well-developed theory of mind, and ability to nurture secure attachment to one's own children in later life.

Deviations from secure attachment, as assayed by the "strange situations test" that tests a child's behavior toward its mother when subject to short separations, take a small set of forms (1) avoidant attachment, whereby children with unmet expectations of attachment security come to at least provisionally reject significant others, (2) anxious/ambivalent attachment, with unmet solicitation leading to "escalation" of distress and behavior characterized by contact-seeking combined with anger and ambivalence, and (3) disorganized attachment, with lack of a coherent, organized "strategy" for interacting with the caregiver (e.g., Shaver and Mikulincer 2002). These deviations have been interpreted in the context of developmental responses by the child to variation in caregiver sensitivity, that is, provision of consistent physical and psychological support, in contrast to neglectful, hostile, or inconsistent care.

The framework for interpretation of childhood attachment patterns has developed in the combined contexts of post-Freudian psychodynamics, evolutionary-ethological constructs for the study of animal behavior, and psychological theories of stages and processes in child social development, such as the social-behavioral internalization theories of Vygotsky (Bretherton 1992; Thompson 2008). In her book *Mother Nature*, Hrdy (1999) first conceptualized an evolutionary-genetic basis for understanding central aspects of attachment, unappreciated by previous work, that follow directly from W.D. Hamilton's inclusive fitness theory. Due ultimately to genetic relatedness between mothers and children of only one-half, mother–child interactions are expected to comprise complex mixtures of cooperation and conflict, with children having been selected to solicit higher levels of behavioral as well as nutritional investment than mothers have been selected to provide. The theory underlying parent–offspring conflict has been well supported by empirical studies (Bowlby 1969, p. 203; Haig 1993; Hinde and Kilner 2007), and Hrdy (1999) interprets a broad swath of human-specific childhood phenotypes, from high levels of neonatal fat, to precocious neurological development of eye contact, facial expression, and vocalization, as subject to a long history of selection in the context of child signaling of vigor and solicitation of increased energetic and psychological investment. Childhood attachment to mother – from placenta, to breast, and to psychological development – is thus expected to be centrally mediated by both cooperation and conflict, which should be expressed in patterns of child attachment behaviors that represent largely adaptive responses to the behavior of the mother, who is in physical control of investment. The major patterns of child attachment have indeed been interpreted by attachment theorists as conditionally adaptive responses of children to sensitive, hostile, neglectful, or inconsistent mothering, though not in terms of strategies grounded by the fundamentals of evolutionary genetic and epigenetics.

Parent–offspring conflict theory applies to autosomal genes with conditional, temporally restricted effects in children, and autosomal genes expressed in mothers. The primary implication of this theory is that evolved systems of mother–child interaction (and father–child interaction, given some degree of paternal care) should be characterized in part by conflicts – mainly centered on increased demands from the child, and responses from mother conditioned on marginal benefits to her from incremental investment in child versus benefits from other fitness-accruing activities. Haig (1993) describes evidence of such dynamics in the context of human maternal–fetal interactions, as do Wells (2003) and Soltis (2004), for suckling and crying; these authors also demonstrate how the major disorders of food provision via placenta and breast, including intrauterine growth restriction, pre-eclampsia, gestational diabetes, excess post-natal weight gain, failure to thrive, and colic, can usefully be understood in part as forms and effects of dysregulation to systems of evolved mother–child conflict – conflicts that are revealed most clearly in cases of genetic or environmental perturbation from "normal" development. Mother's primary form of investment in children beyond food is, of course, psychological training and guidance, and mother–child conflicts in this arena are expected to exhibit constrained-conflict dynamics squarely manifest in attachment, with disorders of mental health, for the grown child, more likely to result when dynamics are perturbed (Berry et al. 2007, 2008; Lyons-Ruth 2008).

To understand the expected role of imprinted genes in attachment, conflicts due to imprinted genes must be conceptually distinguished from, and related to, conflicts between parents and offspring. Imprinted-gene conflicts are thus expected, from the kinship theory of imprinting, to involve interactions between paternally expressed genes and maternally expressed genes in the child. As such, imprinted genes are predicted, through the integration of their effects, to influence the child's "set level" of resource demand imposed upon the mother. An example of such an economic system, in a physiological situation, is provided by expression of the imprinted gene *Cdnk1c* in fetal mouse development: levels of its protein product, *p57kip2*, have been experimentally demonstrated to act as a "rheostat" for embryonic growth, with ultimate levels of growth determined by the balance between fetal demand and maternal supply (Andrews et al. 2007). In the context of child psychology and behavior, imprinted genes are expected to similarly mediate levels of imposed demand, here for psychological time and energy; more generally, they should exert effects that result, by any mechanism, in higher or lower, longer or shorter, levels of investment from the mother. Small alterations to such systems, toward, for example, stronger effects from paternal gene expression that lead to higher investment, are expected to benefit the child, and his or her paternally expressed imprinted genes, at a small cost to the mother and to the child's maternally expressed imprinted genes. In contrast, large alterations, which like any large genetic or epigenetic effects surmount the homeostatic effects of canalized development, are expected to result in disorders of psychological development that are detrimental to both mother and child, and to all genomic parties concerned. The nature of such disorders, however, provides useful tests of evolutionary theory involving genomically based conflicts, and insights into strategies for therapy, prevention, and research (Crespi 2008b; Crespi et al. 2009).

These considerations from attachment theory, parent–offspring conflict theory, and the kinship theory of imprinting generate a simple conceptual framework for understanding normal and dysregulated social-behavioral interactions between mothers and small children (Fig. 8.2). From birth, young children exhibit some level of social-behavioral "demand", manifest in solicitations of interaction via facial and auditory cues, as well as in the contexts of crying, fussing, and suckling. Such levels are expected to vary between children, and over time in response to levels and forms of reciprocal and unsolicited maternal behavior. Child-specific, dynamic "demand" is matched, less or more, by levels of maternal sensitivity and responsiveness to such cues – varying from neglect, to solicitous, attentive care, and to controlling over-involvement.

Evolutionary histories of parent–offspring conflict, and imprinted-gene conflict, have generated conditional behavioral adaptations, in child and in mother, that potentiate the possibility of mismatches between demand and response, which may result in maladaptation for one or both parties. Thus, relatively low social-behavioral demand from the child may delay or dysregulate social-brain development, but provide marginal benefits to the mother in terms of her lifetime inclusive fitness.

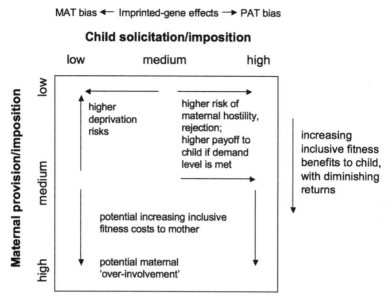

Fig. 8.2 A simple model for potential interactions of levels of maternal social-behavioral provision/imposition with levels of child social-behavioral solicitation/imposition

In contrast, relatively high demands may, if matched by supply, provide benefits to the child at some cost to mother; if not matched or if too insistent, however, such demands may provoke neglect, ambivalence, or even hostility, if they interfere sufficiently with a given mother's perceived optimal life-history trajectory. Levels of maternal "supply" higher than child demand – "over-involvement" – may, in contrast, come to interfere with the child's ability to explore and increasingly detach, physically and social-emotionally, from its secure base of the controlling maternal brain, to individuate its own psyche. This conceptual framework can help to explain the surprisingly low rates of secure attachment in children (not much over 50%), with anxious attachment representing, in part, attempts to solicit increased investment and improve one's lot, whereas avoidant attachment may involve a form of defensive strategy to, in part, avoid making matters any worse.

The outcomes of parent–offspring and imprinting-mediated conflicts are difficult to predict a priori, but they should depend upon the relative fitness costs and benefits to the child and mother of the alternative behaviors, and the degree to which each party controls aspects of the interaction. Thus, tactics available to young children include auditory and facial expressions of positive and negative affect, crying, suckling intensity, and physical movement varying with age; in contrast, mothers control access to breast and physical presence, and provision of information and social interaction crucial to the child's affective and cognitive development. Indeed, as Bowlby (1951, p. 53) noted:

> "*In dealing here with the embryology of the human mind one is struck by a similarity with the embryological development of the human body, during the course of which*

undifferentiated tissues respond to the influence of chemical organizers. If growth is to proceed smoothly, the tissues must be exposed to the influence of the appropriate organizer at certain critical periods. In the same way, if mental development is to proceed smoothly, it would appear necessary for the undifferentiated psyche to be exposed during certain critical periods to the influence of the psychic organizer – the mother". Thus, during infancy and early childhood, *"she is his ego and his super-ego."*

The primary usefulness of a Keynesian, supply–demand model for attachment is that it provides a framework, compatible with both developmental psychology and evolutionary-genetic theory, that generates novel explanations and predictions for alternative patterns of social-brain development. The model can be conceptualized as a developmental landscape, canalized to secure attachment and its sequelae but with different optimal trajectories for mother and child, and for child's paternal and maternal imprinted genes. Child development along the landscape initially proceeds via basic emotional-behavioral attachment mediated in part by paternal imprinted-gene effects, which serve as an affective-attentional scaffold upon which the social, maternal brain is gradually built, via maternal-gene effects and interactions with the mother and other caregivers. Actual trajectories for any child are determined by some dynamic integration of genetic, epigenetic, and environmental inputs into social-brain development, and into mother–child interaction; most importantly for mental health, relatively large genetic, epigenetic, or environmental alterations to this system are expected to generate predictable consequences, manifest in major disorders of the social brain, such as schizophrenia, depression, and autism. The assumptions and predictions of the model can be evaluated using information from human imprinted-gene syndromes, and studies on the etiology of schizophrenia and autism, in the contexts of attachment and evolutionary-genetic theory.

8.5 Prader–Willi Syndrome

Haig and Wharton (2003) describe how the complacent nature of Prader–Willi infants (with low levels of crying and wakefulness), and their compulsive self-foraging for food after the usual age of weaning, can be interpreted in the context of reduced demands on mothers, as expected under imprinted-gene biases involving loss of paternal-gene expression. Prader–Willi syndrome is known to centrally involve hypothalamic alterations and relatively low levels of oxytocin (Swaab et al. 1995; Holland et al. 2003; Höybye 2004; Goldstone 2006), which is consistent with the oxytocin-reducing effects of *Ndn* gene knockouts in mice (Davies et al. 2008a, b) and the expected behavioral effects of lower oxytocin levels – reduced motivation toward social bonding behavior. These considerations suggest that Prader–Willi syndrome should involve insecure attachment in children, especially among cases due to maternal uniparental disomy in which the genomic deviations toward maternal imprinted-gene effects are more extensive. This suite of behavioral and other alterations in Prader–Willi syndrome may involve, in part, disruptions to genes that underlie a human-lineage trajectory toward earlier weaning and shorter interbirth intervals (Sellen 2007; Haig 2009; Humphrey 2009), a transition expected to impose strong selection in the context of maternal-offspring and imprinted-gene conflicts given generally high rates of early-childhood mortality.

The extensions of attachment theory described here provide a simple, novel hypothesis to help explain one of the other major features of Prader–Willi syndrome: the extremely high levels of affective psychosis upon reaching adolescence (Soni et al. 2008; Webb et al. 2008). By this hypothesis, Prader–Willi infants and children may essentially undergo a process of self-induced maternal deprivation, whereby their low levels of care solicitation lead to reduced interaction with the mother and dysregulated social-emotional development. The primary line of evidence supporting this hypothesis, in addition to the theory and data described above, is that maternal deprivation, due to diverse causes including reduced physical care, temporary early separation, or permanent loss, is a well-documented, highly penetrant causal factor in the etiologies of depression (e.g., Pesonen et al. 2007; Tyrka et al. 2008; Liu et al. 2009), schizophrenia (reviewed in Read and Gumley 2008), and schizotypy (Anglin et al. 2008). Convergent evidence for interactions of maternal deprivation with imprinted-gene expression comes from a study of mice, where 2 (5.4%) of 37 genes significantly upregulated in the hypothalamic paraventricular nucleus of young mice in response to maternal deprivation were imprinted (*Gtl2* and *Ipw*), a higher proportion than expected given an approximate 1.2% (120 of 10,000) (http://igc.otago.ac.nz/ table.html) of brain-expressed genes imprinted in the mouse genome ($P < 0.05$).

To the extent that affective psychosis in Prader–Willi syndrome is mediated by gene–environment interaction in this context, alterations to early maternal-social environments, and facilitation of early bonding via behavioral and hormonal therapies, may help to alleviate the psychiatric sequelae of this large-scale epigenetic disruption. Similar considerations should apply to genetic and epigenetic alterations that yield phenotypes overlapping with Prader–Willi syndrome (Crespi 2008a) and, perhaps, to effects from reduced size of the paraventricular nucleus in patients with bipolar disorder and major depression, compared to controls (Manaye et al. 2005). More generally, an evolutionary trajectory toward earlier weaning and shorter interbirth intervals in humans might be expected to have increased vulnerability to affective-psychotic conditions, unless attachment through alloparents and fathers (Hrdy 2009) compensates for abbreviated maternal care.

8.6 Angelman Syndrome

In contrast to children with Prader–Willi syndrome, children with Angelman syndrome are highly active, with reduced duration of sleep, frequent suckling attempts, and enhanced levels of socially directed positive affect (Cohen et al. 2005; Oliver et al. 2007). These diverse phenotypes have been interpreted as reflecting increased behavioral and energetic demands on the mother, as predicted by the direction of imprinted-gene deviation, toward reduced relative effects from the maternally expressed imprinted gene *UBE3A* (Oliver et al. 2007). Such an increased "set level" of demands imposed on mothers might be expected to lead to insecure forms of attachment, unless the demands are met, whereupon social-emotional development should proceed as normally as possible under the circumstances of severe intellectual disability that characterize this syndrome. A high prevalence of autistic traits in Angelman syndrome (Sahoo et al. 2006; Bonati et al. 2007; Jedele 2007) has also been interpreted in the context of selectively reduced social-brain development and high demands imposed on the mother in the context of paternal imprinted-gene bias (Brown and Consedine 2004; Isles et al. 2006; Crespi and Badcock 2008).

8.7 Schizophrenia and Attachment

Schizophrenia represents a set of conditions, due to diverse causes, with some combination of symptoms that may include hallucinations, delusions, thought disorder, flat affect, and anhedonia (Read et al. 2004a, b). An attachment-theory perspective on schizophrenia was first provided by Bowlby (1973, pages 174–177, 318–319), in his description of continuities between forms of abusive and dysfunctional psychological treatment of children by parents and the later development of specific schizophrenic symptoms. Systematic analyses of attachment in relation to aspects of schizotypy and schizophrenia (Berry et al. 2007, 2008; Gumley et al. 2008; Tiliopoulos and Goodall 2009) have documented higher than normal levels of insecure attachment in these conditions, with general support for Bowlby's prediction of linkages between childhood experiences and psychotic-behavioral profiles. Thus, in nonclinical populations avoidant attachment has been associated with negative schizoptypal traits, and anxious attachment with positive schizotypy (Wilson and Costanzo 1996; Berry et al. 2006); insecure attachment has also been linked with paranoia in schizophrenia (Pickering et al. 2008), and disorganized attachment may be related to dissociative cognitive states that accompany schizophrenia in some patients (Berry et al. 2008; Liotti and Gumley 2008).

One of the best-replicated patterns reported in families with an adolescent or young-adult schizophrenic offspring is high levels of "expressed emotion" – some mix of parental hostility, criticism, and over-involvement (Read et al. 2004a, b), which commonly occurs in the context of emotional over-involvement by one or both parents but low levels of actual care. Higher expressed-emotion predicts higher rates of relapse after a first psychotic episode and also appears to be linked with the initial development of schizophrenic symptoms themselves (Read and Gumley 2008; Read et al. 2004a, b). The causal bases for such associations have puzzled psychiatrists for many years, but perspectives from attachment theory and genomic conflict offer novel, testable insights. Thus, parental over-involvement might be expected to involve attempted control over offspring behavior, interfering with the usual processes of physical and emotional separation of the child from attachment figures, which becomes most pronounced in adolescence (Harrop and Trower 2001). Moreover, extended controlling influences on the offspring psyche by the mother – the "maternal brain" of genomic imprinting theory (Badcock 2009, pages 154–157) – as expressed in the mother's behavior and in maternal-gene influences on development within her child – are expected to engender notably higher risk of schizophrenia. Such a prediction is broadly compatible with maternal imprinted-gene biases, and their correlates, being differentially associated with higher schizophrenia risk (Crespi 2008a; Crespi and Badcock 2008), but additional, targeted tests are required for robust evaluation. More generally, evolutionary theory provides clear, specific predictions regarding the presence and causes of conflicts within families (Emlen 1995, 1997; Surbey 1998), which underpin and complement psychodynamic and socioeconomic perspectives on such conflicts, as well as providing a basis for understanding conflicts within the minds of normal "individuals", and those beset with such conditions as schizophrenia or depression (Read et al. 2004a, b; Haig 2006b; Badcock 2009). As Laing and Esterson (1970, p. 12) inquired, "are the experiences and behaviour that psychiatrists take as symptoms and signs of schizophrenia more socially intelligible than has come to be supposed?"

Long-term prospective studies, using high-risk populations, are required to evaluate patterns of cause and effect in relating childhood experiences and attachment patterns to the risks and forms of depression, schizophrenia, and other conditions. Evolutionary theory provides a conceptual framework to guide such studies, a framework that is fully compatible with both a psychoanalytic focus on childhood social-brain development in the family context and a strong role for interactive genetic and epigenetic effects in modulation of risk. In this context, the mother represents the primary environment of the child from conception until well past weaning, an environment that intimately modifies gene expression, and neurodevelopment, in the growing child. As such, supportive public-health interventions during early child development and in adolescence, which are sensitive to the main causes of conflicts within families, are expected to yield disproportionate returns in reducing the incidence, severity, and recurrence of schizophrenia and depression, and more generally increase emotional well-being in society (e.g., Gumley et al. 2008).

8.8 Autism and Attachment

Idiopathic autism represents a spectrum of related conditions, with many genetic, epigenetic and environmental causes, characterized by differential underdevelopment of the social brain from earliest infancy (Kanner 1943; Happé 1994; Abrahams and Geschwind 2008). A central focus in attachment-theory research on autism has been whether or not autistic children can indeed develop secure attachment with the mother, given that Kanner's (1943) original description of autism posited lack or disturbance of affective contact as a central feature. Rutgers et al. (2004) reviewed 16 studies of attachment in autistic children, finding that autism was associated with lower levels of secure attachment overall, but that this difference "disappeared in samples of children with higher mental development" or less severe symptoms, suggesting that attachment security is compatible with at least relatively high-functioning autism. In contrast, van Ijzendoorn et al. (2007) and Rutter et al. (2009) question the applicability and validity of attachment theory itself to autism, given the unusual nature of social relationships in this condition and uncertainties concerning whether autistics can develop internal working models of self and others, which form the bases for linguistic discourse. Psychological perspectives based in Vygotsky's work indicate, for example, that linguistic inter-actions with mother mediate childhood progress from listening, to private speech, and eventually to inner speech as thoughts (Fernyhough 1996), a process that is absent or underdeveloped in autism but may by contrast, be dysregulated via "re-expansion" in the auditory hallucinations of schizophrenia (Fernyhough 2004).

A general view of autism posits that under-development of the social brain should, as described by Kanner, centrally involve weak social-emotional connec-tions with other individuals. Such differential social deficits, however, need not preclude relatively basic forms of attachment to the mother, as described by Bowlby for mother–offspring relations across most mammals. Indeed, from the perspective of parent–offspring conflicts and genomic imprinting, some subset of autism cases might also be considered to involve pathological overexpression of increased levels of demand imposed on mothers by offspring (Badcock and Crespi 2006; Crespi and Badcock 2008). Such demand may be imposed either directly, through behaviors that solicit forms of investment as in Angelman syndrome, or indirectly, through self-oriented, nonsocial behavior that precludes or delays phys-ical independence, requiring mothers or others to provide longer-term, more highly intensive care. This hypothesis is concordant with several lines of evidence, including (1) accelerated brain and body growth in young children with autism and increased relative effects from paternally expressed imprinted genes (Crespi and Badcock 2008), (2) imprinted-gene effects on reaction to novelty, and dis-persal, in mice (Isles et al. 2002; Plagge et al. 2005), (3) a higher incidence of autism in males, who are more costly than females to rear (Gibson and Mace 2003; Rickard et al. 2007; Tamimi et al. 2003), (4) myriad reports of close and sustained, if atypical, relationships between mothers and their autistic children (e.g., Hoffman et al. 2009), and (5) temperaments of autistic children that involve higher rates of activity, impulsivity, and noncompliance (e.g., Garon et al. 2009).

The degree to which autism spectrum traits in nonclinical populations actually engender higher levels of early maternal or biparental investment has yet to be investigated, and indeed, many childhood social abilities are expected to have evolved in the context of soliciting higher investment from mother via providing her with positive-affect emotional benefits contingent on social skill development (e.g., Hrdy 1999), in addition to imposing negative-affect costs through behaviors such as refusal, tantrums, and, perhaps, insistence on sameness. For analyzing behavioral interactions between mothers and offspring, it is crucial to bear in mind that "disorders" such as autism are postulated to represent sequelae to dysregulation of mechanisms that evolved in contexts of both conflict and cooperation, with evolutionary and behavioral conflicts potentiating increased levels of risk (Crespi 2010).

A primary implication of attachment theory, and behavioral-evolutionary genetics, for elucidating the causes of autism, is that early-childhood social motivation, in the context of "demands" imposed on mothers via physical, social-emotional, and linguistic interactions, should drive cascading effects on social-brain development that are either normal or deviate toward autistic phenotypes. The neurological and endocrine bases for social motivation and affective bonding in infants (e.g., Bowlby 1969 p. 203–204; Moriceau and Sullivan 2005; Grossmann et al. 2008) and children (e.g., Bartz and Hollander 2008) have been much less studied than those in mothers (e.g., Strathearn et al. 2009), though their relevance for understanding mother–child interactions should be no less consequential. Studies of plasma oxytocin levels in autism have yielded unusual results: two studies found lower plasma oxytocin in children with autism (Modahl et al. 1998; Green et al. 2001), but unexpectedly, oxytocin levels were positively associated with degree of social impairment (Modahl et al. 1998); in the single study of adults, autistic individuals showed significantly higher levels of plasma oxytocin than did controls (Jansen et al. 2006). Might oxytocin in autistics subserve, to some degree, positive reinforcement of nonsocial stimuli, or might epigenetically based reduction of oxytocin receptor expression (Gregory et al. 2009) follow from early social-interaction deficits?

The μ-opioid system represents another important candidate mechanism, in addition to oxytocin, for neuroendocrine regulation of attachment, given links of allelic variants in the μ-opioid receptor gene *OPRM1* with attachment patterns, sensitivity to social rejection, drug dependence, and risk of schizophrenia (Insel 2003; Barr et al. 2008; Way et al. 2009; Mague and Blendy 2010; Serý et al. 2010) and evidence for parent-of-origin effects influencing phenotypic effects of this gene (Lemire 2005).

8.9 An Imprinted-Gene Network for Attachment of the Social Brain

Three lines of evidence (1) demonstrations that imprinted-gene expression and coexpression centrally mediate prenatal and postnatal growth, (2) diverse forms of data on imprinted-gene expression effects in the brain, and (3) expectations from theory that mother–offspring interactions should involve genomic conflicts, lead to the prediction that a brain-specific imprinted-gene coexpression network should exist, and should modulate aspects of human mother–child attachment. The presence of such a network in humans was evaluated by testing statistically for differentially frequent coexpression of brain-expressed imprinted genes, compared to expression of imprinted genes with other genes independent of imprinting status. For each of the 64 verified human imprinted genes (http://igc.otago.ac.nz/table. html), a set of highly coexpressed genes were generated using the Gemma coexpression database (http://www.chibi.ubc.ca/Gemma/searchCoexpression.html). These sets of coexpressed genes were combined to generate a list of genes that were highly coexpressed with four or more imprinted genes. The list comprised 188 genes in all, of which approximately 0.6% (64/~10,000 total brain-expressed genes) should be imprinted under a null model of coexpression random with regard to imprinting status. Six (3.1%) of the 188 coexpressed genes were imprinted, an approximate fivefold excess ($P < 0.001$). The highly coexpressed imprinted genes included *PEG3* and *NDN*, two genes that mediate development of oxytocin-secreting neurons (Davies et al. 2008a, b); *NDN* may also be involved in the risk of schizophrenia (Le-Niculescu et al. 2007), and both *PEG3* and *NDN* are members of a network of genes differentially coexpressed in the prefrontal cortex of schizophrenics (module 16 of Torkamani et al. 2010). Additional relatively highly coexpressed genes in the network included three genes with genetic-association or copy-number variation links to both autism and schizophrenia, *CNTNAP2*, *NRXN1*, and *BOLA2* (reviewed in Crespi et al. 2010; coexpressed with 6, 7, and 11 imprinted genes, respectively). Additional data implicating this network, and imprinting effects, in autism and schizophrenia include (1) the presence of parent-of-origin effects for the associations of *CNTNAP2* with autism (Arking et al. 2008) and for the speech-language associated gene *FOXP2* (Feuk et al. 2006) that interacts directly with *CNTNAP2* (Vernes et al. 2008), and (2) colocalization of the imprinted, schizophrenia-associated gene *LRRTM1* (Francks et al. 2007) with *NRXN1* at glutamatergic synapses (Brose 2009).

This analysis requires replication using other datasets, and more detailed bioinformatic dissection of coexpression patterns, but it provides preliminary evidence of interactions between brain-expressed imprinted genes that mediate aspects of mother–offspring interaction and social-brain disorders. The existence and structure of brain-specific imprinted-gene network should have important implications for pharmacological interventions; for example, of the 11 genes most highly altered in expression from treatment of mice with the mood-stabilizer drug valproic acid (Chetcuti et al. 2006), two are imprinted (*Peg3* and *Sfmbt2*), one is predicted to be imprinted (*Zic1*)(Luedi et al. 2007), one interacts directly with the imprinted gene *Wt1* (*Par-4*)(Richard et al. 2001), and one (*Kcna1*) interacts directly with *Cntnap2* (Strauss et al. 2006). Such a striking concentration of imprinted-gene related expression changes is consistent with the molecular function of valproic acid as a histone deacetylase inhibitor, an agent that exhibits differential epigenetic effects on imprinted genes (e.g., Baqir and Smith 2006); moreover, valproic acid during human or rodent pregnancy is a highly penetrant cause of autism in offspring (Rinaldi et al. 2008; Dufour-Rainfray et al. 2010), and valproic acid partially restores levels of MeCP2 in a mouse model of Rett syndrome (Vecsler et al. 2010). Might such epigenetic treatments exert their effects though canalizing or decanalizing neurological-pathway functions of interacting imprinted genes?

8.10   Conclusions

Understanding human social development requires integration of theory and data from diverse, highly specialized, disciplines, including genetics, development, neuroscience, psychology, and psychiatry. Conrad Waddington's still-nascent science of epigenetics serves as a conceptual and experimental platform to connect social-environmental variation with the gene-expression patterns that drive development, as genes and family, especially the mother, jointly sculpt developing brains. Like other traits, epigenetic landscapes of social development have evolved, subject to the conflicts and confluences of genetic interest that form the cornerstone of modern evolutionary theory. Effects of parent–offspring conflicts, and the intragenomic conflicts of imprinting, are predicted from such theory to modulate normal development and to potentiate specific directions and forms of maladaptive trajectory, due to genetic, epigenetic, and social-environmental perturbations. As such, dovetailing of predictions from evolutionary genetics and epigenetics with the conceptual constructs and experimental tools of developmental psychology, neuroscience, and epigenetics should yield novel insights into the evolutionary underpinnings of the human social brain and its disorders, and the strategies of the genes involved.

Acknowledgments I am grateful to Christopher Badcock, David Haig, Sarah Hrdy, and Felicity Larson for comments, and Paul Pavlidis for advice.

References

Abrahams BS, Geschwind DH (2008) Advances in autism genetics: on the threshold of a new neurobiology. Nat Rev Genet 9:341–355

Allen ND, Logan K, Lally G et al (1995) Distribution of parthenogenetic cells in the mouse brain and their influence on brain development and behavior. Proc Natl Acad Sci USA 92:10782–10786

Andrews SC, Wood MD, Tunster SJ et al (2007) Cdkn1c (p57Kip2) is the major regulator of embryonic growth within its imprinted domain on mouse distal chromosome 7. BMC Dev Biol 7:53

Angiolini E, Fowden A, Coan P et al (2006) Regulation of placental efficiency for nutrient transport by imprinted genes. Placenta 27:S98–S102

Anglin DM, Cohen PR, Chen H (2008) Duration of early maternal separation and prediction of schizotypal symptoms from early adolescence to midlife. Schizophr Res 103:143–150

Arima T, Kamikihara T, Hayashida T et al (2005) ZAC, LIT1 (KCNQ1OT1) and p57KIP2 (CDKN1C) are in an imprinted gene network that may play a role in Beckwith-Wiedemann syndrome. Nucleic Acids Res 33:2650–2660

Arking DE, Cutler DJ, Brune CW et al (2008) A common genetic variant in the neurexin superfamily member CNTNAP2 increases familial risk of autism. Am J Hum Genet 82:160–164

Badcock C (2009) The imprinted brain. Jessica Kingsley, London

Badcock C, Crespi B (2006) Imbalanced genomic imprinting in brain development: an evolutionary basis for the aetiology of autism. J Evol Biol 19:1007–1032

Baqir S, Smith LC (2006) Inhibitors of histone deacetylases and DNA methyltransferases alter imprinted gene regulation in embryonic stem cells. Cloning Stem Cells 8:200–213

Barr CS, Schwandt ML, Lindell SG, Higley JD, Maestripieri D, Goldman D, Suomi SJ, Heilig M (2008) Variation at the mu-opioid receptor gene (OPRM1) influences attachment behavior in infant primates. Proc Natl Acad Sci USA 105:5277–5281

Bartz JA, Hollander E (2008) Oxytocin and experimental therapeutics in autism spectrum disorders. Prog Brain Res 170:451–462

Berry K, Wearden AJ, Barrowclough C, Liversidge T (2006) Attachment styles, interpersonal relationships and psychotic phenomena in a non-clinical student sample. Pers Indiv Diff 41:707–718

Berry K, Barrowclough C, Wearden A (2007) A review of the role of adult attachment style in psychosis: unexplored issues and questions for further research. Clin Psychol Rev 27:458–745

Berry K, Barrowclough C, Wearden A (2008) Attachment theory: a framework for understanding symptoms and interpersonal relationships in psychosis. Behav Res Ther 46:1275–1282

Blissett J, Harris G, Kirk J (2001) Feeding problems in Silver-Russell syndrome. Dev Med Child Neurol 43:39–44

Bonati MT, Russo S, Finelli P et al (2007) Evaluation of autism traits in Angelman syndrome: a resource to unfold autism genes. Neurogenetics 8:169–178

Bowlby J (1951) Maternal care and mental health. Schocken, New York

Bowlby J (1969) Attachment and loss: attachment, vol 1. Basic Books, New York

Bressan FF, De Bem TH, Perecin F et al (2009) Unearthing the roles of imprinted genes in the placenta. Placenta 30:823–834

Bretherton I (1992) The origins of attachment theory: John Bowlby and Mary Ainsworth. Devel Psychol 28:759–775

Bretherton I (1997) Bowlby's legacy to developmental psychology. Child Psychiatry Hum Dev 28:33–43

Brose N (2009) Synaptogenic proteins and synaptic organizers: "many hands make light work". Neuron 61:650–652

Brown WM, Consedine NS (2004) Just how happy is the happy puppet? An emotion signaling and kinship theory perspective on the behavioral phenotype of children with Angelman syndrome. Med Hypotheses 63:377–385

Burt A, Trivers RL (2006) Genes in conflict: the biology of selfish genetic elements. Belknap, Cambridge

Champagne FA, Curley JP, Swaney WT et al (2009) Paternal influence on female behavior: the role of Peg3 in exploration, olfaction, and neuroendocrine regulation of maternal behavior of female mice. Behav Neurosci 123:469–480

Charalambous M, da Rocha ST, Ferguson-Smith AC (2007) Genomic imprinting, growth control and the allocation of nutritional resources: consequences for postnatal life. Curr Opin Endocrinol Diabetes Obes 14:3–12

Chetcuti A, Adams LJ, Mitchell PB, Schofield PR (2006) Altered gene expression in mice treated with the mood stabilizer sodium valproate. Int J Neuropsychopharmacol 9:267–276

Cohen MM Jr (2005) Beckwith-Wiedemann syndrome: historical, clinicopathological, and etiopathogenetic perspectives. Pediatr Dev Pathol 8:287–304

Cohen D, Pichard N, Tordjman S et al (2005) Specific genetic disorders and autism: clinical contribution towards their identification. J Autism Dev Disord 35:103–116

Crespi B (2008a) Genomic imprinting in the development and evolution of psychotic spectrum conditions. Biol Rev Camb Philos Soc 83:441–493

Crespi B (2008b) Turner syndrome and the evolution of human sexual dimorphism. Evol Appl 1:449–461

Crespi B (2010) The origins and evolution of genetic disease risk in modern humans. Ann N Y Acad Sci 1206:80–109

Crespi B, Badcock C (2008) Psychosis and autism as diametrical disorders of the social brain. Behav Brain Sci 31:241–261, discussion 261–320

Crespi B, Summers K, Dorus S (2009) Genomic sister-disorders of neurodevelopment: an evolutionary approach. Evol Appl 2:81–100

Crespi B, Stead P, Elliot M (2010) Comparative genomics of autism and schizophrenia. Proc Natl Acad Sci USA 107 Suppl 1:1736–1741

Curley JP, Barton S, Surani A, Keverne EB (2004) Coadaptation in mother and infant regulated by a paternally expressed imprinted gene. Proc Biol Sci 271:1303–1309

Davies W, Isles AR, Humby T, Wilkinson LS (2008a) What are imprinted genes doing in the brain? Adv Exp Med Biol 626:62–70

Davies W, Lynn PM, Relkovic D, Wilkinson LS (2008b) Imprinted genes and neuroendocrine function. Front Neuroendocrinol 29:413–427

Dudley O, Muscatelli F (2007) Clinical evidence of intrauterine disturbance in Prader–Willi syndrome, a genetically imprinted neurodevelopmental disorder. Early Hum Dev 83:471–478

Dufour-Rainfray D, Vourc'h P, Le Guisquet AM et al (2010) Behavior and serotonergic disorders in rats exposed prenatally to valproate: a model for autism. Neurosci Lett 470:55–59

Eggermann T (2009) Silver-Russell and Beckwith-Wiedemann syndromes: opposite (epi)mutations in 11p15 result in opposite clinical pictures. Horm Res 71(Suppl 2):30–35

Eggermann T, Eggermann K, Schönherr N (2008) Growth retardation versus overgrowth: Silver-Russell syndrome is genetically opposite to Beckwith-Wiedemann syndrome. Trends Genet 24:195–204

Emlen ST (1995) An evolutionary theory of the family. Proc Natl Acad Sci USA 92:8092–8099

Emlen ST (1997) The evolutionary study of human family systems. Soc Sci Inf 36:563–589

Fauque P, Ripoche MA, Tost J et al (2010) Modulation of imprinted gene network in placenta results in normal development of in vitro manipulated mouse embryos. Hum Mol Genet 19:1779–1790

Fernyhough C (1996) The dialogic mind: a dialogic approach to the higher mental functions. New Ideas In Psychol 14:47–62

Fernyhough C (2004) Alien voices and inner dialogue: towards a developmental account of auditory verbal hallucinations. New Ideas In Psychol 22:49–68

Feuk L, Kalervo A, Lipsanen-Nyman M et al (2006) Absence of a paternally inherited FOXP2 gene in developmental verbal dyspraxia. Am J Hum Genet 79:965–972

Fox M, Sear R, Beise J et al (2010) Grandma plays favourites: X-chromosome relatedness and sex-specific childhood mortality. Proc Biol Sci 277:567–573

Francks C, Maegawa S, Laurén J et al (2007) LRRTM1 on chromosome 2p12 is a maternally suppressed gene that is associated paternally with handedness and schizophrenia. Mol Psychiatry 12:1129–1139, 1057

Frith CD (2008) Social cognition. Philos Trans R Soc Lond B Biol Sci 363:2033–2039

Gabory A, Ripoche MA, Le Digarcher A et al (2009) H19 acts as a trans regulator of the imprinted gene network controlling growth in mice. Development 136:3413–3421

Garon N, Bryson SE, Zwaigenbaum L et al (2009) Temperament and its relationship to autistic symptoms in a high-risk infant sib cohort. J Abnorm Child Psychol 37:59–78

Geneviève D, Sanlaville D, Faivre L et al (2005) Paternal deletion of the GNAS imprinted locus (including Gnasxl) in two girls presenting with severe pre- and post-natal growth retardation and intractable feeding difficulties. Eur J Hum Genet 13:1033–1039

Gibson MA, Mace R (2003) Strong mothers bear more sons in rural Ethiopia. Proc Biol Sci 270 (suppl 1):S108–S109

Goldstone AP (2006) The hypothalamus, hormones, and hunger: alterations in human obesity and illness. Prog Brain Res 153:57–73

Green L, Fein D, Modahl C, Feinstein C, Waterhouse L, Morris M (2001) Oxytocin and autistic disorder: alterations in peptide forms. Biol Psychiatry 50:609–613

Gregory SG, Connelly JJ, Towers AJ et al (2009) Genomic and epigenetic evidence for oxytocin receptor deficiency in autism. BMC Med 7:62

Grossmann T, Johnson MH, Lloyd-Fox S et al (2008) Early cortical specialization for face-to-face communication in human infants. Proc Biol Sci 275:2803–2811

Gumley AI, Schwannauer M, MacBeth A, Read J (2008) Emotional recovery and staying well after psychosis: an attachment based conceptualisation. Attachment 2:127–148

Haig D (1993) Genetic conflicts in human pregnancy. Q Rev Biol 68:495–532

Haig D (1997) The social gene. In: Krebs JR, Davies NB (eds) Behavioural ecology: an evolutionary approach. Blackwell, London, pp 284–304

Haig D (2002) Genomic imprinting and kinship. Rutgers University Press, New Brunswick, NJ

Haig D (2004a) The (dual) origin of epigenetics. Cold Spring Harb Symp Quant Biol 69:1–4

Haig D (2004b) Genomic imprinting and kinship: how good is the evidence? Annu Rev Genet 38:553–585

Haig D (2006a) Intragenomic politics. Cytogenet Genome Res 113:68–74

Haig D (2006b) Intrapersonal conflict. In: Jones MK, Fabian AC (eds) Conflict. Cambridge University Press, Cambridge, pp 8–22

Haig D (2009) Transfers and transitions: Parent–offspring conflict, genomic imprinting, and the evolution of human life history. Proc Natl Acad Sci USA 107:1731–1735

Haig D, Graham C (1991) Genomic imprinting and the strange case of the insulin-like growth factor-II receptor. Cell 64:1045–1046

Haig D, Wharton R (2003) Prader–Willi syndrome and the evolution of human childhood. Am J Hum Biol 15:320–329

Hamilton WD (1964) The genetical evolution of social behaviour I and II. J Theor Biol 7:1–16, 17–52

Hamilton WD (1996) Narrow roads of gene land vol. 1: Evolution of social behaviour. Oxford University Press, Oxford. ISBN 0-7167-4530-5

Happé F (1994) Autism: an introduction to psychological theory. UCL Press, London

Harrop C, Trower P (2001) Why does schizophrenia develop at late adolescence? Clin Psychol Rev 21:241–265

Hinde CA, Kilner RM (2007) Negotiations within the family over the supply of parental care. Proc Biol Sci 274:53–60

Hoffman CD, Sweeney DP, Hodge D (2009) Parenting stress and closeness in mothers of typically developing children and mothers of children with autism. Focus on Autism and other Developmental Disabilities 24:178–187

Holland A, Whittington J, Hinton E (2003) The paradox of Prader–Willi syndrome: a genetic model of starvation. Lancet 362:989–991

Höybye C (2004) Endocrine and metabolic aspects of adult Prader–Willi syndrome with special emphasis on the effect of growth hormone treatment. Growth Horm IGF Res 14:1–15

Hrdy S (1999) Mother nature: a history of mothers, infants, and natural selection. Pantheon Books, New York

Hrdy S (2009) Mothers and others: the evolutionary origins of mutual understanding. Harvard University Press, Harvard

Humphrey LT (2009) Weaning behaviour in human evolution. Semin Cell Dev Biol 21:453–461

Insel TR (2003) Is social attachment an addictive disorder? Physiol Behav 79:351–357

Isles AR, Holland AJ (2005) Imprinted genes and mother-offspring interactions. Early Hum Dev 81:73–77

Isles AR, Baum MJ, Ma D, Szeto A, Keverne EB, Allen ND (2002) A possible role for imprinted genes in inbreeding avoidance and dispersal from the natal area in mice. Proc Biol Sci 269:665–670

Isles AR, Davies W, Wilkinson LS (2006) Genomic imprinting and the social brain. Philos Trans R Soc Lond B Biol Sci 361:2229–2237

Jansen LMC, Gispen-de Wied CC, Wiegant VM (2006) Autonomic and neuroendocrine responses to a psychosocial stressor in adults with autistic spectrum disorder. J Autism Devel Dis 36:891–899

Jedele KB (2007) The overlapping spectrum of Rett and Angelman syndromes: a clinical review. Semin Pediatr Neurol 14:108–117

Joseph B, Wallén-Mackenzie A, Benoit G et al (2003) p57(Kip2) cooperates with Nurr1 in developing dopamine cells. Proc Natl Acad Sci USA 100:15619–15624

Kanner L (1943) Autistic disturbances of affective contact. Nerv Child 2:217–250

Kelsey G (2007) Genomic imprinting – roles and regulation in development. Endocr Dev 12:99–112

Kernohan KD, Jiang Y, Tremblay DC, Bonvissuto AC, Eubanks JH, Mann MR, Bérubé NG (2010) ATRX partners with cohesin and MeCP2 and contributes to developmental silencing of imprinted genes in the brain. Dev Cell 18:191–202

Keverne EB (2001a) Genomic imprinting and the maternal brain. Prog Brain Res 133:279–285

Keverne EB (2001b) Genomic imprinting, maternal care, and brain evolution. Horm Behav 40: 146–155

Keverne EB, Fundele R, Narasimha M et al (1996) Genomic imprinting and the differential roles of parental genomes in brain development. Brain Res Dev Brain Res 92:91–100

Laing RD, Esterson A (1970) Sanity, madness and the family. Tavistock, London

Lemire M (2005) A simple nonparametric multipoint procedure to test for linkage through mothers or fathers as well as imprinting effects in the presence of linkage. BMC Genet 6(6 Suppl 1):S159

Le-Niculescu H, Balaraman Y, Patel S et al (2007) Towards understanding the schizophrenia code: an expanded convergent functional genomics approach. Am J Med Genet B Neuropsychiatr Genet 144B:129–158

Ling JQ, Hoffman AR (2007) Epigenetics of long-range chromatin interactions. Pediatr Res 61:11R–16R

Liotti L, Gumley A (2008) An attachment perspective on schizophrenia: the role of disorganized attachment, dissociation and mentalization. In: Moskowitz A, Schafer I, Dorahy MJ (eds) Psychosis, trauma and dissociation. Wiley, New York, pp 117–133

Liu Z, Li X, Ge X (2009) Left too early: the effects of age at separation from parents on Chinese rural children's symptoms of anxiety and depression. Am J Public Health 99:2049–2054

Luedi PP, Dietrich FS, Weidman JR, Bosko JM, Jirtle RL, Hartemink AJ (2007) Computational and experimental identification of novel human imprinted genes. Genome Res 17:1723–1730

Lui JC, Finkielstain GP, Barnes KM, Baron J (2008) An imprinted gene network that controls mammalian somatic growth is down-regulated during postnatal growth deceleration in multiple organs. Am J Physiol Regul Integr Comp Physiol 295:R189–R196

Lyons-Ruth K (2008) Contributions of the mother–infant relationship to dissociative, borderline, and conduct symptoms in young adulthood. Infant Ment Health J 29:203–218

Macdonald K, Macdonald TM (2010) The peptide that binds: a systematic review of oxytocin and its prosocial effects in humans. Harv Rev Psychiatry 18:1–21

Maestripieri D (2002) Parent–offspring conflict in primates. Int J Primatol 23:923–951

Mague SD, Blendy JA (2010) OPRM1 SNP (A118G): Involvement in disease development, treatment response, and animal models. Drug Alcohol Depend 108:172–182

Manaye KF, Lei DL, Tizabi Y et al (2005) Selective neuron loss in the paraventricular nucleus of hypothalamus in patients suffering from major depression and bipolar disorder. J Neuropathol Exp Neurol 64:224–229

McMinn J, Wei M, Schupf N et al (2006) Unbalanced placental expression of imprinted genes in human intrauterine growth restriction. Placenta 27:540–549

Miyano M, Horike S, Cai S, Oshimura M, Kohwi-Shigematsu T (2008) DLX5 expression is monoallelic and Dlx5 is up-regulated in the Mecp2-null frontal cortex. J Cell Mol Med 12:1188–1191

Modahl C, Green L, Fein D et al (1998) Plasma oxytocin levels in autistic children. Biol Psychiatry 43:270–277

Moriceau S, Sullivan RM (2005) Neurobiology of infant attachment. Dev Psychobiol 47:230–242

Oliver C, Horsler K, Berg K et al (2007) Genomic imprinting and the expression of affect in Angelman syndrome: what's in the smile? J Child Psychol Psychiatry 48:571–579

Owen MJ, Craddock N, Jablensky A (2007) The genetic deconstruction of psychosis. Schizophr Bull 33:905–911

Pesonen AK, Räikkönen K, Heinonen K et al (2007) Depressive symptoms in adults separated from their parents as children: a natural experiment during World War II. Am J Epidemiol 166:1126–1133

Pickering L, Simpson J, Bentall RP (2008) Insecure attachment predicts proneness to paranoia but not hallucinations. Pers Individ Diff 44:1212–1224

Plagge A, Gordon E, Dean W et al (2004) The imprinted signaling protein XL alpha s is required for postnatal adaptation to feeding. Nat Genet 36:818–826

Plagge A, Isles AR, Gordon E et al (2005) Imprinted Nesp55 influences behavioral reactivity to novel environments. Mol Cell Biol 25:3019–3026

Read J, Gumley AI (2008) Can attachment theory help explain the relationship between childhood adversity and psychosis? Attachment: New Directions in Psychotherapy and Relational Psychoanalysis 2:1–35

Read J, Seymour F, Mosher LR (2004a) Unhappy families. In: Read J, Bentall R, Mosher L (eds) Models of madness: psychological, social and biological approaches to schizophrenia. Brunner-Routledge, Hove, England, pp 253–268

Read J, Mosher L, Bentall R (2004b) Models of madness: psychological, social and biological approaches to schizophrenia. Routledge, Basingstoke, UK

Reik W, Davies K, Dean W et al (2001) Imprinted genes and the coordination of fetal and postnatal growth in mammals. Novartis Found Symp 237:19–31, discussion 31–42

Renfree MB, Hore TA, Shaw G et al (2009) Evolution of genomic imprinting: insights from marsupials and monotremes. Annu Rev Genomics Hum Genet 10:241–262

Richard DJ, Schumacher V, Royer-Pokora B, Roberts SG (2001) Par4 is a coactivator for a splice isoform-specific transcriptional activation domain in WT1. Genes Dev 15:328–339

Rickard IJ, Russell AF, Lummaa V (2007) Producing sons reduces lifetime reproductive success of subsequent offspring in pre-industrial Finns. Proc Biol Sci 274:2981–2988

Rinaldi T, Perrodin C, Markram H (2008) Hyper-connectivity and hyper-plasticity in the medial prefrontal cortex in the valproic acid animal model of autism. Front Neural Circuits 2:4

Ross HE, Young LJ (2009) Oxytocin and the neural mechanisms regulating social cognition and affiliative behavior. Front Neuroendocrinol 30:534–547

Royle NJ, Hartley IR, Parker GA (2004) Parental investment and family dynamics: interactions between theory and empirical tests. Pop Ecol 46:231–241

Rutgers AH, Bakermans-Kranenburg MJ, van Ijzendoorn MH, van Berckelaer-Onnes IA (2004) Autism and attachment: a meta-analytic review. J Child Psychol Psychiatry 45:1123–1134

Rutter M, Kreppner J, Sonuga-Barke E (2009) Emanuel Miller Lecture: attachment insecurity, disinhibited attachment, and attachment disorders: where do research findings leave the concepts? J Child Psychol Psychiatry 50:529–543

Sahoo T, Peters SU, Madduri NS et al (2006) Microarray based comparative genomic hybridization testing in deletion bearing patients with Angelman syndrome: genotype-phenotype correlations. J Med Genet 43:512–516

Sandhu KS, Shi C, Sjölinder M et al (2009) Nonallelic transvection of multiple imprinted loci is organized by the H19 imprinting control region during germline development. Genes Dev 23:2598–2603

Sellen DW (2007) Evolution of infant and young child feeding: implications for contemporary public health. Annu Rev Nutr 27:123–148

Serý O, Prikryl R, Castulík L, St'astný F (2010) A118G polymorphism of OPRM1 gene is associated with schizophrenia. J Mol Neurosci 41:219–222

Shaver PR, Mikulincer M (2002) Attachment-related psychodynamics. Attach Hum Dev 4:133–161

Sigurdsson MI, Jamshidi N, Jonsson JJ, Palsson BO (2009) Genome-scale network analysis of imprinted human metabolic genes. Epigenetics 4:43–46

Smiseth PT, Wright J, Kölliker M (2008) Parent–offspring conflict and co-adaptation: behavioural ecology meets quantitative genetics. Proc Biol Sci 275:1823–1830

Smits G, Kelsey G (2006) Imprinting weaves its web. Dev Cell 11:598–599

Soltis J (2004) The signal functions of early infant crying. Behav Brain Sci 27:443–458, discussion 459–490

Soni S, Whittington J, Holland AJ et al (2008) The phenomenology and diagnosis of psychiatric illness in people with Prader–Willi syndrome. Psychol Med 38:1505–1514

Strathearn L, Li J, Fonagy P, Montague PR (2008) What's in a smile? Maternal brain responses to infant facial cues. Pediatrics 122:40–51

Strauss KA, Puffenberger EG, Huentelman MJ et al (2006) Recessive symptomatic focal epilepsy and mutant contactin-associated protein-like 2. N Engl J Med 354:1370–1377

Surbey MK (1998) Parent and offspring strategies in the transition at adolescence. Hum Nat 9:67–94

Swaab DF, Purba JS, Hofman MA (1995) Alterations in the hypothalamic paraventricular nucleus and its oxytocin neurons (putative satiety cells) in Prader–Willi syndrome: a study of five cases. J Clin Endocrinol Metab 80:573–579

Tamimi RM, Lagiou P, Mucci LA et al (2003) Average energy intake among pregnant women carrying a boy compared with a girl. Br Med J 326:1245–1246

Thompson RA (2008) Attachment-related mental representations: introduction to the special issue. Attach Hum Devel 10:347–358

Tiliopoulos N, Goodall K (2009) The neglected link between adult attachment and schizotypal personality traits. Pers Individ Diff 47:299–304

Torkamani A, Dean B, Schork NJ, Thomas EA (2010) Coexpression network analysis of neural tissue reveals perturbations in developmental processes in schizophrenia. Genome Res 20:403–412

Trivers RL (1974) Parent–offspring conflict. Am Zool 14:249–264

Tsai TF, Armstrong D, Beaudet AL (1999) Necdin-deficient mice do not show lethality or the obesity and infertility of Prader–Willi syndrome. Nat Genet 22:15–16

Tyrka AR, Wier L, Price LH et al (2008) Childhood parental loss and adult psychopathology: effects of loss characteristics and contextual factors. Int J Psychiatry Med 38:329–344

van Ijzendoorn MH, Rutgers AH, Bakermans-Kranenburg MJ et al (2007) Parental sensitivity and attachment in children with autism spectrum disorder: comparison with children with mental retardation, with language delays, and with typical development. Child Dev 78:597–608

Varrault A, Gueydan C, Delalbre A et al (2006) Zac1 regulates an imprinted gene network critically involved in the control of embryonic growth. Dev Cell 11:711–722

Vecsler M, Simon AJ, Amariglio N et al (2010) MeCP2 deficiency downregulates specific nuclear proteins that could be partially recovered by valproic acid in vitro. Epigenetics 5:61–67

Vernes SC, Newbury DF, Abrahams BS et al (2008) A functional genetic link between distinct developmental language disorders. N Engl J Med 359:2337–2345

Waddington C (1957) The strategy of the genes. Macmillan, New York

Wagner A (2000) Robustness against mutations in genetic networks of yeast. Nat Genet 24:355–361

Wagschal A, Feil R (2006) Genomic imprinting in the placenta. Cytogenet Genome Res 113:90–98

Way BM, Taylor SE, Eisenberger NI (2009) Variation in the mu-opioid receptor gene (OPRM1) is associated with dispositional and neural sensitivity to social rejection. Proc Natl Acad Sci USA 106:15079–15084

Webb T, Maina EN, Soni S et al (2008) In search of the psychosis gene in people with Prader–Willi syndrome. Am J Med Genet A 146:843–853

Weinstein LS, Liu J, Sakamoto A et al (2004) Minireview: GNAS: normal and abnormal functions. Endocrinology 145:5459–5464

Wells JC (2003) Parent–offspring conflict theory, signaling of need, and weight gain in early life. Q Rev Biol 78:169–202

Wilkinson LS, Davies W, Isles AR (2007) Genomic imprinting effects on brain development and function. Nat Rev Neurosci 8:832–843

Wilson JS, Costanzo PR (1996) A preliminary study of attachment, attention, and schizotypy in early adulthood. J Soc Clin Psychol 15:231–260

Zhao Z, Tavoosidana G, Sjölinder M et al (2006) Circular chromosome conformation capture (4C) uncovers extensive networks of epigenetically regulated intra- and interchromosomal interactions. Nat Genet 38:1341–1347

Chapter 9
Genomic Imprinting Effects on Brain and Behavior: Future Directions

Anthony R. Isles and Lawrence S. Wilkinson

Abstract Studies over the last 15 years have indicated that genomic imprinting is important for brain function. However, much of the focus has been on the role that imprinted genes play in mediating fetal and early postnatal growth, and maternal behavior. Nevertheless, there is now a growing body of evidence to suggest that many imprinted genes are expressed in many different areas of the adult brain. Moreover, these genes also influence a wide range of behavior and aspects of cognition. Here, we provide an overview of these data and give pointers to interesting new aspects of imprinted gene function in the brain. We also discuss how genomic imprinting may have evolved in the human brain and the extent to which imprinted genes impact on mental illness.

Keywords Epigenetics · Evolution · Imprinted genes · Monoamines · Neurodevelopment

9.1 Introduction

Unlike the majority of genes where there is equivalent expression from both inherited copies of a gene (alleles), imprinted genes are subjected to epigenetic modifications during germ cell development that lead to paternal and maternal alleles having different levels of activity. This means that despite the presence of a maternal and paternal allele in the DNA, one of these parental alleles is essentially silenced and expression is monoallelic. This silencing is robust and stable across generations; for instance, the imprinted gene *Necdin* is always expressed only

A.R. Isles (✉) and L.S. Wilkinson
Behavioural Genetics Group, MRC Centre for Neuropsychiatric Genetics and Genomics, Schools of Medicine and Psychology, Cardiff University, Henry Wellcome Building, Heath Park Campus, 14 4XN Cardiff, UK
e-mail: IslesAR1@cardiff.ac.uk; WilkinsonL@cardiff.ac.uk

A. Petronis and J. Mill (eds.), *Brain, Behavior and Epigenetics*,
Epigenetics and Human Health, DOI 10.1007/978-3-642-17426-1_9,
© Springer-Verlag Berlin Heidelberg 2011

from the paternal allele. Although imprinted gene representation in mammalian genomes is small (there are currently ~130 recognized imprinted genes in mice), they are absolutely crucial for normal development and function. Mouse embryos manipulated to have either only a paternal or only a maternal genome are malformed and die before mid-gestation (Barton et al. 1984; McGrath and Solter 1984). Since this early pioneering work, individual imprinted genes have been characterized and it is now clear that imprinted genes play a key role in three major areas: placental physiology, fetal, and preweaning growth (Constancia et al. 2004); energy metabolism (Smith et al. 2006); and brain development and behavior (Wilkinson et al. 2007).

9.1.1   Evolution of Genomic Imprinting

Despite their apparent rarity in the genome, genes that are subjected to imprinting are (at least part of the time) effectively haploid, thus negating the apparent benefits of diploidy (increased genetic diversity and reduced exposure to deleterious alleles) (Goddard et al. 2005; Orr 1995). This is an evolutionary conundrum, and consequently, why imprinting has evolved is subject to much debate and several theories have been put forward (Curley et al. 2004; Hurst and McVean 1997, 1998; Moore and Haig 1991; Varmuza and Mann 1994; Wolf and Hager 2006). Two of these – the "intragenomic conflict" and "coadaptation" theories – provide an explanation for many of the widely observed physiological roles of imprinted genes (Keverne and Curley 2008; Moore and Haig 1991; Wolf and Hager 2006).

The intragenomic conflict theory, which was developed with kinship ideas in mind and is an extension of the classic "parent–offspring" conflict (Trivers 1974), suggests that where asymmetries of relatedness between maternal and paternal genes exist, there will be a conflict of interests between parental genomes over certain aspects of physiology (Haig 1997). These asymmetries of relatedness occur in developing fetuses as a consequence of multiple paternities, either within or between pregnancies. Consequently, maternally derived genes are always shared between siblings, but this is not necessarily true for paternal genes. Within an offspring, paternal genes would be predicted to attempt to increase resources from the mother, whereas maternally derived genes would limit any effect as this would not maximize the mother's (and therefore the maternal genes) overall reproductive output (Moore and Haig 1991). This imbalance leads to an "arms race" involving expression levels of maternal and paternal copies of a gene, ultimately resulting in the silencing of one parental allele. This intragenomic conflict can also be seen at a physiological level, as illustrated in the mouse by the $Igf2–Igf2r$ system. The insulin-like growth factor type 2 ($Igf2$) is a paternally expressed growth enhancer, whereas the insulin-like growth factor type 2 receptor ($Igf2r$) is a maternally expressed growth inhibitor that binds Igf2 and targets it for degradation (Haig and Graham 1991).

By contrast, the coadaptation theory suggests that genomic imprinting occurs in mammals as a means to coordinate the evolution of provisioning of offspring pre- and postnatally. In this context, the monoallelic expression of imprinted genes is a means by which their "evolvability" is accelerated (Keverne and Curley 2008). This is because haploid expression, while increasing exposure to deleterious alleles, also has the advantage over diploid expression of rapid fixation of an advantageous trait in a population (Greig and Travisano 2003); although this effect is presumably lessened by the fact that monoallelic expression results in higher than average recombination rates (Necsulea et al. 2009). It is thought that the development of a placenta and maternal care in mammals is an area of function where such rapid fixation of any selective advantage is important, leading to the evolution of imprinted genes influencing these aspects of physiology (Keverne and Curley 2008; Wolf and Hager 2006).

This idea was originally developed in light of the identification of two separate paternally expressed genes in the mouse (*Paternally expressed 1* and *Paternally expressed 3*), both of which were found to effect placental function and fetal growth, and maternal care in adult females (Lefebvre et al. 1998; Li et al. 1999). Further analysis also revealed that *Peg3* was not only important for mothers providing postnatal care and feeding, but was also involved in the neonates' ability to suckle (Curley et al. 2004). The idea proposed was that the high turnover of the genes down the paternal line would provide the platform for the rapid coadaptation of these in utero and postnatal provisioning and care (Keverne and Curley 2008). Recently, a similar argument, based on the adaptive integration of offspring and maternal genomes, has been made for the evolution of maternally expressed imprinted genes (Wolf and Hager 2006).

Both of these theories provide an explanation for a large proportion of the observed physiological effects of imprinted gene; although no one theory can account for all occurrences. However, with regards to the adult brain, at present, the coadaptation theory offers only an explanation for the role of imprinted genes in the hypothalamus controlling maternal behavior (something the intragenomic conflict theory struggles with) and yet imprinted genes are now known to be expressed in many brain regions and influence many other behaviors.

9.2   Imprinted Gene Expression in the Brain

9.2.1   Early Findings

Seminal mouse studies in the mid 1990s revealed that imprinted genes are likely to contribute significantly to brain development, and also indicated potentially dissociable (and possibly antagonistic) influences of paternally and maternally expressed genes on this process. Briefly, chimeric mice were created, which contained either a mixture of androgenetic (AG) (containing two paternal genomes but no maternal genome) and normal cells, or a mixture of parthenogenetic/gyno-genetic (PG/GG) (containing two maternal genomes but no paternal genome) and normal cells. "PG/GG chimeras" displayed relatively large brain:body ratios, whereas "AG chimeras" displayed relatively small brain:body size ratios, implying that one or more imprinted genes have profound effects on brain size (Allen et al. 1995; Keverne et al. 1996a). Specifically, the data seem to indicate that the overall effect of maternally expressed genes is to enhance brain size, whereas the combined effect of paternally expressed genes is to limit brain growth. More interesting perhaps, was the fact that the distribution of the PG/GG and AG cells in the two types of chimera was reciprocal, with PG/GG cells contributing mainly to the neocortex, and AG cells contributing more to the hypothalamic, septal, and preoptic areas. This provided the first suggestion that imprinted genes of different parental origins may have differential "interests" with regards to the brain. These effects may represent either the combined effects of many paternally and maternally expressed imprinted genes, or the actions of one or two imprinted genes of major effect. If the former is the case, we may expect maternally expressed imprinted genes to be disproportionately expressed in neocortical regions and paternally expressed imprinted genes to be disproportionately expressed in hypothalamic and septal regions; this is not exactly the case (Davies et al. 2005b) and the answer is probably somewhere in between. In reality, the distribution of AG and PG/GG cells in the two types of chimera probably points to where the interests of maternal- and paternal-imprinted genes in the brain lie when unfettered by the action of opposing parental alleles.

9.2.2 New Genes

Since those pioneering experiments, many imprinted genes (~90%) have been shown to be brain expressed. We have published a number of reviews detailing the characteristics of imprinted genes in the brain (Davies et al. 2005b) and also have produced a freely accessible online database of imprinted genes expressed in the brain (Davies et al. 2007). However, a number of new brain-expressed imprinted genes have recently been identified, partly due to the development of new screening methods (Schulz et al. 2006). Many of these have been identified in humans, often via the study of neurodevelopmental (Francks et al. 2003, 2007; Wawrzik et al. 2010) or psychiatric disease (Francks et al. 2003, 2007); the possible importance of this is discussed later.

One criticism that is often leveled at the imprinting community is that despite their developmental importance, there is a relative paucity of imprinted genes in the mammalian genome. Although a number of imprinted microRNAs have recently been identified, the overall number of imprinted gene still remains low, being around 130 (Beechey et al. 2003). In light of this criticism, it will be interesting to see the impact of more focused association studies aimed at identifying traits and diseases showing parent of origin effects (Kong et al. 2009). However, probably more important to the discovery of novel imprinted genes is the development of next-generation sequencing methods (Mardis 2008). It has been known for some time that a number of imprinted genes, particularly in the brain, show complex patterns of epigenetic regulation (Albrecht et al. 1997; Yamasaki et al. 2003). The result of this is that some genes are only imprinted in certain tissues (or brain regions) and/or certain developmental time points, while being expressed in a biallelic manner in others (Davies et al. 2005b). In the past, this subtle regulation would have been a hindrance to the identification of new imprinted genes. However, next-generation sequencing technologies are capable of producing tens of millions of sequence reads from very little input material. This is expected to revolutionize how we analyze gene expression and would, for instance, allow the quantification of allelic expression from discrete tissue samples.

9.2.3 Filling in the Details

In addition to identifying new candidates, interest in the physiological function of imprinted genes continues to grow within the imprinting community. This has led to the gaps in our knowledge of the expression patterns and neural function of previously known brain-expressed imprinted genes being filled. In particular, the neural and biochemical role of a number of imprinted genes of relevance to disease, such as *Ube3a* (Greer et al. 2010; van Woerden et al. 2007; Yashiro et al. 2009) and *Necdin* (Kuwajima et al. 2006; Kuwako et al. 2005; Zanella et al. 2008), have been studied in some detail.

One striking recent finding is the relative importance of two paternally expressed brain-specific small nucleolar (sno)RNA molecules, *snord115* and *snord116* (formerly known as *mbii-52* and *mbii-85*, respectively). snoRNAs are noncoding and thought to negatively regulate posttranscriptional modification (alternate splicing and RNA editing) of other pre-RNA species (Kishore and Stamm 2006). *snord116* is strongly expressed in the hypothalamus, suggesting a role in regulating feeding and metabolism. Although its target genes have not been identified, a knockout of *snord116* has demonstrated that its loss has important consequences for early postnatal survival and homeostasis and therefore makes it a key candidate for the imprinting disorder Prader–Willi syndrome (PWS) (Ding et al. 2008). More recently, a study of a clinical case has confirmed that loss of *SNORD116* is the main (but probably not sole – Peters 2008) contributor to the phenotype of the imprinting disorder PWS (Sahoo et al. 2008).

The second snoRNA, *SNORD115*, is also part of the PWS-imprinting cluster, but unlike *SNORD116*, its targets and mode of action are much better understood. *SNORD115* has a clear complimentary region for serotonin 2C receptor (*5htr2c*) pre-RNA exon Vb, a region that is subjected to both RNA editing and alternate splicing (Cavaille et al. 2000) and shows a reasonable overlap in expression with *5htr2c* found in cortical regions, the hippocampus, striatum and hypothalamus (Vitali et al. 2005). Loss of *snord115* in a mouse model for PWS results in increased

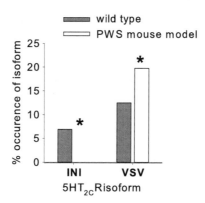

Fig. 9.1 Predicted pattern of two key serotonin 2C receptor protein isoforms in PWS mouse model brain. Data are based on the pattern of RNA editing as revealed by sequencing analysis (Doe et al. 2009). The INI isoform results as a consequence of no RNA editing, and is completely absent in PWS mouse brain. The VSV is the most abundant in brain and results as a consequence of editing at most of the five potential sites in the *5htr2c* pre-RNA. This is significantly increased in PWS mouse brain

levels of RNA editing across the five edited sites in exon Vb of the *5htr2c* pre-RNA. Such adenosine-to-inosine editing has consequences for the receptor protein function as inosine behaves like a guanine in translation, resulting in altered amino acid sequence. Bioinformatic analysis indicates that the pattern of serotonin receptor protein isoforms in the PWS mouse model brain is significantly altered, with a decrease in functional, and an increase in less function variants (Fig. 9.1).

9.2.3.1 Genomic Imprinting and the Monoamine System

More detailed analysis of imprinted genes expressed in the brain has thrown up the beginnings of an interesting pattern relating to monoamine system. A number of imprinted genes are now known to influence the function of one or more of the members of the monoamines (see Table 9.1). Some genes, such as *Necdin*, may be having general neurodevelopmental effects (Zanella et al. 2008) or they are not centrally important to monoamine function like *Ddc* (Menheniott et al. 2008). However, many more others, such as *Th*, *5htr2a*, and the snoRNA *snord115* described above, are directly linked to the efficacy of monoamine function in the brain.

Most interesting of all perhaps is the overlap in expression of *Dlk1*, *Nesp*, and *Grb10* in the brain (Jensen et al. 2001; Plagge et al. 2005). All three of these genes are expressed in discrete regions of the brain, but show important overlap in the locus ceoreleus and raphe nuclei. These two midbrain regions are important for noradrenergic and serotonergic projections to forebrain. Furthermore, *Dlk1* and *Grb10* are also expressed in the dopaminergic ventral tegmental area and the substantia nigra. This striking overlap in expression ties all three of these imprinted

Table 9.1 Imprinted gene involvement in the monoamine system

Gene(s)	Parental expression	Relation to monoamine system	References
Dlk1	Paternal	Expressed in areas with monoaminergic projections to forebrain. Involved in dopamine neuron differentiation	Jacobs et al. (2009)
Nesp	Maternal	Expressed in areas with monoaminergic projections to forebrain, including locus coeruleus and dorsal raphe nucleus	Plagge et al. (2005)
Grb10	Paternal	Expressed in areas with monoaminergic projections to forebrain, including locus coeruleus, dorsal raphe nucleus, and striatum	
Th	Maternal	Tyrosine hydroxylase; upstream enzyme in the production of dopamine and noradrenaline important in many aspects of monamine mediated behavior	Palmiter (2008)
CDKN1C	Maternal	Cooperates with Nurr1 in directing dopaminergic neuron differentiation	Joseph et al. (2003)
H19-IGF2	Maternal and paternal	Many of the genes in this interval are highly expressed in dopaminergic progenitor cells	Freed et al. (2008)
5HTR2A	Maternal	Serotonin receptor 2A	Bunzel et al. (1998), Kato et al. (1996)
Magel2	Paternal	Mice lacking *magel2* show altered serotonin metabolism in the cortex and reduced dopamine in hypothalamus	Mercer et al. (2009)
snord115	Paternal	Regulates posttranscriptional modification of the serotonin 2C receptor	Doe et al. (2009)
Ddc	Paternal	Dopa decarboxylase; imprinted in heart	Menheniott et al. (2008)
Necdin	Paternal	Modulation of seronergic innervation of respiratory system	Zanella et al. (2008)

genes (two paternally and one maternally expressed) to key areas in monoaminergic function. Nevertheless, thus far, only *Dlk1* has been explicitly shown to be important in dopamine neuron differentiation (Christophersen et al. 2007; Jacobs et al. 2009; Jensen et al. 2001). Although loss of *Nesp* and *Grb10* results in behavioral changes (Plagge et al. 2005), it is not clear as yet whether these behavioral changes are due to specific alterations in monoamines.

9.3 Behavior

Much of the original work on imprinted genes in the brain has centered on mother–pup interactions. Deficits were seen in two mouse models, null for *Peg1* and *Peg3*. In addition to mothering deficits in the adults, *Peg3* null pups also show poor postnatal development, such as soliciting suckling and homeostasis

(Curley et al. 2004). This pattern of physiological deficit has been seen in a number of other imprinted gene mutants (Plagge et al. 2004; Skryabin et al. 2007) and is also seen in the children with PWS (Haig and Wharton 2003). Whether these early life deficits have knock-on effects for adult behavior is a distinct possibility (Francis et al. 1999) and has been suggested as a possible cause of the psychiatric problems seen in genomic imprinting syndromes such as PWS (Isles and Holland 2005).

However, just as it has become increasingly recognized that imprinted genes are expressed in the adult brain, it has become clear that many may also directly influence other adult behaviors. Apart from the *Peg1* and *Peg3* studies, much work has focused on those imprinted genes within the PWS cluster. Many of these genes are expressed primarily in the hypothalamus, and the behavioral studies reflect this. As such, in addition to maternal behavior, we now know that imprinted genes influence sexual behavior (Swaney et al. 2007), circadian rhythms (Kozlov et al. 2007), feeding, and homeostasis (Ding et al. 2008). Nevertheless, as we have outlined earlier, imprinted genes are also found in many other brain regions, including the prefrontal cortex, hippocampus, striatum, and areas of importance for mediating neurotransmitter innervations of cortical regions.

9.3.1 Attention, Impulsivity, and Behavioral Flexibility

There is a growing body of work demonstrating that imprinted genes are also important for aspects of cognition. This includes some molecules with well-established roles in learning and memory such as the ubiquitin protein ligase E3A encoded by the maternally expressed *Ube3a* gene (Jiang et al. 1998), and the paternally expressed Ras signaling molecule *Grf1* (Brambilla et al. 1997; Giese et al. 2001).

Given increasing prominence of imprinted genes in monoamine function, it is not unsurprising that genomic imprinting has also been found to impact on other discrete aspects of cognition. Recently, independent studies of people with PWS and a mouse model for PWS have demonstrated deficits in executive function. Typically, individuals with PWS have mild learning difficulties as indicated by a general reduction in IQ scores (Whittington et al. 2004). Although explicit psychological testing is limited, it is known that there is a reduced ability in attention and visuoperceptual organization in the PWS subjects when compared with the normal population (Jauregi et al. 2007) and even when corrected for general intellectual ability (Woodcock et al. 2009). The work on the animal model for PWS used the 5-choice serial reaction time task (5-CSRTT), which is a form of continuous performance task, assays components of executive functioning, taxing aspects of visuospatial attention and inhibitory control, and has been extensively characterized as a valid cross-species behavioral test (Humby et al. 1999; Robbins 2002). The findings from the 5-CSRTT point to reduced attentional capabilities in the PWS mice. Although the animals could acquire the task to our criteria levels, their baseline performance was impaired across three main measures: with PWS animals showing decreased accuracy, increased omissions, and slower correct reaction times. Moreover, under a task manipulation considered to tax attentional functioning (reduced stimulus duration), the PWS mice displayed increased deficits relative to controls. These animal data are coupled with clinical findings demonstrate a specific contribution of the paternally expressed genes in the PWS interval to attention.

Another aspect of cognition upon which genomic imprinting impacts is response control, or the processes that are involved in what is more generally known as impulsivity and behavioral flexibility. In fact, genomic imprinting has been linked with impulsive behavior previously, though not explicitly (Higley and Linnoila 1997; Higley et al. 1993). However, recent work has now unambiguously linked genomic imprinting with different aspects of response control. This includes the maternally expressed Nesp55, which when deleted reduces the willingness of mice to explore a novel environment (Plagge et al. 2005); and studies of mice monosomic for the X chromosome, which have shown that lack of a paternal X gives rise to deficits in behavioral flexibility on a reversal learning task (Davies et al. 2005a).

Nevertheless, thus far, only one study has really explored the impact of an imprinted gene on the neural substrates of impulsive behavior. As outlined earlier, the snoRNA *snord115* plays an important role in the regulation of posttranscriptional modification of the *5htr2c* pre-RNA. Consequently, in a mouse model of PWS that lacks expression *snord115*, there is an increase in abundance of the less functional isoforms of serotonin 2C receptor ($5HT_{2C}R$) (Fig. 9.1). The $5HT_{2C}R$ plays an important role in modulating aspects of response control, which when measured in the 5-CSRTT is due to its specific effects on dopamine release in the nucleus accumbens (Robinson et al. 2008). When behavior of mice lacking *snord115* in the 5-CSRTT is probed with $5HT_{2C}R$ selective drugs, an enhanced increase in impulsivity is seen relative to controls (Doe et al. 2009). This effect is specific, as drugs for $5HT_{2A}R$ have no differential effect. This work indicates that the paternally expressed *snord115* is an important factor in mediating $5HT_{2C}R$ controlled impulsivity.

9.4 Evolution of Imprinted Genes in the Human Brain

The development of genomic imprinting in animals (true genomic imprinting has also evolved independently in plants – Kinoshita et al. 1999) seems to be linked with the evolution of mammals (Renfree et al. 2009). This suggests that key aspects of being mammalian, namely in utero development, a placenta, and postnatal parental care, were the original driving forces in the evolution of imprinting; the extensive role of imprinted genes in these functions (Constancia et al. 2004) would point to this being true. However, recent data from parental expression and/or epigenetic marking studies of imprinted genes known to influence in utero growth in rodents indicate that many have lost their monoallelic status in humans (Isles 2009). This would imply that the selective pressure on maintenance of the imprinting status of genes in the placenta and developing fetus is reduced or absent in humans. Thus far, two explanations for this have been suggested, namely the fact that human reproductive strategies have change (Monk et al. 2006) and that increased resourcing of the later stage fetus is not desirable due to our bipedalism (Isles 2009).

Nevertheless, while the importance of imprinted genes in the placenta and prenatal growth in humans is diminished, the opposite may be true of imprinted genes in the brain. Certainly, a key area where imprinted genes exert an influence is the early postnatal period. Several studies in mice (Curley et al. 2004; Ding et al. 2005; Plagge et al. 2004; Shiura et al. 2005; Skryabin et al. 2007) and human disorders (Haig and Wharton 2003) have indicated that in addition to in utero, imprinted genes can also impact upon nutrient acquisition and growth while the offspring are still dependent on their mother for feeding. Indeed, the rapid increase in body weight and size over the first year of life (Bluestone 2005), coupled with the extended dependence of human offspring for nutritional support (Sellen 2007), make postnatal feeding an important arena for imprinted genes (Haig 2010). Moreover, the acquisition of "social resources" (in addition to nutritional resources) from the mother (Horsler and Oliver 2006; Isles and Holland 2005; Oliver et al. 2007) during this crucial neurodevelopmental period may also be an important substrate for the evolution of genomic imprinting; these ideas are developed further elsewhere within this book (Bernard Crespi 2010). However, it is increasingly clear that some imprinted genes have an important role in the brain beyond this mother–offspring interaction. Furthermore, although much of the work on these adult brain expressed imprinted genes has been carried out in rodents, there is a suggestion that this role may be increasingly important in humans.

Although it is highly likely that the driving force behind the evolution of genomic imprinting was the development of an extended pregnancy and parental care, once established other selective pressures may have led genomic imprinting to be co-opted to act on other functions, such as brain and behavior. There is some evidence for this; a number of brain expressed imprinted genes such as *Neuronatin* (Evans et al. 2005) and Nesp (Gavin Kelsey pers. comm.) appear only later in the Eutherian mammalian lineages. Interestingly, there appears to be even more enrichment in humans, with the genes *LRRTM1*, *C15ORF2*, and *5HTR2A* only occurring or being imprinted in the human brain (Francks et al. 2003, 2007; Wawrzik et al. 2010).

Although these data are limited, they do provide a tantalizing suggestion that genomic imprinting in the brains of humans may be particularly important. Obviously, of direct relevance to this question is the analysis of imprinted genes in other species of primates; unfortunately much of the data we have simply allows a comparison between mouse and human. However, two separate studies of brain-expressed imprinted genes have directly addressed the question of whether these genes are particularly important for humans. As mentioned earlier, paternally expressed *C15ORF2* is only found in man, but more detailed analysis has also pointed to the fact that it has been positively selected through human evolution (Wawrzik et al. 2010). Similarly, the maternally expressed *Klf14* has also undergone accelerated evolution in humans (Parker-Katiraee et al. 2007). However, this gene is also present (and imprinted) in mice, suggesting that the positive selection is very much related to some key changes in the human lineage.

What selective pressures have led to this is not clear at present. One idea links back to the original work with mouse chimeras demonstrating differential distribution of PG/GG (maternal genomes only) and AG (paternal genome only) cells in the brain (Keverne et al. 1996b). The distinct brain regions to which PG/GG and AG cells contribute have also evolved differentially in primates. While the frontal cortex and striatal areas have expanded relative to the rest of the brain, the hypothalamus and septum have contracted in size. The forebrain areas that have expanded are thought to have done so due to the selective pressure of living in social groups and all complexities of social behavior which that entails. In the majority of primate societies, the maintenance of social cohesion and group continuity over successive generations is dependent on the matriline; these are also in the "interests" of the maternal genome, which is more likely to be shared among the members of the group. It seems more than coincidental that the areas of brain expansion required for living in social groups are also those to which the maternal genome makes a substantial developmental contribution. In humans, social behavior is taken to another level and so it may be the case that the importance of imprinted genes in the brain has also increased.

9.4.1 Consequences of Genomic Imprinting for Mental Illness

Whether or not they are adaptive, the increased numbers of imprinted genes expressed in the human brain may still be important contributors to abnormal brain function, particularly those with pleiotropic effects where any secondary phenotypes may be suboptimal as a result of the intragenomic conflict (Wilkins 2010). Indeed, there is an increasing evidence to suggest that this is the case not only from imprinting syndromes, such as PWS and Angelman syndrome, but also from other genome-wide studies of mental illness.

The contribution of genomic imprinting to disease may actually be amplified as the tight regulation of imprinted genes means that in addition to classic coding changes, they are also particularly susceptible to any mutations that cause alterations in expression levels. This added vulnerability may occur in two ways: either incorrect epigenetic regulation of the genes or changes in the dosage. The former has not been well explored, although the increased incidence of imprinting syndromes in individuals born as a result assisted reproductive technologies hints at the potential problems (Isles and Wilkinson 2008). The consequences of alterations in gene dosage have recently been revealed in a number of genome-wide studies linking Copy Number Variations (CNVs) with neuropsychiatric problems. Among those areas identified as important contributors to mental illness is the PWS-imprinted gene interval, 15q11–q13. This region has been linked in a number of independent studies to both schizophrenia (Kirov et al. 2009; Stefansson et al. 2008) and autism (Glessner et al. 2009; Sebat et al. 2007), with maternal duplications being particularly problematic (Cook et al. 1997; Schroer et al. 1998).

Note added in proof Some new and exciting results have been published since this article was submitted. Firstly, next-generation sequencing techniques have been used to examine the parent-of-origin specific expression bias in the brains of reciprocal cross F1 mouse sub-strains. These studies revealed existence of approximately 1300 genes showing a parent-of-origin specific bias in their expression (Gregg *et al. Science* **329**:643–8 and *Science* **329**:682–5). Moreover, these studies identified the hypothalamus and monoaminergic regions (noradrenergic locus coeruleus, seroto-nergic dorsal raphe nucleus and dopaminergic Nucleus accumbens and Ventral tegmental area) as being key hotspots for expression of these candidate imprinted genes. Supporting this idea was a recent paper examining the brain expression of the imprinted gene *Grb10*. This too was expressed in these specific brain regions and also appeared to co-localise with the dopamine transporter (Garfield *et al. Nature* **469**:534–38).

References

Albrecht U, Sutcliffe JS, Cattanach BM, Beechey CV, Armstrong D, Eichele G et al (1997) Imprinted expression of the murine Angelman syndrome gene, *Ube3a*, in hippocampal and Purkinje neurons. Nat Genet 17(1):75–78

Allen ND, Logan K, Lally G, Drage DJ, Norris ML, Keverne EB (1995) Distribution of partheno-genetic cells in the mouse-brain and their influence on brain-development and behavior. Proc Natl Acad Sci USA 92(23):10782–10786

Barton SC, Surani MA, Norris ML (1984) Role of paternal and maternal genomes in mouse development. Nature 311(5984):374–376

Beechey CV, Cattanach BM, Blake A, Peters J (2003) World Wide Web Site – Mouse imprinting data and references. Retrieved June, 2004, from http://www.mgu.har.mrc.ac.uk/imprinting/imprinting.html

Bernard Crespi BJ (2010) The strategies of the genes: genomic conflicts, attachment theory and the development of the social brain. In: Petronis A, Mill J (eds) Brain, behaviour and epigenetics. Springer, Berlin

Bluestone CD (2005) Humans are born too soon: impact on pediatric otolaryngology. Int J Pediatr Otorhinolaryngol 69(1):1–8

Brambilla R, Gnesutta N, Minichiello L, White G, Roylance AJ, Herron CE et al (1997) A role for the Ras signalling pathway in synaptic transmission and long-term memory. Nature 390(6657):281–286

Bunzel R, Blumcke I, Cichon S, Normann S, Schramm J, Propping P et al (1998) Polymorphic imprinting of the serotonin-2A (*5-HT2A*) receptor gene in human adult brain. Mol Brain Res 59(1):90–92

Cavaille J, Buiting K, Kiefmann M, Lalande M, Brannan CI, Horsthemke B et al (2000) Identifi-cation of brain-specific and imprinted small nucleolar RNA genes exhibiting an unusual genomic organization. Proc Natl Acad Sci USA 97(26):14311–14316

Christophersen NS, Gronborg M, Petersen TN, Fjord-Larsen L, Jorgensen JR, Juliusson B et al (2007) Midbrain expression of Delta-like 1 homologue is regulated by GDNF and is associated with dopaminergic differentiation. Exp Neurol 204(2):791–801

Constancia M, Kelsey G, Reik W (2004) Resourceful imprinting. Nature 432(7013):53–57

Cook EH, Lindgren V, Leventhal BL, Courchesne R, Lincoln A, Shulman C et al (1997) Autism or atypical autism in maternally but not paternally derived proximal 15q duplication. Am J Hum Genet 60(4):928–934

Curley JP, Barton S, Surani A, Keverne EB (2004) Coadaptation in mother and infant regulated by a paternally expressed imprinted gene. Proc R Soc Lond B Biol Sci 271(1545):1303–1309

Davies W, Isles A, Smith R, Karunadasa D, Burrmann D, Humby T et al (2005a) Xlr3b is a new imprinted candidate for X-linked parent-of-origin effects on cognitive function in mice. Nat Genet 37(6):625–629

Davies W, Isles AR, Wilkinson LS (2005b) Imprinted gene expression in the brain. Neurosci Biobehav Rev 29(3):421–430

Davies W, Isles AR, Humby T, Wilkinson LS (2007) What are imprinted genes doing in the brain? Epigenetics 2(4):201–206

Ding F, Prints Y, Dhar MS, Johnson DK, Garnacho-Montero C, Nicholls RD et al (2005) Lack of Pwcr1/MBII-85 snoRNA is critical for neonatal lethality in Prader-Willi syndrome mouse models. Mamm Genome 16(6):424–431

Ding F, Li HH, Zhang S, Solomon NM, Camper SA, Cohen P et al (2008) SnoRNA Snord116 (Pwcr1/MBII-85) deletion causes growth deficiency and hyperphagia in Mice. PLoS ONE 3(3):e1709

Doe CM, Relkovic D, Garfield AS, Dalley JW, Theobald DE, Humby T et al (2009) Loss of the imprinted snoRNA mbii-52 leads to increased 5htr2c pre-RNA editing and altered 5HT2CR-mediated behaviour. Hum Mol Genet 18(12):2140–2148

Evans HK, Weidman JR, Cowley DO, Jirtle RL (2005) Comparative phylogenetic analysis of Blcap/Nnat reveals eutherian-specific imprinted gene. Mol Biol Evol 22(8):1740–1748

Francis D, Diorio J, Liu D, Meaney MJ (1999) Nongenomic transmission across generations of maternal behavior and stress responses in the rat. Science 286(5442):1155–1158

Francks C, DeLisi LE, Shaw SH, Fisher SE, Richardson AJ, Stein JF et al (2003) Parent-of-origin effects on handedness and schizophrenia susceptibility on chromosome 2p12-q11. Hum Mol Genet 12(24):3225–3230

Francks C, Maegawa S, Lauren J, Abrahams BS, Velayos-Baeza A, Medland SE et al (2007) LRRTM1 on chromosome 2p12 is a maternally suppressed gene that is associated paternally with handedness and schizophrenia. Mol Psychiatry 12(12):1129–1139, 1057

Freed WJ, Chen J, Backman CM, Schwartz CM, Vazin T, Cai J et al (2008) Gene expression profile of neuronal progenitor cells derived from hESCs: activation of chromosome 11p15.5 and comparison to human dopaminergic neurons. PLoS ONE 3(1):e1422

Giese KP, Friedman E, Telliez JB, Fedorov NB, Wines M, Feig LA et al (2001) Hippocampus-dependent learning and memory is impaired in mice lacking the Ras-guanine-nucleotide releasing factor 1 (Ras-GRF1). Neuropharmacology 41(6):791–800

Glessner JT, Wang K, Cai G, Korvatska O, Kim CE, Wood S et al (2009) Autism genome-wide copy number variation reveals ubiquitin and neuronal genes. Nature 459(7246):569–573

Goddard MR, Godfray HC, Burt A (2005) Sex increases the efficacy of natural selection in experimental yeast populations. Nature 434(7033):636–640

Greer PL, Hanayama R, Bloodgood BL, Mardinly AR, Lipton DM, Flavell SW et al (2010) The Angelman Syndrome protein Ube3A regulates synapse development by ubiquitinating arc. Cell 140(5):704–716

Greig D, Travisano M (2003) Evolution. Haploid superiority. Science 299(5606):524–525

Haig D (1997) Parental antagonism, relatedness asymmetries, and genomic imprinting. Proc R Soc Lond B Biol Sci 264(1388):1657–1662

Haig D (2010) Evolution in health and medicine sackler colloquium: transfers and transitions: parent-offspring conflict, genomic imprinting, and the evolution of human life history. Proc Natl Acad Sci USA 107:1731–1735

Haig D, Graham C (1991) Genomic imprinting and the strange case of the insulin-like growth-factor II receptor. Cell 64(6):1045–1046

Haig D, Wharton R (2003) Prader-Willi syndrome and the evolution of human childhood. Am J Hum Biol 15(3):320–329

Higley JD, Linnoila M (1997) Low central nervous system serotonergic activity is traitlike and correlates with impulsive behavior. A nonhuman primate model investigating genetic and environmental influences on neurotransmission. Ann NY Acad Sci 836:39–56

Higley JD, Thompson WW, Champoux M, Goldman D, Hasert MF, Kraemer GW et al (1993) Paternal and maternal genetic and environmental contributions to cerebrospinal fluid monoamine metabolites in rhesus monkeys (Macaca mulatta). Arch Gen Psychiatry 50(8):615–623

Horsler K, Oliver C (2006) Environmental influences on the behavioral phenotype of Angelman syndrome. Am J Ment Retard 111(5):311–321

Humby T, Laird FM, Davies W, Wilkinson LS (1999) Visuospatial attentional functioning in mice: interactions between cholinergic manipulations and genotype. Euro J Neurosci 11(8): 2813–2823

Hurst LD, McVean GT (1997) Growth effects of uniparental disomies and the conflict theory of genomic imprinting. Trends Genet 13(11):436–443

Hurst LD, McVean GT (1998) Do we understand the evolution of genomic imprinting? Curr Opin Genet Dev 8(6):701–708

Isles AR (2009) Evolution of genomic imprinting in humans: does bipedalism have a role? Trends Genet 25(11):495–500

Isles AR, Holland AJ (2005) Imprinted genes and mother–offspring interactions. Early Hum Dev 81(1):73–77

Isles AR, Wilkinson LS (2008) Epigenetics: what is it and why is it important to mental disease? Br Med Bull 85:35–45

Jacobs FM, van der Linden AJ, Wang Y, von Oerthel L, Sul HS, Burbach JP et al (2009) Identification of Dlk1, Ptpru and Klhl1 as novel Nurr1 target genes in meso-diencephalic dopamine neurons. Development 136(14):2363–2373

Jauregi J, Arias C, Vegas O, Alen F, Martinez S, Copet P et al (2007) A neuropsychological assessment of frontal cognitive functions in Prader-Willi syndrome. J Intellect Disabil Res 51(Pt 5):350–365

Jensen CH, Meyer M, Schroder HD, Kliem A, Zimmer J, Teisner B (2001) Neurons in the monoaminergic nuclei of the rat and human central nervous system express FA1/dlk. Neuro-Report 12(18):3959–3963

Jiang YH, Armstrong D, Albrecht U, Atkins CM, Noebels JL, Eichele G et al (1998) Mutation of the angelman ubiquitin ligase in mice causes increased cytoplasmic p53 and deficits of contextual learning and long-term potentiation. Neuron 21(4):799–811

Joseph B, Wallen-Mackenzie A, Benoit G, Murata T, Joodmardi E, Okret S et al (2003) p57(Kip2) cooperates with Nurr1 in developing dopamine cells. Proc Natl Acad Sci USA 100(26): 15619–15624

Kato MV, Shimizu T, Nagayoshi M, Kaneko A, Sasaki MS, Ikawa Y (1996) Genomic imprinting of the human serotonin-receptor (HTR2) gene involved in development of retinoblastoma. Am J Hum Genet 59(5):1084–1090

Keverne EB, Curley JP (2008) Epigenetics, brain evolution and behaviour. Front Neuroendocrinol 29(3):398–412

Keverne EB, Fundele R, Narasimha M, Barton SC, Surani MA (1996a) Genomic imprinting and the differential roles of parental genomes in brain development. Dev Brain Res 92(1):91–100

Keverne EB, Martel FL, Nevison CM (1996b) Primate brain evolution: genetic and functional considerations. Proc R Soc Lond B Biol Sci 263(1371):689–696

Kinoshita T, Yadegari R, Harada JJ, Goldberg RB, Fischer RL (1999) Imprinting of the MEDEA polycomb gene in the Arabidopsis endosperm. Plant Cell 11(10):1945–1952

Kirov G, Grozeva D, Norton N, Ivanov D, Mantripragada KK, Holmans P et al (2009) Support for the involvement of large copy number variants in the pathogenesis of schizophrenia. Hum Mol Genet 18(8):1497–1503

Kishore S, Stamm S (2006) Regulation of alternative splicing by snoRNAs. Cold Spring Harb Symp Quant Biol 71:329–334

Kong A, Steinthorsdottir V, Masson G, Thorleifsson G, Sulem P, Besenbacher S et al (2009) Parental origin of sequence variants associated with complex diseases. Nature 462(7275):868–874

Kozlov SV, Bogenpohl JW, Howell MP, Wevrick R, Panda S, Hogenesch JB et al (2007) The imprinted gene Magel2 regulates normal circadian output. Nat Genet 39 (10):1266–1272

Kuwajima T, Nishimura I, Yoshikawa K (2006) Necdin promotes GABAergic neuron differentiation in cooperation with Dlx homeodomain proteins. J Neurosci 26(20):5383–5392

Kuwako K, Hosokawa A, Nishimura I, Uetsuki T, Yamada M, Nada S et al (2005) Disruption of the paternal necdin gene diminishes TrkA signaling for sensory neuron survival. J Neurosci 25(30):7090–7099

Lefebvre L, Viville S, Barton SC, Ishino F, Keverne EB, Surani MA (1998) Abnormal maternal behaviour and growth retardation associated with loss of the imprinted gene *Mest*. Nat Genet 20(2):163–169

Li LL, Keverne EB, Aparicio SA, Ishino F, Barton SC, Surani MA (1999) Regulation of maternal behavior and offspring growth by paternally expressed *Peg3*. Science 284(5412):330–333

Mardis ER (2008) The impact of next-generation sequencing technology on genetics. Trends Genet 24(3):133–141

McGrath J, Solter D (1984) Completion of mouse embryogenesis requires both the maternal and paternal genomes. Cell 37(1):179–183

Menheniott TR, Woodfine K, Schulz R, Wood AJ, Monk D, Giraud AS et al (2008) Genomic imprinting of Dopa decarboxylase in heart and reciprocal allelic expression with neighboring Grb10. Mol Cell Biol 28(1):386–396

Mercer RE, Kwolek EM, Bischof JM, van Eede M, Henkelman RM, Wevrick R (2009) Regionally reduced brain volume, altered serotonin neurochemistry, and abnormal behavior in mice null for the circadian rhythm output gene Magel2. Am J Med Genet B Neuropsychiatr Genet 150B (8):1085–1099

Monk D, Arnaud P, Apostolidou S, Hills FA, Kelsey G, Stanier P et al (2006) Limited evolutionary conservation of imprinting in the human placenta. Proc Natl Acad Sci USA 103(17): 6623–6628

Moore T, Haig D (1991) Genomic imprinting in mammalian development – a parental tug-of-war. Trends Genet 7(2):45–49

Necsulea A, Semon M, Duret L, Hurst LD (2009) Monoallelic expression and tissue specificity are associated with high crossover rates. Trends Genet 25(12):519–522

Oliver C, Horsler K, Berg K, Bellamy G, Dick K, Griffiths E (2007) Genomic imprinting and the expression of affect in Angelman syndrome: what's in the smile? J Child Psychol Psychiatry 48(6):571–579

Orr HA (1995) Somatic mutation favors the evolution of diploidy. Genetics 139(3):1441–1447

Palmiter RD (2008) Dopamine signaling in the dorsal striatum is essential for motivated behaviors: lessons from dopamine-deficient mice. Ann NY Acad Sci 1129:35–46

Parker-Katiraee L, Carson AR, Yamada T, Arnaud P, Feil R, Abu-Amero SN et al (2007) Identification of the imprinted KLF14 transcription factor undergoing human-specific accelerated evolution. PLoS Genet 3(5):e65

Peters J (2008) Prader-Willi and snoRNAs. Nat Genet 40(6):688–689

Plagge A, Gordon E, Dean W, Boiani R, Cinti S, Peters J et al (2004) The imprinted signaling protein XLalphas is required for postnatal adaptation to feeding. Nat Genet 36(8):818–826

Plagge A, Isles AR, Gordon E, Humby T, Dean W, Gritsch S et al (2005) Imprinted nesp55 influences behavioral reactivity to novel environments. Mol Cell Biol 25(8):3019–3026

Renfree MB, Hore TA, Shaw G, Graves JA, Pask AJ (2009) Evolution of genomic imprinting: insights from marsupials and monotremes. Annu Rev Genomics Hum Genet 10:241–262

Robbins TW (2002) The 5-choice serial reaction time task: behavioural pharmacology and functional neurochemistry. Psychopharmacology (Berl) 163(3–4):362–380

Robinson ES, Dalley JW, Theobald DE, Glennon JC, Pezze MA, Murphy ER et al (2008) Opposing roles for 5-HT2A and 5-HT2C receptors in the nucleus accumbens on inhibitory response control in the 5-choice serial reaction time task. Neuropsychopharmacology 33 (10):2398–2406

Sahoo T, Del Gaudio D, German JR, Shinawi M, Peters SU, Person RE et al (2008) Prader-Willi phenotype caused by paternal deficiency for the HBII-85 C/D box small nucleolar RNA cluster. Nat Genet 40(6):719–721

Schroer RJ, Phelan MC, Michaelis RC, Crawford EC, Skinner SA, Cuccaro M et al (1998) Autism and maternally derived aberrations of chromosome 15q. Am J Med Genet 76(4):327–336

Schulz R, Menheniott TR, Woodfine K, Wood AJ, Choi JD, Oakey RJ (2006) Chromosome-wide identification of novel imprinted genes using microarrays and uniparental disomies. Nucleic Acids Res 34(12):e88

Sebat J, Lakshmi B, Malhotra D, Troge J, Lese-Martin C, Walsh T et al (2007) Strong association of de novo copy number mutations with autism. Science 316(5823):445–449

Sellen DW (2007) Evolution of infant and young child feeding: implications for contemporary public health. Annu Rev Nutr 27:123–148

Shiura H, Miyoshi N, Konishi A, Wakisaka-Saito N, Suzuki R, Muguruma K et al (2005) Meg1/Grb10 overexpression causes postnatal growth retardation and insulin resistance via negative modulation of the IGF1R and IR cascades. Biochem Biophys Res Comm 329(3):909–916

Skryabin BV, Gubar LV, Seeger B, Pfeiffer J, Handel S, Robeck T et al (2007) Deletion of the MBII-85 snoRNA Gene Cluster in Mice Results in Postnatal Growth Retardation. PLoS Genet 3(12):e235

Smith FM, Garfield AS, Ward A (2006) Regulation of growth and metabolism by imprinted genes. Cytogenet Genome Res 113(1–4):279–291

Stefansson H, Rujescu D, Cichon S, Pietilainen OP, Ingason A, Steinberg S et al (2008) Large recurrent microdeletions associated with schizophrenia. Nature 455(7210):232–236

Swaney WT, Curley JP, Champagne FA, Keverne EB (2007) Genomic imprinting mediates sexual experience-dependent olfactory learning in male mice. Proc Natl Acad Sci USA 104(14):6084–6089

Trivers RL (1974) Parent–offspring conflict. Am Zool 14:249–264

van Woerden GM, Harris KD, Hojjati MR, Gustin RM, Qiu S, de Avila Freire R et al (2007) Rescue of neurological deficits in a mouse model for Angelman syndrome by reduction of alphaCaMKII inhibitory phosphorylation. Nat Neurosci 10(3):280–282

Varmuza S, Mann M (1994) Genomic imprinting – defusing the ovarian time bomb. Trends Genet 10(4):118–123

Vitali P, Basyuk E, Le Meur E, Bertrand E, Muscatelli F, Cavaille J et al (2005) ADAR2-mediated editing of RNA substrates in the nucleolus is inhibited by C/D small nucleolar RNAs. J Cell Biol 169(5):745–753

Wawrzik M, Unmehopa UA, Swaab DF, van de Nes J, Buiting K, Horsthemke B (2010) The C15orf2 gene in the Prader-Willi syndrome region is subject to genomic imprinting and positive selection. Neurogenetics 11(2):153–161

Whittington J, Holland A, Webb T, Butler J, Clarke D, Boer H (2004) Cognitive abilities and genotype in a population-based sample of people with Prader-Willi syndrome. J Intellect Disabil Res 48(Pt 2):172–187

Wilkins JF (2010) Antagonistic coevolution of two imprinted loci with pleiotropic effects. Evolution 64:142–151

Wilkinson LS, Davies W, Isles AR (2007) Genomic imprinting effects on brain development and function. Nat Rev Neurosci 8(11):832–843

Wolf JB, Hager R (2006) A maternal–offspring coadaptation theory for the evolution of genomic imprinting. PLoS Biol 4(12):e380

Woodcock KA, Oliver C, Humphreys GW (2009) Task-switching deficits and repetitive behaviour in genetic neurodevelopmental disorders: data from children with Prader-Willi syndrome chromosome 15 q11-q13 deletion and boys with Fragile X syndrome. Cogn Neuropsychol 26(2):172–194

Yamasaki K, Joh K, Ohta T, Masuzaki H, Ishimaru T, Mukai T et al (2003) Neurons but not glial cells show reciprocal imprinting of sense and antisense transcripts of Ube3a. Hum Mol Genet 12(8):837–847

Yashiro K, Riday TT, Condon KH, Roberts AC, Bernardo DR, Prakash R et al (2009) Ube3a is required for experience-dependent maturation of the neocortex. Nat Neurosci 12(6):777–783

Zanella S, Watrin F, Mebarek S, Marly F, Roussel M, Gire C et al (2008) Necdin plays a role in the serotonergic modulation of the mouse respiratory network: implication for Prader-Willi syndrome. J Neurosci 28(7):1745–1755

Chapter 10
Epigenetic Influence of the Social Environment

Frances A. Champagne and James P. Curley

Abstract Social experiences occurring during infancy have been demonstrated to exert persistent effects on neurobiological and behavioral outcomes. This social modulation of the developing brain has been observed in humans and animal models of abuse, neglect, and variation in parental style. Although the mechanisms through which these effects are achieved likely involve diverse cellular and molecular pathways, there is emerging evidence supporting the hypothesis that epigenetic changes, such as DNA methylation and histone modifications, may mediate the effects of early life variations in the social interactions between mothers and infants. Moreover, there may be plasticity within these epigenetic pathways at later developmental time points, such that the social experiences of juveniles and adults may also induce epigenetic change. These findings have implications for behavioral variation observed both within and across generations and highlight the dynamic interactions occurring between genes and environments during the course of development.

Keywords Abuse · Epigenetic · Maternal · Neglect · Neurodevelopment · Parenting · Transgenerational

10.1 Introduction

The quality of the social environment can have a significant impact on physiology, neurobiology, and behavior. There is growing evidence from epidemiological studies in humans for the persistent effects of the early life experience of abuse, neglect, and variations in parenting style, which suggest that multiple neural

F.A. Champagne (✉) and J.P. Curley
Department of Psychology, Columbia University, Schermerhorn Hall, 1190 Amsterdam Avenue, New York, NY 10027, USA
e-mail: fac2105@columbia.edu

A. Petronis and J. Mill (eds.), *Brain, Behavior and Epigenetics*,
Epigenetics and Human Health, DOI 10.1007/978-3-642-17426-1_10,
© Springer-Verlag Berlin Heidelberg 2011

systems may be subjected to modulation via the social context of development. Further, explorations of the mechanisms through which these effects are achieved have focused on experimental paradigms involving primate and rodent models of variation in the social environment, and in particular, disruption of postnatal mother–infant interactions. Although multiple molecular and cellular pathways are implicated in mediating the link between early life experiences and long-term changes in phenotype, recent evidence has highlighted the role of epigenetic mechanisms, such as DNA methylation and posttranslational modifications to histone proteins within the nucleosome. Although shifts in DNA methylation were once thought to be restricted to early embryonic development, studies of nutritional (Lillycrop et al. 2007, 2008), chemical (Onishchenko et al. 2008), and a broad range of environmental exposures (Mueller and Bale 2008; Roth et al. 2009; Weaver et al. 2004) occurring during pre- and postnatal development have implicated epigenetic regulation of gene expression as a critical target of experience-dependent change. In this chapter, we describe the experimental approaches that have been used to explore the long-term effects of early life social experiences; highlight evidence from humans, primates, and rodents for social modulation of the brain; and illustrate the role of epigenetic mechanisms in maintaining the effects of the social environment. Although plasticity in development is typically associated with the perinatal period, there is continued social modulation of gene expression and behavior among juveniles and adults and this plasticity may likewise involve epigenetic modifications. Moreover, the impact of the social environment may not be restricted to within-generation effects and may lead to the transgenerational inheritance of phenotypic variation that involves experience-dependent changes in DNA methylation (Champagne 2008). These findings suggest that an exploration of epigenetic mechanisms may advance our understanding of the complex and dynamic interplay between the genome and the environment.

10.1.1   From Epidemiology to the Laboratory: Strategies for Studying Early Life Social Influences

Epidemiological and longitudinal studies have provided significant support for the hypothesis that the quality of the early life social environment may shape developmental trajectories leading to either risk or resilience to later life psychiatric disorder. In humans, neglect and abuse have been demonstrated to reduce cognitive performance and impair social development (Trickett and McBride-Chang 1995) and is associated with a fourfold increase in personality disorders (Johnson et al. 1999). The severe neglect experienced by institutionalized infants, most recently explored among Romanian orphans, further demonstrates the persistent effects of these experiences. Delays in growth, social, and cognitive development observed in Romanian orphans are associated with later life impairments in attachment, heightened inattention, and increased autistic-like behaviors (Beckett et al. 2002;

MacLean 2003; O'Connor and Rutter 2000; O'Connor et al. 2000; Rutter and O'Connor 2004). Although it is difficult to identify the particular aspect of the neglectful or abusive childhood experience which contributes to this outcome, disruption to the mother–infant relationship, consisting of both physical and emotional contact, associated with these conditions is thought to be critical. Variations in the attachment relationship between mother and infant have been associated with either resilience to psychological distress or increased incidence of psychopathology (Sroufe et al. 1999; Sroufe 2005). Secure attachment, typically assessed by the Strange Situation Task (in which infants' response to separation followed by reintroduction of the mother is measured) is associated with increased social competence and cognitive performance, whereas disorganized attachment patterns predict increased rates of borderline personality disorder, dissociation, and self-harm in adulthood (Carlson 1998; Carlson et al. 2009). Studies using a retrospective assessment of the quality of the mother–infant relationship, such as the Parental Bonding Index (PBI), suggest that low levels of maternal care combined with controlling–overprotective parenting are a significant predictor of adult depression (Parker et al. 1979; Parker 1993). Overall, these studies indicate that disruption to the early social environment, particularly the interactions between mother and infant, can have sustained effects on numerous biobehavioral outcomes in adulthood.

Our understanding of the mechanisms linking these early life experiences to adult outcomes has come from the development of animal models, which incorporate aspects of neglect, abuse, or variation in the quality of the mother–infant interactions' that are evident in human longitudinal studies (see Fig. 10.1). The classic studies of Harry Harlow on the development of rhesus macaques exposed to maternal deprivation provide evidence that the absence of mother–infant interactions during the early phases of development can induce disruptions to social play, hyperactivity, and sensitivity to stressors (Harlow et al. 1965; Seay and Harlow 1965; Suomi et al. 1971). The importance of mother–infant contact is further

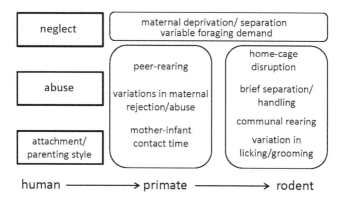

Fig. 10.1 Summary of paradigms used to study social modulation of brain and behavior during postnatal development in humans, primates, and rodents

demonstrated by the persistence of abnormalities in development that emerge in response to peer-rearing (Suomi 1991), where infants have social contact with the peers but not with the mother. In primates, variable foraging demand can also be used to disrupt the quality and quantity of mother–infant interactions (Coplan et al. 2006). When the duration of time that is needed to locate and retrieve sufficient amounts of food is inconsistent across weeks, the sensitivity of mothers to infant cues is disrupted, and consequently, offspring exhibit elevated levels of anxiety-like behavior and are less social in adulthood (Coplan et al. 1995, 2005; Gorman et al. 2002). These variations in mother–infant interaction are also observed to occur naturally among colonies of rhesus and pigtail macaques. Maternal abuse in the form of dragging and stepping-on infants occurs in isolation-reared and group-housed macaques at a frequency of 2–10% (Berman 1990; Carroll and Maestripieri 1998; Maestripieri 1998). Abused infants show a delayed onset in social play and are hyperaggressive in novel environments (McCormack et al. 2006). Abusive mothers also engage in high levels of maternal rejection, where infant attempts to make contact with the mother are rejected, and the experience of high levels of this parenting style may be associated with neurobiological outcomes associated with infant abuse (as discussed in the next section). High levels of mother–infant contact (characteristic of an over-protective parenting style) have also been observed in non-human primates and are associated with decreased exploration of a novel environment when infants are juveniles (Fairbanks and McGuire 1988). Thus, both experimental manipulation of the early social environment and observational studies of naturally occurring variations in mother–infant interactions can be used to explore the persistent effects of social experiences.

Although primate studies provide a useful model for exploring the effects of neglect, abuse, and variations in maternal behavior that may shape the developing brain and behavior, our understanding of the mechanisms through which this is achieved have relied primarily on studies of laboratory rodents. Maternal neglect and deprivation can be experimentally induced by separating pups from the dam for extended periods of time, a manipulation referred to as maternal separation (Rosenfeld et al. 1992), or through rearing pups in complete isolation from the dam, referred to as artificial rearing (Hall 1975). In general, prolonged separation or deprivation from maternal contact induces heightened anxiety-like behaviors, reduced performances on learning and memory tasks, and decreased social behaviors in adulthood (Lehmann et al. 1999; Lovic and Fleming 2004). The duration of separation is an important modulator of this effect, and there is evidence that brief maternal separations (often referred to as "handling") can stimulate maternal behavior and attenuate the stress response (Levine 1957; Meaney et al. 1991). The effects of abusive caregiving can also be studied in rodents. Removal or disruption of the bedding material normally included in the cages of laboratory rats and mice can induce dams to engage in rough handling, stepping-on, and avoidance of pups (Roth and Sullivan 2005). This paradigm has been used primarily for studying the factors influencing attachment to abusive caregivers and may also be a useful approach for studying the effects of early life trauma. Extended periods of maternal separation can also be induced in the laboratory by imposing foraging demands, and evidence from studies in mice suggests that a variable foraging demand on dams is associated with increased anxiety-like responses in male offspring (Bredy et al. 2007; Coutellier et al. 2009). Interestingly, studies of biparental voles indicate that removal of the father can have lasting effects on neurodevelopment (Ahern and Young 2009), though the benefits of multiple caregivers for offspring development is not limited to biparental species. In laboratory mice, communal rearing can be used to study the effects of increased social interactions during the postnatal period (Branchi 2009). In a communal nest, multiple postparturient females are housed together with their own litters or foster pups and the litters are combined and cared for as a group by the lactating dams. When compared with standard reared pups, offspring reared in communal nests are found to exhibit changes in anxiety-like and social behavior that are dependent on the age distribution of pups in the nest and conditions of the testing environment (Branchi and Alleva 2006; Branchi et al. 2009; Curley et al. 2009). This rearing paradigm has been demonstrated to ameliorate many of the behavioral deficits characteristic of the highly anxious BALB/c mouse strain (Curley et al. 2009), suggesting the modulating effect of social experiences on strain differences in behavior.

Individual variation in maternal styles that are observed in humans and primates are also exhibited by laboratory rodents and can likewise be associated with divergent developmental outcomes. In rats and mice, there are individual variations in several aspects of maternal behavior during the first week postpartum (Champagne et al. 2003a, 2007). In particular, there are stable between-dam variations in the frequency of pup licking/grooming (LG). One strategy for studying the long-term influence of mother–infant interactions is to characterize the LG behavior of a cohort of lactating females and compare outcome measures between offspring reared by Low or High LG dams [with Low or High being defined as 1 SD below or above the cohort average LG (Champagne et al. 2003a)]. This approach has been used successfully to study the origins of individual differences in stress response, response to novelty, learning and memory, and numerous indices of social/reproductive behavior (Meaney 2001). Variations in LG during the postnatal period can also be induced by gestational stress (Champagne and Meaney 2006; Moore and Power 1986), postparturient exposure to predator odor (McLeod et al. 2007), and various manipulations of the postnatal and juvenile rearing environment of the dams (Champagne and Meaney 2007; Lovic et al. 2001), with consequences for offspring development. Thus, plasticity in maternal behavior in response to environmental conditions is one route through which the quality of the environment can shape offspring physiology, brain, and behavior.

10.1.2 Social Modulation of the Developing Brain

The rodent and primate models of neglect, abuse, and variations in mother–infant interaction described in the previous section have been used to explore the neurobiological impact of the social environment and have yielded target neural systems, which have been subsequently explored in human cohorts. Disruption to the early life environment has been demonstrated to exert persistent effects on the hypothalamic–pituitary–adrenal (HPA) response to stress (for recent reviews see Korosi and Baram 2009; Lupien et al. 2009). Elevations in glucocorticoids associated with exposure to stress is achieved via release of corticotropin-releasing hormone (CRH) from the paraventricular nucleus (PVN) of the hypothalamus that acts on CRH receptors within the pituitary to trigger the release of adrenocorticotropin hormone (ACTH) and consequent release of glucocorticoids from the adrenal cortex. This HPA activity can be potentiated by neuropeptides such as vasopressin (AVP) and down-regulated through a negative feedback loop involving hippocampal glucocorticoid receptors (GR). In early development, social experiences that promote increased levels of mother–infant tactile stimulation generally lead to long-term reduction in HPA stress reactivity. Adult rats that were reared by High LG dams or exposed to postnatal handling have attenuated stress responsivity, reduced CRH mRNA expression in the PVN, and higher expression of GR in the hippocampus (Francis et al. 1999; Liu et al. 1997; Meaney and Aitken 1985; Meaney et al. 1985, 1989; Viau et al. 1993). In contrast, postnatal maternal separation induces increased stress reactivity associated with reduced GR expression in the hypothalamus and hippocampus, and regional changes in CRH receptor expression (Ladd et al. 2004; Plotsky and Meaney 1993). Thus, neural circuits involved in emotionality are susceptible to modulation in response to early life experiences, particularly those experiences affecting the frequency of mother–infant interactions.

The influence of the social environment is not limited to neuroendocrine pathways, which are primarily involved in regulating the stress response. However, it should be noted that most investigations of the neurobiological consequences of experimental manipulations of the early life environment use a target gene/neural system approach such that the specificity vs. breadth of the effects of particular manipulations are not well elucidated. Maternal separation is associated with increased dopamine (DA) in the striatum of mice (Ognibene et al. 2008). Moreover, compared with individuals who were handled during the first 2 weeks of life, adults who experienced postnatal maternal separation have increased dopamine D1 receptor binding levels in the nucleus accumbens (NAc) core and caudate putamen, increased D3 receptor mRNA in the NAc shell, and decreased levels of dopamine transporter (DAT – which uptakes DA from the synapse) (Brake et al. 2004). Maternally separated rat pups have decreased 5-HIAA and HVA (serotonin (5-HT) metabolites) levels in the amygdala and increased stress-induced 5-HT and 5-HIAA levels (Arborelius and Eklund 2007). Similar increases in 5-HT levels are found in the prefrontal cortex, hippocampus, and striatum of mice that are maternally separated during the first week postpartum (Ognibene et al. 2008). Handling-induced increases in gamma-aminobutyric acid (GABA) A central benzodiazepine (CBZ) receptors have been detected in the medial prefrontal cortex (mPFC), hippocampus, and amygdala (Bodnoff et al. 1987; Caldji et al. 2000; Weizman et al. 1999). Extended periods of maternal separation in rats have been reported to cause reductions in the expression of the hippocampal N-methyl-D-aspartic acid (NMDA) and α-amino-3-hydroxyl-5-methyl-4-isoxazole-propionate (AMPA) receptor subunits (Bellinger et al. 2006; Pickering et al. 2006;

Roceri et al. 2002). Postnatal maternal separation has also generally been associated with elevated AVP immunoreactivity and mRNA in the PVN (Vazquez et al. 2006; Veenema et al. 2006; Veenema and Neumann 2007), though some studies only find this increase in subjects undergoing a subsequent exposure to stress (Veenema et al. 2006). Maternal separation leads to increased vasopressin V1A receptor (V1Ar) binding in the lateral septum (LS) of juvenile males (Lukas et al. 2010). Maternally separated male rats have lower oxytocin receptor (OTR) binding in the LS and caudate putamen, and higher OTR binding in the medial preoptic area (MPOA) and ventro-medial hypothalamus (VMH) (Lukas et al. 2010). Overall, these studies illustrate the broad effects of early life manipulations achieved through long and brief maternal separations.

Similarly, variations in maternal behavior have been demonstrated to exert long-term influences on dopaminergic, GABAergic, glutamatergic, oxytocin and vasopressin neuropeptide systems, and brain-derived neurotrophic factor (BDNF). Offspring of Low LG dams have elevated stress-induced dopamine release within the mPFC (Zhang et al. 2005). Variations in maternal behavior in the rat and between different strains of mice have been shown to regulate GABAA receptor subunit composition with implications for its receptor pharmacology (Caldji et al. 2000, 2003, 2004). Offspring of Low LG dams exhibit a deficit in NMDA hippo-campal subunit mRNA expression as adults (Bredy et al. 2003, 2004; Liu et al. 2000). Similarly, in biparental species, reduced paternal contact results in increased NR2A and decreased NR2B NMDA subunit mRNA expression in the hippocampus (Bredy et al. 2007). Male offspring of High LG rat dams have elevated levels of V1Ar in the amygdala (Francis et al. 2002b), whereas communally reared female mice have reduced V1Ar binding in the LS (Curley et al. 2009). Communally rearing and the experience of High LG are associated with elevations in hypotha-lamic OTR of female offspring (Champagne et al. 2001; Curley et al. 2009; Francis et al. 2000). Finally, hippocampal levels of BDNF have been demonstrated to decrease in response to maternal separation and complete maternal deprivation (Burton et al. 2007; Roceri et al. 2002), and increase in response to communal rearing in mice (Branchi et al. 2006a, b) and high LG in rats (Liu et al. 2000). Social modulation of these target systems has implications for response to novelty, anxiety-like and social behavior, and cognition, such that these early life experi-ences can achieve diverse developmental effects that persist into adulthood.

The translation of these laboratory-based findings to primate and human studies has provided further support for the impact of social experiences on brain region-specific activation, neuropeptide/neurotransmitter levels, and variations in gene expression. As it is the case for early deprivation paradigms in rodents, reductions in mother–infant contact in primates have a profound impact on the HPA response to stress. Heightened stress-induced cortisol and decreased rhythmicity in basal cortisol release are common features of rhesus monkeys reared in the absence of maternal stimulation, typically using a peer-rearing strategy (Barr et al. 2004; Suomi 1991). Compared with mother-reared rhesus monkeys, peer-reared infants showed increases in the volume of stress-sensitive brain regions, such as the dorsomedial prefrontal cortex and dorsal anterior cingulate cortex (ACC), in later life (Spinelli et al. 2009). Peer-reared infants also have decreased serotonin trans-porter binding in the hypothalamus, caudate and putamen, globus pallidum, anterior cingulate gyrus, amygdala, and hippocampus (Ichise et al. 2006); decreased CSF 5-HIAA concentrations (Shannon et al. 2005); and an altered density of 5-HT1A receptors (Spinelli et al. 2010). Exposure of infant marmosets to repeated separations from parents is associated with long-term changes in gene expression, with particular effects on 5-HT1A mRNA levels within the ACC and hippocampus (Law et al. 2009a, b). Comparisons between nursery- and mother-reared infants indicate decreased CSF oxytocin levels in maternally deprived rhesus monkeys, which may account for the decreased social behavior observed in nursery-reared infants (Winslow 2005). Disruptions of mother–infant interactions, through use of a variable foraging demand, have been demonstrated to increase CSF levels of CRH (when exposure occurs in infancy; Coplan et al. 2001), induce elevations in CSF 5-HIAA and HVA (Coplan et al. 1998), and alter metabolism within the ACC (Mathew et al. 2003). Likewise, natural variation in maternal rejection rates is associated with altered serotonergic activity in offspring (Maestripieri et al. 2005, 2006). Thus, studies in primates have confirmed the neurobiological pathways that had previously been implicated in rodent models of abuse, neglect, and variation in parental behavior.

Advances in the development of noninvasive strategies for studying the impact of early life experiences on neural systems in humans have provided opportunities for translational studies on social modulation of the brain. Childhood neglect and abuse are associated with increased HPA activity and increased pituitary volume (Fries et al. 2008; Gerra et al. 2008; Neigh et al. 2009). CSF levels of 5-HIAA and HVA have been show to be negatively correlated with retrospective self-report scores of childhood emotional neglect (Roy 2002). Reduced levels of plasma BDNF associated with childhood neglect have also been reported in depressed patients and may account for cognitive impairments observed in these subjects (Grassi-Oliveira et al. 2008). Neuroimaging studies of Romanian adoptees that experienced severe neglect associated with institutionalization in infancy have indicated decreased overall white- and gray-matter volume and increased amygdala volume (Mehta et al. 2009). Positron emission tomography (PET) analysis indicates decreased metabolic activity within the orbital frontal gyrus, the infralimbic pre-frontal cortex, amygdala, hippocampus, the lateral temporal cortex, and the brain stem of Romanian orphans (Chugani et al. 2001). Levels of vasopressin and oxytocin have also been found to be blunted in children who experienced early neglect (Fries et al. 2005). Variations in retrospective reports of parental care have also yielded significant negative associations with cerebrospinal levels of CRH (Lee et al. 2006). In nonclinical subjects, high levels of maternal care are associated with reduced trait anxiety and decreased salivary cortisol in response to stress, whereas low levels of maternal care are associated with increased DA release in the ventral striatum in response to stress (Pruessner et al. 2004). Other studies using the PBI have found a positive relationship between gray matter volume in the left dorsolateral prefrontal cortex (DLPFC) and paternal care score, whereas paternal and maternal overprotection were negatively correlated with the volume of this region (Narita et al. 2010). In a longitudinal study, observational ratings of parental nurturance at age 4 predicted hippocampal volume in adolescence (Rao et al. 2010). These neurobiological studies of the effect of early life adversity suggest the persistent influence of these experiences on neural systems that regulate anxiety, social behavior, and cognition with implications for risk of later life psychiatric disorders.

10.1.3 Epigenetic Mechanisms and the Long-Term Effects of Social Experiences

The biological pathways, though which early life social experiences exert such a profound neurobiological and behavioral impact, are being explored within many of the rodent, primate, and human experimental designs described in the previous sections. Although there may certainly be neuroanatomical alterations through which these effects are achieved, one approach to advancing our understanding of the association between the social environment and phenotypic variation comes from experimental designs incorporating the study of epigenetic regulation of gene activity. This epigenetic regulation of transcription is a critical feature of the link between genotype and phenotype and refers to those factors which control accessibility of DNA to transcription and which can alter the levels of gene expression (either silencing genes or increasing transcriptional activity) without altering the sequence of DNA. The molecular mechanisms through which these epigenetic effects are achieved include, but are not exclusive to, histone protein modifications and DNA methylation (Feng et al. 2007; Razin 1998). Within the cell nucleus, DNA is wrapped around a core of histone proteins, which can undergo multiple post-translational modifications including methylation, acetylation, and ubiquination (Peterson and Laniel 2004; Zhang and Reinberg 2001). These modifications alter the dynamic interactions between the histones and DNA, which either reduce or enhance the accessibility of DNA to transcription factors and RNA polymerase. In particular, histone acetylation is associated with increased transcriptional activity, whereas histone deacetylation or methylation is typically associated with transcriptional repression. Acetylation of histones is mediated by the enzyme histone acetyltransferase (HAT), whereas histone deacetylase (HDAC) promotes removal of the acetyl group from the histone tails. Thus, through alterations in the conformation of histones, the accessibility of DNA can be rapidly and reversibly altered. In contrast, DNA methylation has the potential to be a more stable and enduring modification to the activity of genes. DNA methylation occurs when cytosine nucleotides, usually located in CpG islands, are converted to 5-methylcytosine. This process is mediated by methyltransferases, which promote either maintenance (i.e., DNMT1) or de novo DNA methylation (i.e., DNMT3) (Feng et al. 2007; Razin 1998; Turner 2001). The conversion to 5-methylcytosine does not alter the DNA sequence, but can alter the likelihood that the gene will be transcribed and reduce transcription factor-mediated responses, particularly when methylation occurs within gene promoter regions. Methylated DNA attracts methyl-binding proteins, such as MeCP2, which further reduce the accessibility of the gene and are associated with transcriptional repression (Fan and Hutnick 2005). The stability of DNA methylation patterns within the genome permits the stable regulation of gene expression associated with cellular differentiation and the heritability of this modification can be observed during mitotic cell divisions (Fukuda and Taga 2005).

Investigations of the role of epigenetic mechanisms in maintaining changes in gene expression induced by the early social environment have been explored in rodent experimental designs that model maternal abuse, maternal separation, and variations in mother–infant interactions during postnatal development (see Fig. 10.2). Daily exposure to abusive social interactions leads to reduced expression of BDNF in the prefrontal cortex in adulthood associated with increased DNA methylation within the BDNF IV promoter region (Roth et al. 2009). The functional importance of DNA methylation in mediating the long-term effects of abuse is further supported by findings that central administration of zebularine, a compound that reduces DNA methylation, leads to increased BDNF expression in maltreated rats such that BDNF levels are equivalent among abused and nonabused offspring. Daily and prolonged maternal separation has effects on a broad range of neurotransmitter and neuropeptide systems, and in a recent study, significant increases in AVP mRNA in the parvocellular neurons of the PVN was explored in maternally separated mice (Murgatroyd et al. 2009). Within the AVP gene, there are four regions rich in CpG islands that may regulate gene expression through DNA methylation. Analysis of PVN tissue indicated that at one of the four regions (CGI3), maternally separated males have significantly reduced DNA methylation

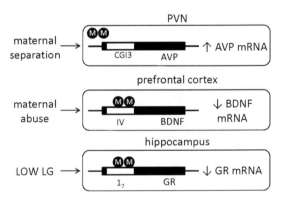

Fig. 10.2 Epigenetic effects of postnatal environmental experiences. In rodents, postnatal maternal separation is associated with decreased DNA methylation within the AVP promoter region leading to increased AVP mRNA in the PVN (Murgatroyd et al. 2009), whereas maternal abuse is associated with increased methylation within the BDNF promoter in the prefrontal cortex leading to decreased BDNF expression (Roth et al. 2009) and the experience of low levels of LG in infancy is associated with increased methylation in the GR promoter region leading to decreased hippocampal GR expression (Weaver et al. 2004)

compared with control males at 6 weeks, 3 months, and 1 year of age. Furthermore, this hypomethylation was significantly correlated with increased mRNA expression, and these effects were brain region-specific as no changes in AVP mRNA or DNA methylation were found between maternally separated and control males in the supraoptic nucleus (SON). Analysis of the time course of the molecular changes involved in this differential methylation suggests that short-term activation of MeCP2 may be critical within the pathways leading to AVP hypomethylation and increased AVP mRNA levels within the PVN (Murgatroyd et al. 2009). Conversely, in response to brief maternal separation (handling), reductions in CRH mRNA in the parvocellular neurons of the PVN can be observed as early as PN9 (Korosi et al. 2010). Within the regulatory region of the CRH gene, there is a binding element for the repressor neuron-restrictive silencer factor (NRSF) (Seth and Majzoub 2001). This factor recruits cofactors and other enzymes/proteins involved in epigenetic regulation leading to the repression of gene expression (Zheng et al. 2009). Among handled offspring, protein levels of NRSF are dramatically higher in PVN tissue at PN9 and throughout adulthood, suggesting a possible mechanism for the initiation and maintenance of reduced CRH gene expression in response to handling-induced stimulation of mother–infant interactions.

Natural variations in postnatal maternal LG in the rat are associated with changes in numerous receptor pathways, with effects on hippocampal GR being implicated in the high levels of HPA reactivity observed among offspring of Low LG dams (Liu et al. 1997). Analysis of the GR 1_7 promoter region suggests that low levels of LG are associated with increased GR 1_7 methylation, decreased GR expression and an increased HPA response to stress. Time course analysis has indicated that these maternally induced epigenetic profiles emerge during the postnatal period and are sustained into adulthood (Weaver et al. 2004). The pathways through which these effects are achieved are currently being elucidated and it appears likely that maternal LG mediated up-regulation of nerve growth factor-inducible protein A (NGFI-A) in infancy may be critical to activating GR transcription and maintaining low levels of DNA methylation within the GR 1_7 promoter among the offspring of High LG dams (Weaver et al. 2007). These experience-dependent shifts in epigenetic regulation of target genes within HPA stress pathways have also been observed to emerge prenatally in response to maternal exposure to chronic variable stress. Male offspring of mice exposed to gestational stress have decreased DNA methylation of the CRH gene promoter and increased methylation of the GR exon 1_7 promoter region in hypothalamic tissue (Mueller and Bale 2008). These epigenetic modifications are associated with exposure to stress during the early stages of prenatal development and may involve dysregulation of placental gene expression. These findings complement studies in humans illustrating that methylation status of the GR promoter, particularly at the NGFI-A-binding site, in cord blood mononuclear cells of infants is associated with exposure to third trimester maternal depressed mood. Maternal depression was found to be associated with increased GR 1F promoter methylation in fetal blood samples and these methylation patterns predicted HPA reactivity in infants at 3 months of age (Oberlander et al. 2008). The susceptibility of HPA responses to social modulation suggests that genes within these stress-sensitive pathways may be the target of epigenetic dysregulation associated with many forms of early life adversity.

10.1.4 Beyond Infancy: Epigenetic Effects of Juvenile and Adult Social Experiences

Although social modulation of brain and behavior has been primarily explored in response to early social experiences, and in particular, mother–infant interactions, there continues to be plasticity in response to social experiences occurring during juvenile development and into adulthood. Social isolation during the postweaning period has generally been found to increase anxiety-like responses, though this may not involve the same neuroendocrine pathways targeted by earlier social experiences (Francis et al. 2002a; Lukkes et al. 2009). In rodents, postweaning social isolation has been associated with decreased expression of several 5-HT receptor subtypes in the prefrontal cortex, hypothalamus, and midbrain (Bibancos et al. 2007); latent elevations in DA levels in the NAc (Shao et al. 2009); reduced GABAA/CBZ receptor binding (Insel 1989; Miachon et al. 1990); decreased neuronal plasticity associated with glutamatergic hypofunction (Lu et al. 2003; Silva-Gomez et al. 2003; Stranahan et al. 2006); and sex-specific effects on the numbers of OT-positive neurons in the PVN (Grippo et al. 2007a, b). This cascade of neuroendocrine changes is associated with a phenotype referred to as an "isolation syndrome," which can be attenuated by treatment with antidepressants (Heritch et al. 1990). In contrast, juvenile environmental enrichment (typically involving both physical and social environmental complexity) in rodents attenuates the HPA response to stress with a concomitant decrease in basal corticosterone levels (Belz et al. 2003), and there is evidence for enrichment-induced elevations in hippocampal NGFI-A and GR (Olsson et al. 1994). In addition, social enrichment during juvenile development is associated with increased levels of the DAT within the NAc (Zakharova et al. 2009), increased GAD enzyme activity and extracellular GABA concentrations within the hippocampus (Frick et al. 2003; Segovia et al. 2006), increased AMPA receptor expression in the hippocampus (Bredy et al. 2003, 2004), and elevated OTR binding in a number of forebrain and hypothalamic areas including the central nucleus of the amygdala (Champagne and Meaney 2007). The social enrichment paradigm has been used to reverse deficits associated with pre- and postnatal environmental exposures (Francis et al. 2002a; Laviola et al. 2004; Morley-Fletcher et al. 2003) and augment phenotypes associated with targeted genetic manipulations (Jankowsky et al. 2005; van Dellen et al. 2000). Interestingly, recovery of memory deficits induced through p25-mediated neuronal loss can be achieved through exposure to complex housing environments and this enrichment is associated with increased histone (H3 and H4) acetylation in the hippocampus and cortex (Fischer et al. 2007). Moreover, treatment with histone deacetylase inhibitors can mimic the effects of environmental enrichment on learning and synaptic plasticity. These findings suggest the role of epigenetic mechanisms in shifting gene expression and behavior at these later stages of development.

In adulthood, chronic social defeat has been used to illustrate the continued influence of social experiences on neurobiological outcomes. This form of social stress, in which an individual has prolonged exposure to agonistic behavioral encounters, is associated with disruptions in social and emotional responding (Keeney and Hogg 1999). In adulthood, even a single social defeat is associated with prolonged alterations to the HPA stress response and changes to the expression of CRH receptors (Buwalda et al. 1999; Cooper and Huhman 2007). Social defeat results in transient changes in GABA receptor levels in cortex, cerebellum, and hypothalamus (Miller et al. 1987); increases in NMDA and decreases in AMPA receptor binding in the hippocampus (Krugers et al. 1993); and increases in expression of AVP mRNA in the PVN (Erhardt et al. 2009). Exploration of the epigenetic pathways linking the experience of social defeat to the behavioral phenotype that emerges in response to this adult social stressor has focused primarily on BDNF, which serves as a trophic factor that is a common downstream mediator of the effects of the multiple neurotransmitter and neuropeptide systems. BNDF gene expression is significantly decreased in the hippocampus of socially defeated male mice and this effect appears to be mediated by specific decreases in the BDNF III and IV transcripts (Tsankova et al. 2006). These effects are observed a month following exposure to the social stress, indicating a persistent effect on gene expression. Chromatin immunoprecipitation (ChIP) analysis indicates increased histone H3-K27 dimethylation at the BDNF III and IV promoters among socially defeated males, which may account for the reduced BDNF expression. Histone deacetylase (HDAC5) mRNA levels are also found to be decreased in socially defeated males (Tsankova et al. 2006) and HDAC5 appears to be important in mediating the effects of antidepressant treatment in males exposed to chronic social stress (Renthal et al. 2007). The differential levels of histone H3-K27 dimethylation are also found across the genome within the NAc, both in response to chronic social defeat and prolonged adult social isolation (Wilkinson et al. 2009). Analysis of histone acetylation in the NAc indicates that H3-K14 acetylation is initially decreased and then increased following chronic social defeat associated with decreases in HDAC2 levels. These studies suggest that though there is plasticity beyond the postnatal period, and that epigenetic mechanisms are responsive to juvenile and adult social experiences, dynamic histone modifications may be more evident in response to these later life experiences.

10.1.5   Transgenerational Epigenetic Effects

Although use of the term "epigenetic" has its origin in the study of development and the notion that divergent gene activity plays a critical role in phenotypic variation, more recent conceptualizations of "epigenetic" are derived from the root "genetic" meaning the study of the units of heritable material (Jablonka and Lamb 2002). The notion that meiotic inheritance can be considered outside the realm of the DNA sequence is an area of growing philosophical and scientific interest, and there are two distinct pathways via which epigenetic modifications are currently believed to be involved in the transmission of traits across generations. The first pathway, often referred to as epigenetic inheritance, involves incorporation of an epigenetic mark into the DNA which is then transmitted and perpetuated in subsequent generations through the germline (Morgan et al. 1999). The second pathway builds on the role of experience-dependent epigenetic modifications in developmental plasticity illustrated in the previous sections. Through these pathways, DNA methylation has been demonstrated to play a critical role in the transgenerational impact of early life experiences. The role of social experiences in shaping transgenerational effects is associated with experience-depended changes in the activity of genes that will, in adulthood, alter the reproductive behavior of females, leading to variations in the quantity and quality of mother–infant interactions (Champagne 2008). Natural variations in postnatal maternal care have been associated with altered gene expression and receptor levels within the MPOA, a brain region that is critical for maternal behavior (Fleming 1986). Females reared by Low LG dams have a reduced sensitivity to estrogen-mediated increases in neuronal activation within the MPOA (Champagne et al. 2001, 2003b) and analysis of levels of ERα in the offspring of High and Low LG dams suggest that differences in estrogen sensitivity are mediated by variations in ERα levels such that expression of ERα in the MPOA of both lactating and nonlactating female offspring of Low LG dams is significantly reduced (Champagne et al. 2003b). Analysis of levels of DNA methylation within the 1B promoter region of the ERα gene in MPOA tissue indicates that the experience of High LG is associated with decreased promoter methylation, whereas Low LG is associated with increased promoter methylation, leading to reduced gene expression and an attenuated response to hormonally primed behaviors (Champagne et al. 2006). ChIP assays demonstrate that this differential DNA methylation has consequences for the binding of transcription factors such as STAT5a to the 1B promoter. Maternal LG is associated with increased levels of STAT5a during the postnatal period and the increased levels of this factor may lead to sustained activation of transcription and reduced DNA methylation (Champagne et al. 2006). As a consequence of these epigenetic modifications, individual differences in maternal LG are transmitted from mother to offspring (F1 generation) and to grand-offspring (F2 generation) (Champagne and Meaney 2007; Champagne 2008). A similar experience-dependent transmission of behavior is observed in response to exposure to abuse. Female rat pups exposed to abusive caregiving in infancy engage in abusive caregiving toward their own offspring and F2 offspring of these F1 females have elevated levels of methylation within the BDNF promoter in the PFC and hippocampus (Roth et al. 2009). Interestingly, postnatal cross-fostering of F2 females to nonabusive dams did not reverse these epigenetic effects, suggesting that there may be prenatal factors that contribute to the generational transmission of altered DNA methylation patterns. The transgenerational inheritance of stable individual differences in behavior, mediated through epigenetic mechanisms, provides an alternative route of inheritance of phenotype that may allow for the environmental conditions and social experiences of previous generations to influence development.

10.1.6   Concluding Remarks

Development occurs within a social context and there is increasing evidence that epigenetic mechanisms may play a critical role in linking experiences to long-term neurobiological changes. Although much of the evidence supporting the hypotheses that DNA methylation and histone modifications are altered by the social environment has come from studies in rodents, translational studies are emerging, which suggest that, for example, the experience of abuse in infancy can lead to epigenetic variation in the human brain (McGowan et al. 2008, 2009). Thus, the animal models of abuse, neglect, and variation in parental care that have been used to study social modulation of the developing brain can continue to inform and inspire hypothesis-driven epigenetic research in humans. Given the brain region specificity of many of the gene expression changes that have been observed in these models, one critical question that must be addressed relates to the ability to predict epigenetic changes in the brain using peripheral markers of transcriptional activity measured in blood lymphocytes. Establishing this relationship will enable the application of an epigenetic approach to longitudinal studies in humans where in vivo changes in DNA methylation and histone modifications can be associated with variations in social experience. In addition, the plasticity of the epigenome in response to both behavioral and pharmacological intervention in later life that has been observed in rodent studies (Roth et al. 2009; Weaver et al. 2004, 2005) may provide a novel therapeutic approach to the treatment of disorders related to early life adversity. The dynamic yet stable nature of epigenetic variation may be a critical feature of both within- and across-generation individual differences in phenotype that expand our concept of the origins of variation in brain and behavior.

Acknowledgment   This work was supported by Grant Number DP2OD001674 from the Office of the Director, National Institutes of Health.

References

Ahern TH, Young LJ (2009) The impact of early life family structure on adult social attachment, alloparental behavior, and the neuropeptide systems regulating affiliative behaviors in the monogamous prairie vole (*Microtus ochrogaster*). Front Behav Neurosci 3:17

Arborelius L, Eklund MB (2007) Both long and brief maternal separation produces persistent changes in tissue levels of brain monoamines in middle-aged female rats. Neuroscience 145:738–750

Barr CS, Newman TK, Lindell S, Becker ML, Shannon C, Champoux M, Suomi SJ, Higley JD (2004) Early experience and sex interact to influence limbic-hypothalamic-pituitary-adrenal-axis function after acute alcohol administration in rhesus macaques (*Macaca mulatta*). Alcohol Clin Exp Res 28:1114–1119

Beckett C, Bredenkamp D, Castle J, Groothues C, O'Connor TG, Rutter M (2002) Behavior patterns associated with institutional deprivation: a study of children adopted from Romania. J Dev Behav Pediatr 23:297–303

Bellinger FP, Davidson MS, Bedi KS, Wilce PA (2006) Ethanol prevents NMDA receptor reduction by maternal separation in neonatal rat hippocampus. Brain Res 1067:154–157

Belz EE, Kennell JS, Czambel RK, Rubin RT, Rhodes ME (2003) Environmental enrichment lowers stress-responsive hormones in singly housed male and female rats. Pharmacol Biochem Behav 76:481–486

Berman C (1990) Intergenerational transmission of maternal rejection rates among free-ranging rheus monkeys on Cayo Santiago. Anim Behav 44:247–258

Bibancos T, Jardim DL, Aneas I, Chiavegatto S (2007) Social isolation and expression of serotonergic neurotransmission-related genes in several brain areas of male mice. Genes Brain Behav 6:529–539

Bodnoff SR, Suranyi-Cadotte B, Quirion R, Meaney MJ (1987) Postnatal handling reduces novelty-induced fear and increases [3H]flunitrazepam binding in rat brain. Eur J Pharmacol 144:105–107

Brake WG, Zhang TY, Diorio J, Meaney MJ, Gratton A (2004) Influence of early postnatal rearing conditions on mesocorticolimbic dopamine and behavioural responses to psychostimulants and stressors in adult rats. Eur J Neurosci 19:1863–1874

Branchi I (2009) The mouse communal nest: investigating the epigenetic influences of the early social environment on brain and behavior development. Neurosci Biobehav Rev 33:551–559

Branchi I, Alleva E (2006) Communal nesting, an early social enrichment, increases the adult anxiety-like response and shapes the role of social context in modulating the emotional behavior. Behav Brain Res 172:299–306

Branchi I, D'Andrea I, Fiore M, Di Fausto V, Aloe L, Alleva E (2006a) Early social enrichment shapes social behavior and nerve growth factor and brain-derived neurotrophic factor levels in the adult mouse brain. Biol Psychiatry 60:690–696

Branchi I, D'Andrea I, Sietzema J, Fiore M, Di Fausto V, Aloe L, Alleva E (2006b) Early social enrichment augments adult hippocampal BDNF levels and survival of BrdU-positive cells while increasing anxiety- and "depression"-like behavior. J Neurosci Res 83:965–973

Branchi I, D'Andrea I, Cirulli F, Lipp HP, Alleva E (2009) Shaping brain development: mouse communal nesting blunts adult neuroendocrine and behavioral response to social stress and modifies chronic antidepressant treatment outcome. Psychoneuroendocrinology 35:743–751

Bredy TW, Humpartzoomian RA, Cain DP, Meaney MJ (2003) Partial reversal of the effect of maternal care on cognitive function through environmental enrichment. Neuroscience 118:571–576

Bredy TW, Zhang TY, Grant RJ, Diorio J, Meaney MJ (2004) Peripubertal environmental enrichment reverses the effects of maternal care on hippocampal development and glutamate receptor subunit expression. Eur J Neurosci 20:1355–1362

Bredy TW, Brown RE, Meaney MJ (2007) Effect of resource availability on biparental care, and offspring neural and behavioral development in the California mouse (*Peromyscus californicus*). Eur J Neurosci 25:567–575

Burton CL, Chatterjee D, Chatterjee-Chakraborty M, Lovic V, Grella SL, Steiner M, Fleming AS (2007) Prenatal restraint stress and motherless rearing disrupts expression of plasticity markers and stress-induced corticosterone release in adult female Sprague-Dawley rats. Brain Res 1158:28–38

Buwalda B, de Boer SF, Schmidt ED, Felszeghy K, Nyakas C, Sgoifo A, Van der Vegt BJ, Tilders FJ, Bohus B, Koolhaas JM (1999) Long-lasting deficient dexamethasone suppression of hypothalamic-pituitary-adrenocortical activation following peripheral CRF challenge in socially defeated rats. J Neuroendocrinol 11:513–520

Caldji C, Francis D, Sharma S, Plotsky PM, Meaney MJ (2000) The effects of early rearing environment on the development of GABAA and central benzodiazepine receptor levels and novelty-induced fearfulness in the rat. Neuropsychopharmacology 22:219–229

Caldji C, Diorio J, Meaney MJ (2003) Variations in maternal care alter GABA(A) receptor subunit expression in brain regions associated with fear. Neuropsychopharmacology 28:1950–1959

Caldji C, Diorio J, Anisman H, Meaney MJ (2004) Maternal behavior regulates benzodiazepine/ GABAA receptor subunit expression in brain regions associated with fear in BALB/c and C57BL/6 mice. Neuropsychopharmacology 29:1344–1352

Carlson EA (1998) A prospective longitudinal study of attachment disorganization/disorientation. Child Dev 69:1107–1128

Carlson EA, Egeland B, Sroufe LA (2009) A prospective investigation of the development of borderline personality symptoms. Dev Psychopathol 21:1311–1334

Carroll KA, Maestripieri D (1998) Infant abuse and neglect in monkeys–a discussion of definitions, epidemiology, etiology, and implications for child maltreatment: reply to Cicchetti (1998) and Mason (1998). Psychol Bull 123:234–237

Champagne FA (2008) Epigenetic mechanisms and the transgenerational effects of maternal care. Front Neuroendocrinol 29:386–397

Champagne FA, Meaney MJ (2006) Stress during gestation alters postpartum maternal care and the development of the offspring in a rodent model. Biol Psychiatry 59:1227–1235

Champagne FA, Meaney MJ (2007) Transgenerational effects of social environment on variations in maternal care and behavioral response to novelty. Behav Neurosci 121:1353–1363

Champagne F, Diorio J, Sharma S, Meaney MJ (2001) Naturally occurring variations in maternal behavior in the rat are associated with differences in estrogen-inducible central oxytocin receptors. Proc Natl Acad Sci USA 98:12736–12741

Champagne FA, Francis DD, Mar A, Meaney MJ (2003a) Variations in maternal care in the rat as a mediating influence for the effects of environment on development. Physiol Behav 79:359–371

Champagne FA, Weaver IC, Diorio J, Sharma S, Meaney MJ (2003b) Natural variations in maternal care are associated with estrogen receptor alpha expression and estrogen sensitivity in the medial preoptic area. Endocrinology 144:4720–4724

Champagne FA, Weaver IC, Diorio J, Dymov S, Szyf M, Meaney MJ (2006) Maternal care associated with methylation of the estrogen receptor-alpha1b promoter and estrogen receptor-alpha expression in the medial preoptic area of female offspring. Endocrinology 147:2909–2915

Champagne FA, Curley JP, Keverne EB, Bateson PP (2007) Natural variations in postpartum maternal care in inbred and outbred mice. Physiol Behav 91:325–334

Chugani HT, Behen ME, Muzik O, Juhasz C, Nagy F, Chugani DC (2001) Local brain functional activity following early deprivation: a study of postinstitutionalized Romanian orphans. Neuroimage 14:1290–1301

Cooper MA, Huhman KL (2007) Corticotropin-releasing factor receptors in the dorsal raphe nucleus modulate social behavior in Syrian hamsters. Psychopharmacology (Berl) 194:297–307

Coplan JD, Rosenblum LA, Gorman JM (1995) Primate models of anxiety. Longitudinal perspectives. Psychiatr Clin North Am 18:727–743

Coplan JD, Trost RC, Owens MJ, Cooper TB, Gorman JM, Nemeroff CB, Rosenblum LA (1998) Cerebrospinal fluid concentrations of somatostatin and biogenic amines in grown primates reared by mothers exposed to manipulated foraging conditions. Arch Gen Psychiatry 55:473–477

Coplan JD, Smith EL, Altemus M, Scharf BA, Owens MJ, Nemeroff CB, Gorman JM, Rosenblum LA (2001) Variable foraging demand rearing: sustained elevations in cisternal cerebrospinal fluid corticotropin-releasing factor concentrations in adult primates. Biol Psychiatry 50: 200–204

Coplan JD, Altemus M, Mathew SJ, Smith EL, Sharf B, Coplan PM, Kral JG, Gorman JM, Owens MJ, Nemeroff CB, Rosenblum LA (2005) Synchronized maternal-infant elevations of primate CSF CRF concentrations in response to variable foraging demand. CNS Spectr 10:530–536

Coplan JD, Smith EL, Altemus M, Mathew SJ, Perera T, Kral JG, Gorman JM, Owens MJ, Nemeroff CB, Rosenblum LA (2006) Maternal-infant response to variable foraging demand in nonhuman primates: effects of timing of stressor on cerebrospinal fluid corticotropin-releasing factor and circulating glucocorticoid concentrations. Ann NY Acad Sci 1071:525–533

Coutellier L, Friedrich AC, Failing K, Marashi V, Wurbel H (2009) Effects of foraging demand on maternal behaviour and adult offspring anxiety and stress response in C57BL/6 mice. Behav Brain Res 196:192–199

Curley JP, Davidson S, Bateson P, Champagne FA (2009) Social enrichment during postnatal development induces transgenerational effects on emotional and reproductive behavior in mice. Front Behav Neurosci 3:25

Erhardt A, Muller MB, Rodel A, Welt T, Ohl F, Holsboer F, Keck ME (2009) Consequences of chronic social stress on behaviour and vasopressin gene expression in the PVN of DBA/2OlaHsd mice–influence of treatment with the CRHR1-antagonist R121919/NBI 30775. J Psychopharmacol 23:31–39

Fairbanks LA, McGuire MT (1988) Long-term effects of early mothering behavior on responsiveness to the environment in vervet monkeys. Dev Psychobiol 21:711–724

Fan G, Hutnick L (2005) Methyl-CpG binding proteins in the nervous system. Cell Res 15:255–261

Feng J, Fouse S, Fan G (2007) Epigenetic regulation of neural gene expression and neuronal function. Pediatr Res 61:58R–63R

Fischer A, Sananbenesi F, Wang X, Dobbin M, Tsai LH (2007) Recovery of learning and memory is associated with chromatin remodelling. Nature 447:178–182

Fleming A (1986) Psychobiology of rat maternal behavior: how and where hormones act to promote maternal behavior at parturition. Ann NY Acad Sci 474:234–251

Francis D, Diorio J, Liu D, Meaney MJ (1999) Nongenomic transmission across generations of maternal behavior and stress responses in the rat. Science 286:1155–1158

Francis DD, Champagne FC, Meaney MJ (2000) Variations in maternal behaviour are associated with differences in oxytocin receptor levels in the rat. J Neuroendocrinol 12:1145–1148

Francis DD, Diorio J, Plotsky PM, Meaney MJ (2002a) Environmental enrichment reverses the effects of maternal separation on stress reactivity. J Neurosci 22:7840–7843

Francis DD, Young LJ, Meaney MJ, Insel TR (2002b) Naturally occurring differences in maternal care are associated with the expression of oxytocin and vasopressin (V1a) receptors: gender differences. J Neuroendocrinol 14:349–353

Frick KM, Stearns NA, Pan JY, Berger-Sweeney J (2003) Effects of environmental enrichment on spatial memory and neurochemistry in middle-aged mice. Learn Mem 10:187–198

Fries AB, Ziegler TE, Kurian JR, Jacoris S, Pollak SD (2005) Early experience in humans is associated with changes in neuropeptides critical for regulating social behavior. Proc Natl Acad Sci USA 102:17237–17240

Fries AB, Shirtcliff EA, Pollak SD (2008) Neuroendocrine dysregulation following early social deprivation in children. Dev Psychobiol 50:588–599

Fukuda S, Taga T (2005) Cell fate determination regulated by a transcriptional signal network in the developing mouse brain. Anat Sci Int 80:12–18

Gerra G, Leonardi C, Cortese E, Zaimovic A, Dell'Agnello G, Manfredini M, Somaini L, Petracca F, Caretti V, Baroni C, Donnini C (2008) Adrenocorticotropic hormone and cortisol plasma levels directly correlate with childhood neglect and depression measures in addicted patients. Addict Biol 13:95–104

Gorman JM, Mathew S, Coplan J (2002) Neurobiology of early life stress: nonhuman primate models. Semin Clin Neuropsychiatry 7:96–103

Grassi-Oliveira R, Stein LM, Lopes RP, Teixeira AL, Bauer ME (2008) Low plasma brain-derived neurotrophic factor and childhood physical neglect are associated with verbal memory impairment in major depression – a preliminary report. Biol Psychiatry 64:281–285

Grippo AJ, Cushing BS, Carter CS (2007a) Depression-like behavior and stressor-induced neuroendocrine activation in female prairie voles exposed to chronic social isolation. Psychosom Med 69:149–157

Grippo AJ, Gerena D, Huang J, Kumar N, Shah M, Ughreja R, Carter CS (2007b) Social isolation induces behavioral and neuroendocrine disturbances relevant to depression in female and male prairie voles. Psychoneuroendocrinology 32:966–980

Hall WG (1975) Weaning and growth of artificially reared rats. Science 190:1313–1315

Harlow HF, Dodsworth RO, Harlow MK (1965) Total social isolation in monkeys. Proc Natl Acad Sci USA 54:90–97

Heritch AJ, Henderson K, Westfall TC (1990) Effects of social isolation on brain catecholamines and forced swimming in rats: prevention by antidepressant treatment. J Psychiatr Res 24:251–258

Ichise M, Vines DC, Gura T, Anderson GM, Suomi SJ, Higley JD, Innis RB (2006) Effects of early life stress on [11C]DASB positron emission tomography imaging of serotonin transporters in adolescent peer- and mother-reared rhesus monkeys. J Neurosci 26:4638–4643

Insel TR (1989) Decreased in vivo binding to brain benzodiazepine receptors during social isolation. Psychopharmacology (Berl) 97:142–144

Jablonka E, Lamb MJ (2002) The changing concept of epigenetics. Ann NY Acad Sci 981:82–96

Jankowsky JL, Melnikova T, Fadale DJ, Xu GM, Slunt HH, Gonzales V, Younkin LH, Younkin SG, Borchelt DR, Savonenko AV (2005) Environmental enrichment mitigates cognitive deficits in a mouse model of Alzheimer's disease. J Neurosci 25:5217–5224

Johnson JG, Cohen P, Brown J, Smailes EM, Bernstein DP (1999) Childhood maltreatment increases risk for personality disorders during early adulthood. Arch Gen Psychiatry 56:600–606

Keeney AJ, Hogg S (1999) Behavioural consequences of repeated social defeat in the mouse: preliminary evaluation of a potential animal model of depression. Behav Pharmacol 10:753–764

Korosi A, Baram TZ (2009) The pathways from mother's love to baby's future. Front Behav Neurosci 3:27

Korosi A, Shanabrough M, McClelland S, Liu ZW, Borok E, Gao XB, Horvath TL, Baram TZ (2010) Early-life experience reduces excitation to stress-responsive hypothalamic neurons and reprograms the expression of corticotropin-releasing hormone. J Neurosci 30:703–713

Krugers HJ, Koolhaas JM, Bohus B, Korf J (1993) A single social stress-experience alters glutamate receptor-binding in rat hippocampal CA3 area. Neurosci Lett 154:73–77

Ladd CO, Huot RL, Thrivikraman KV, Nemeroff CB, Plotsky PM (2004) Long-term adaptations in glucocorticoid receptor and mineralocorticoid receptor mRNA and negative feedback on the hypothalamo-pituitary-adrenal axis following neonatal maternal separation. Biol Psychiatry 55:367–375

Laviola G, Rea M, Morley-Fletcher S, Di Carlo S, Bacosi A, De Simone R, Bertini M, Pacifici R (2004) Beneficial effects of enriched environment on adolescent rats from stressed pregnancies. Eur J Neurosci 20:1655–1664

Law AJ, Pei Q, Feldon J, Pryce CR, Harrison PJ (2009a) Gene expression in the anterior cingulate cortex and amygdala of adolescent marmoset monkeys following parental separations in infancy. Int J Neuropsychopharmacol 12:761–772

Law AJ, Pei Q, Walker M, Gordon-Andrews H, Weickert CS, Feldon J, Pryce CR, Harrison PJ (2009b) Early parental deprivation in the marmoset monkey produces long-term changes in hippocampal expression of genes involved in synaptic plasticity and implicated in mood disorder. Neuropsychopharmacology 34:1381–1394

Lee RJ, Gollan J, Kasckow J, Geracioti T, Coccaro EF (2006) CSF corticotropin-releasing factor in personality disorder: relationship with self-reported parental care. Neuropsychopharmacology 31:2289–2295

Lehmann J, Pryce CR, Bettschen D, Feldon J (1999) The maternal separation paradigm and adult emotionality and cognition in male and female Wistar rats. Pharmacol Biochem Behav 64:705–715

Levine S (1957) Infantile experience and resistance to physiological stress. Science 126:405

Lillycrop KA, Slater-Jefferies JL, Hanson MA, Godfrey KM, Jackson AA, Burdge GC (2007) Induction of altered epigenetic regulation of the hepatic glucocorticoid receptor in the offspring of rats fed a protein-restricted diet during pregnancy suggests that reduced DNA methyltransferase-1 expression is involved in impaired DNA methylation and changes in histone modifications. Br J Nutr 97:1064–1073

Lillycrop KA, Phillips ES, Torrens C, Hanson MA, Jackson AA, Burdge GC (2008) Feeding pregnant rats a protein-restricted diet persistently alters the methylation of specific cytosines in the hepatic PPAR alpha promoter of the offspring. Br J Nutr 100:278–282

Liu D, Diorio J, Tannenbaum B, Caldji C, Francis D, Freedman A, Sharma S, Pearson D, Plotsky
    PM, Meaney MJ (1997) Maternal care, hippocampal glucocorticoid receptors, and hypotha-
    lamic-pituitary-adrenal responses to stress. Science 277:1659–1662
Liu D, Diorio J, Day JC, Francis DD, Meaney MJ (2000) Maternal care, hippocampal synaptogen-
    esis and cognitive development in rats. Nat Neurosci 3:799–806
Lovic V, Fleming AS (2004) Artificially-reared female rats show reduced prepulse inhibition and
    deficits in the attentional set shifting task–reversal of effects with maternal-like licking
    stimulation. Behav Brain Res 148:209–219
Lovic V, Gonzalez A, Fleming AS (2001) Maternally separated rats show deficits in maternal care
    in adulthood. Dev Psychobiol 39:19–33
Lu L, Bao G, Chen H, Xia P, Fan X, Zhang J, Pei G, Ma L (2003) Modification of hippocampal
    neurogenesis and neuroplasticity by social environments. Exp Neurol 183:600–609
Lukas M, Bredewold R, Neumann ID, Veenema AH (2010) Maternal separation interferes with
    developmental changes in brain vasopressin and oxytocin receptor binding in male rats.
    Neuropharmacology 58:78–87
Lukkes JL, Watt MJ, Lowry CA, Forster GL (2009) Consequences of post-weaning social
    isolation on anxiety behavior and related neural circuits in rodents. Front Behav Neurosci 3:18
Lupien SJ, McEwen BS, Gunnar MR, Heim C (2009) Effects of stress throughout the lifespan on
    the brain, behaviour and cognition. Nat Rev Neurosci 10:434–445
MacLean K (2003) The impact of institutionalization on child development. Dev Psychopathol
    15:853–884
Maestripieri D (1998) Parenting styles of abusive mothers in group-living rhesus macaques. Anim
    Behav 55:1–11
Maestripieri D, Lindell SG, Ayala A, Gold PW, Higley JD (2005) Neurobiological characteristics
    of rhesus macaque abusive mothers and their relation to social and maternal behavior. Neurosci
    Biobehav Rev 29:51–57
Maestripieri D, Higley JD, Lindell SG, Newman TK, McCormack KM, Sanchez MM (2006) Early
    maternal rejection affects the development of monoaminergic systems and adult abusive
    parenting in rhesus macaques (Macaca mulatta). Behav Neurosci 120:1017–1024
Mathew SJ, Shungu DC, Mao X, Smith EL, Perera GM, Kegeles LS, Perera T, Lisanby SH,
    Rosenblum LA, Gorman JM, Coplan JD (2003) A magnetic resonance spectroscopic imaging
    study of adult nonhuman primates exposed to early-life stressors. Biol Psychiatry 54:727–735
McCormack K, Sanchez MM, Bardi M, Maestripieri D (2006) Maternal care patterns and
    behavioral development of rhesus macaque abused infants in the first 6 months of life. Dev
    Psychobiol 48:537–550
McGowan PO, Sasaki A, Huang TC, Unterberger A, Suderman M, Ernst C, Meaney MJ, Turecki
    G, Szyf M (2008) Promoter-wide hypermethylation of the ribosomal RNA gene promoter in
    the suicide brain. PLoS ONE 3:e2085
McGowan PO, Sasaki A, D'Alessio AC, Dymov S, Labonte B, Szyf M, Turecki G, Meaney MJ
    (2009) Epigenetic regulation of the glucocorticoid receptor in human brain associates with
    childhood abuse. Nat Neurosci 12:342–348
McLeod J, Sinal CJ, Perrot-Sinal TS (2007) Evidence for non-genomic transmission of ecological
    information via maternal behavior in female rats. Genes Brain Behav 6:19–29
Meaney MJ (2001) Maternal care, gene expression, and the transmission of individual differences
    in stress reactivity across generations. Annu Rev Neurosci 24:1161–1192
Meaney MJ, Aitken DH (1985) The effects of early postnatal handling on hippocampal glucocor-
    ticoid receptor concentrations: temporal parameters. Brain Res 354:301–304
Meaney MJ, Aitken DH, Bodnoff SR, Iny LJ, Tatarewicz JE, Sapolsky RM (1985) Early postnatal
    handling alters glucocorticoid receptor concentrations in selected brain regions. Behav Neu-
    rosci 99:765–770
Meaney MJ, Aitken DH, Viau V, Sharma S, Sarrieau A (1989) Neonatal handling alters adreno-
    cortical negative feedback sensitivity and hippocampal type II glucocorticoid receptor binding
    in the rat. Neuroendocrinology 50:597–604

Meaney MJ, Mitchell JB, Aitken DH, Bhatnagar S, Bodnoff SR, Iny LJ, Sarrieau A (1991) The effects of neonatal handling on the development of the adrenocortical response to stress: implications for neuropathology and cognitive deficits in later life. Psychoneuroendocrinology 16:85–103

Mehta MA, Golembo NI, Nosarti C, Colvert E, Mota A, Williams SC, Rutter M, Sonuga-Barke EJ (2009) Amygdala, hippocampal and corpus callosum size following severe early institutional deprivation: the English and Romanian Adoptees study pilot. J Child Psychol Psychiatry 50:943–951

Miachon S, Manchon M, Fromentin JR, Buda M (1990) Isolation-induced changes in radioligand binding to benzodiazepine binding sites. Neurosci Lett 111:246–251

Miller LG, Thompson ML, Greenblatt DJ, Deutsch SI, Shader RI, Paul SM (1987) Rapid increase in brain benzodiazepine receptor binding following defeat stress in mice. Brain Res 414:395–400

Moore CL, Power KL (1986) Prenatal stress affects mother-infant interaction in Norway rats. Dev Psychobiol 19:235–245

Morgan HD, Sutherland HG, Martin DI, Whitelaw E (1999) Epigenetic inheritance at the agouti locus in the mouse. Nat Genet 23:314–318

Morley-Fletcher S, Rea M, Maccari S, Laviola G (2003) Environmental enrichment during adolescence reverses the effects of prenatal stress on play behaviour and HPA axis reactivity in rats. Eur J Neurosci 18:3367–3374

Mueller BR, Bale TL (2008) Sex-specific programming of offspring emotionality after stress early in pregnancy. J Neurosci 28:9055–9065

Murgatroyd C, Wigger A, Frank E, Singewald N, Bunck M, Holsboer F, Landgraf R, Spengler D (2004) Impaired repression at a vasopressin promoter polymorphism underlies overexpression of vasopressin in a rat model of trait anxiety. J Neurosci 24:7762–7770

Murgatroyd C, Patchev AV, Wu Y, Micale V, Bockmuhl Y, Fischer D, Holsboer F, Wotjak CT, Almeida OF, Spengler D (2009) Dynamic DNA methylation programs persistent adverse effects of early-life stress. Nat Neurosci 12:1559–1566

Narita K, Takei Y, Suda M, Aoyama Y, Uehara T, Kosaka H, Amanuma M, Fukuda M, Mikuni M (2010) Relationship of parental bonding styles with gray matter volume of dorsolateral prefrontal cortex in young adults. Prog Neuropsychopharmacol Biol Psychiatry 34:624–631

Neigh GN, Gillespie CF, Nemeroff CB (2009) The neurobiological toll of child abuse and neglect. Trauma Violence Abuse 10:389–410

O'Connor TG, Rutter M (2000) Attachment disorder behavior following early severe deprivation: extension and longitudinal follow-up. English and Romanian Adoptees Study Team. J Am Acad Child Adolesc Psychiatry 39:703–712

O'Connor TG, Rutter M, Beckett C, Keaveney L, Kreppner JM (2000) The effects of global severe privation on cognitive competence: extension and longitudinal follow-up. English and Romanian adoptees study team. Child Dev 71:376–390

Oberlander TF, Weinberg J, Papsdorf M, Grunau R, Misri S, Devlin AM (2008) Prenatal exposure to maternal depression, neonatal methylation of human glucocorticoid receptor gene (NR3C1) and infant cortisol stress responses. Epigenetics 3:97–106

Ognibene E, Adriani W, Caprioli A, Ghirardi O, Ali SF, Aloe L, Laviola G (2008) The effect of early maternal separation on brain derived neurotrophic factor and monoamine levels in adult heterozygous reeler mice. Prog Neuropsychopharmacol Biol Psychiatry 32:1269–1276

Olsson T, Mohammed AH, Donaldson LF, Henriksson BG, Seckl JR (1994) Glucocorticoid receptor and NGFI-A gene expression are induced in the hippocampus after environmental enrichment in adult rats. Brain Res Mol Brain Res 23:349–353

Onishchenko N, Karpova N, Sabri F, Castren E, Ceccatelli S (2008) Long-lasting depression-like behavior and epigenetic changes of BDNF gene expression induced by perinatal exposure to methylmercury. J Neurochem 106:1378–1387

Parker G (1993) Parental rearing style: examining for links with personality vulnerability factors for depression. Soc Psychiatry Psychiatr Epidemiol 28:97–100

Parker G, Tupling H, Brown LB (1979) A parental bonding instrument. Br J Med Psychol 52:1–10

Peterson CL, Laniel MA (2004) Histones and histone modifications. Curr Biol 14:R546–R551

Pickering C, Gustafsson L, Cebere A, Nylander I, Liljequist S (2006) Repeated maternal separa-tion of male Wistar rats alters glutamate receptor expression in the hippocampus but not the prefrontal cortex. Brain Res 1099:101–108

Plotsky PM, Meaney MJ (1993) Early, postnatal experience alters hypothalamic corticotropin-releasing factor (CRF) mRNA, median eminence CRF content and stress-induced release in adult rats. Brain Res Mol Brain Res 18:195–200

Pruessner JC, Champagne F, Meaney MJ, Dagher A (2004) Dopamine release in response to a psychological stress in humans and its relationship to early life maternal care: a positron emission tomography study using [11C]raclopride. J Neurosci 24:2825–2831

Rao H, Betancourt L, Giannetta JM, Brodsky NL, Korczykowski M, Avants BB, Gee JC, Wang J, Hurt H, Detre JA, Farah MJ (2010) Early parental care is important for hippocampal matura-tion: evidence from brain morphology in humans. Neuroimage 49:1144–1150

Razin A (1998) CpG methylation, chromatin structure and gene silencing-a three-way connection. EMBO J 17:4905–4908

Renthal W, Maze I, Krishnan V, Covington HE 3rd, Xiao G, Kumar A, Russo SJ, Graham A, Tsankova N, Kippin TE, Kerstetter KA, Neve RL, Haggarty SJ, McKinsey TA, Bassel-Duby R, Olson EN, Nestler EJ (2007) Histone deacetylase 5 epigenetically controls behavioral adaptations to chronic emotional stimuli. Neuron 56:517–529

Roceri M, Hendriks W, Racagni G, Ellenbroek BA, Riva MA (2002) Early maternal deprivation reduces the expression of BDNF and NMDA receptor subunits in rat hippocampus. Mol Psychiatry 7:609–616

Rosenfeld P, Wetmore JB, Levine S (1992) Effects of repeated maternal separations on the adrenocortical response to stress of preweanling rats. Physiol Behav 52:787–791

Roth TL, Sullivan RM (2005) Memory of early maltreatment: neonatal behavioral and neural correlates of maternal maltreatment within the context of classical conditioning. Biol Psychia-try 57:823–831

Roth TL, Lubin FD, Funk AJ, Sweatt JD (2009) Lasting epigenetic influence of early-life adversity on the BDNF gene. Biol Psychiatry 65:760–769

Roy A (2002) Self-rated childhood emotional neglect and CSF monoamine indices in abstinent cocaine-abusing adults: possible implications for suicidal behavior. Psychiatry Res 112:69–75

Rutter M, O'Connor TG (2004) Are there biological programming effects for psychological development? Findings from a study of Romanian adoptees. Dev Psychol 40:81–94

Seay B, Harlow HF (1965) Maternal separation in the rhesus monkey. J Nerv Ment Dis 140:434–441

Segovia G, Yague AG, Garcia-Verdugo JM, Mora F (2006) Environmental enrichment promotes neurogenesis and changes the extracellular concentrations of glutamate and GABA in the hippocampus of aged rats. Brain Res Bull 70:8–14

Seth KA, Majzoub JA (2001) Repressor element silencing transcription factor/neuron-restrictive silencing factor (REST/NRSF) can act as an enhancer as well as a repressor of corticotropin-releasing hormone gene transcription. J Biol Chem 276:13917–13923

Shannon C, Schwandt ML, Champoux M, Shoaf SE, Suomi SJ, Linnoila M, Higley JD (2005) Maternal absence and stability of individual differences in CSF 5-HIAA concentrations in rhesus monkey infants. Am J Psychiatry 162:1658–1664

Shao F, Jin J, Meng Q, Liu M, Xie X, Lin W, Wang W (2009) Pubertal isolation alters latent inhibition and DA in nucleus accumbens of adult rats. Physiol Behav 98:251–257

Silva-Gomez AB, Rojas D, Juarez I, Flores G (2003) Decreased dendritic spine density on prefrontal cortical and hippocampal pyramidal neurons in postweaning social isolation rats. Brain Res 983:128–136

Spinelli S, Chefer S, Suomi SJ, Higley JD, Barr CS, Stein E (2009) Early-life stress induces long-term morphologic changes in primate brain. Arch Gen Psychiatry 66:658–665

Spinelli S, Chefer S, Carson RE, Jagoda E, Lang L, Heilig M, Barr CS, Suomi SJ, Higley JD, Stein EA (2010) Effects of early-life stress on serotonin(1A) receptors in juvenile rhesus monkeys measured by positron emission tomography. Biol Psychiatry 67:1146–1153

Sroufe LA (2005) Attachment and development: a prospective, longitudinal study from birth to adulthood. Attach Hum Dev 7:349–367

Sroufe LA, Carlson EA, Levy AK, Egeland B (1999) Implications of attachment theory for developmental psychopathology. Dev Psychopathol 11:1–13

Stranahan AM, Khalil D, Gould E (2006) Social isolation delays the positive effects of running on adult neurogenesis. Nat Neurosci 9:526–533

Suomi SJ (1991) Early stress and adult emotional reactivity in rhesus monkeys. Ciba Found Symp 156:171–183

Suomi SJ, Harlow HF, Kimball SD (1971) Behavioral effects of prolonged partial social isolation in the rhesus monkey. Psychol Rep 29:1171–1177

Trickett P, McBride-Chang C (1995) The developmental impact of different forms of child abuse and neglect. Dev Rev 15:11–37

Tsankova NM, Berton O, Renthal W, Kumar A, Neve RL, Nestler EJ (2006) Sustained hippocampal chromatin regulation in a mouse model of depression and antidepressant action. Nat Neurosci 9:519–525

Turner B (2001) Chromatin and gene regulation. Blackwell Science Ltd, Oxford

van Dellen A, Blakemore C, Deacon R, York D, Hannan AJ (2000) Delaying the onset of Huntington's in mice. Nature 404:721–722

Vazquez DM, Bailey C, Dent GW, Okimoto DK, Steffek A, Lopez JF, Levine S (2006) Brain corticotropin-releasing hormone (CRH) circuits in the developing rat: effect of maternal deprivation. Brain Res 1121:83–94

Veenema AH, Neumann ID (2007) Neurobiological mechanisms of aggression and stress coping: a comparative study in mouse and rat selection lines. Brain Behav Evol 70:274–285

Veenema AH, Blume A, Niederle D, Buwalda B, Neumann ID (2006) Effects of early life stress on adult male aggression and hypothalamic vasopressin and serotonin. Eur J Neurosci 24:1711–1720

Viau V, Sharma S, Plotsky PM, Meaney MJ (1993) Increased plasma ACTH responses to stress in nonhandled compared with handled rats require basal levels of corticosterone and are associated with increased levels of ACTH secretagogues in the median eminence. J Neurosci 13:1097–1005

Weaver IC, Cervoni N, Champagne FA, D'Alessio AC, Sharma S, Seckl JR, Dymov S, Szyf M, Meaney MJ (2004) Epigenetic programming by maternal behavior. Nat Neurosci 7:847–854

Weaver IC, Champagne FA, Brown SE, Dymov S, Sharma S, Meaney MJ, Szyf M (2005) Reversal of maternal programming of stress responses in adult offspring through methyl supplementation: altering epigenetic marking later in life. J Neurosci 25:11045–11054

Weaver IC, D'Alessio AC, Brown SE, Hellstrom IC, Dymov S, Sharma S, Szyf M, Meaney MJ (2007) The transcription factor nerve growth factor-inducible protein a mediates epigenetic programming: altering epigenetic marks by immediate-early genes. J Neurosci 27:1756–1768

Weizman R, Lehmann J, Leschiner S, Allmann I, Stoehr T, Heidbreder C, Domeney A, Feldon J, Gavish M (1999) Long-lasting effect of early handling on the peripheral benzodiazepine receptor. Pharmacol Biochem Behav 64:725–729

Wilkinson MB, Xiao G, Kumar A, LaPlant Q, Renthal W, Sikder D, Kodadek TJ, Nestler EJ (2009) Imipramine treatment and resiliency exhibit similar chromatin regulation in the mouse nucleus accumbens in depression models. J Neurosci 29:7820–7832

Winslow JT (2005) Neuropeptides and non-human primate social deficits associated with pathogenic rearing experience. Int J Dev Neurosci 23:245–251

Zakharova E, Miller J, Unterwald E, Wade D, Izenwasser S (2009) Social and physical environment alter cocaine conditioned place preference and dopaminergic markers in adolescent male rats. Neuroscience 163:890–897

Zhang Y, Reinberg D (2001) Transcription regulation by histone methylation: interplay between different covalent modifications of the core histone tails. Genes Dev 15:2343–2360

Zhang TY, Chretien P, Meaney MJ, Gratton A (2005) Influence of naturally occurring variations in maternal care on prepulse inhibition of acoustic startle and the medial prefrontal cortical dopamine response to stress in adult rats. J Neurosci 25:1493–1502

Zheng D, Zhao K, Mehler MF (2009) Profiling RE1/REST-mediated histone modifications in the human genome. Genome Biol 10:R9

Chapter 11
Toward an Understanding of the Dynamic Interdependence of Genes and Environment in the Regulation of Phenotype

Nurturing our Epigenetic Nature

Ian C.G. Weaver

Abstract Developmental plasticity refers to the potential for intraindividual change. Traditionally, the relationship between the human genome and the environment has been presented under the framework of gene–environment interactions. However, adaptive phenotypic plasticity emerges from more than just genotype. In humans and nonhuman primates, the nature of mother–infant interactions early in life has a profound role in mediating variation in offspring phenotype, including emotional and cognitive development, which is endured through life. One critical question: How is this "environmental programming" established and maintained in the offspring? Evidence from rodent studies suggests that maternal care in the first week of postnatal life establishes diverse and stable phenotypes in the offspring through epigenetic modification of genes expressed in the brain, which shape neuroendocrine and behavioral stress responsivity throughout life. This research demonstrates that the epigenetic state of a gene can be established through early in life experience and is potentially reversible in adulthood. These findings may well form the molecular basis for understanding potential mechanisms of environmental and developmental determinates of individual differences in human stress reactivity and health outcomes. Henceforth, epigenetic modifications of specific genomic regions in response to variations in environmental conditions might serve as a major source of variation in biological and behavioral phenotypes.

Keywords Chromatin · DNA methylation · Glucocorticoid receptor · Hippocampus · Maternal care · Stress · Transgenerational inheritance

I.C.G. Weaver
Krembil Family Epigenetics Laboratory, Department of Epigenetics, Centre for Addiction and Mental Health, 250 College Street, Toronto, ON M5T 1R8, Canada
e-mail: ian_weaver@camh.net

A. Petronis and J. Mill (eds.), *Brain, Behavior and Epigenetics*,   209
Epigenetics and Human Health, DOI 10.1007/978-3-642-17426-1_11,
© Springer-Verlag Berlin Heidelberg 2011

11.1 Early Life Development: Making an Intraindividual Difference

The study of development is an examination of adaptation and therein the biological basis of variation among alternative phenotypes. Phenotype is maintained through multifarious interactions between the dynamics of cellular-level function in response to intrinsic and extrinsic (environmental) cues. The cells of an organism contain the same genotype but are structurally, functionally, and phenotypically heterogeneous in response to different spatial and temporal regulation of gene expression profiles influencing multiple cellular functions including differentiation and morphogenesis (Baccarelli and Bollati 2009; Dempfle et al. 2008; Ishibe and Kelsey 1997; Kraft and Hunter 2005; London and Romieu 2009). The generation of different degrees of individual adaptive modification from a single genome in response to changes in the environment – either stochastic or predictable – forms the basis for "phenotypic plasticity", which is apparent across all froms of life.

In altricial species such as humans, the transition from embryo to adulthood is a lengthy process, and its evolutionary development has been long and complex (Saccheri and Hanski 2006). Embryonic development manifests as a series of changes in cellular programs that mark the transitions from the totipotent zygote to increasingly more differentiated cells with specialized morphology and function. As an individual progresses through prenatal (embryonic–fetal combined), neonatal, infancy, childhood, juvenile, puberty, adolescence, prime, and senescence – from dependency to increasing autonomy – physiological and neurodevelopmental systems continually receive, transform, and update information regarding the demands of the environment (Oli and Dobson 2003; Roff 2002). The physiological homeostatic set points of the internal environment of an individual are controlled by multiple systems (cytokines, growth factors, hormone secretion, and neurotransmitter release), and these interactions apply to the brain.

The stability of a child's early life conditions both before birth and in infancy has profound effects on their long-term physical and mental health outcomes. The relationship between the quality of early environment and long-term developmental programming appears to be mediated, in part, by the closeness or degree of positive attachment in parent–infant bonding and parental investment during early life (Canetti et al. 1997). Critical phases in early life are characterized by dynamic responses to chemical, biological, and physical stimuli (i.e., nutritional restriction, gestational diabetes, and maternal stress) that permanently alter (or "program") gene expression profiles contributing to the organization and function of neural circuits and molecular pathways supporting biological mechanisms (intrauterine growth, physiology, and metabolism) and psychological processes (socialization and intellectual maturation) in the offspring (Barker et al. 2002; Fowden et al. 2006; Huizink et al. 2004; Mousseau and Fox 1998). The ability of the early environment to modify adult phenotypes (neuroendocrine, behavioral, emotional, metabolic, and cognitive) via alterations in mother–infant interactions allows the transmission of information involved in enhanced survival to be passed on to offspring without having to go through the slow processes of random mutation and natural selection. This implies that plasticity early in life provides the individual with an evolutionary advantageous ability to adjust physiologically and hone specific biological defensive systems for survival and reproductive success to promote establishment and persistence in the present environment (Bradshaw 1965).

Depending on how close the plastic response is to the new favored phenotypic optimum dictates whether directional selection will cause adaptive divergence between populations (Robinson et al. 2008). Plasticity can become maladaptive under conditions where environmental stimuli programs physiological systems to function outside their normal range, which increases the biological systems "wear and tear" (or allostatic load) and risk for diseases that occur with greater frequency with aging (McEwen 2004). Herein, developmental programming mediates the effects of experience on vulnerability (and resilience) to the emergence of certain metabolic disorder phenotypes in the later stages of life (Coe and Lubach 2005; Gluckman et al. 2008). This begs the question of how the individual is capable of adapting to these developmental or environmental cues at the level of the genome, including the biological mechanism(s) through which these responses are established and maintained.

Genetic variation for phenotypic plasticity has been demonstrated in a number of different species, suggesting that it is open to the forces of natural selection, and that adaptive phenotypic plasticity can evolve (West-Eberhard 2005). However, phenotypic plasticity is more than the simple property of genotype. Indeed, there are multiple potential mechanisms of inheritance, involving the passage of epigenetic marks through the germ line (Chong and Whitelaw 2004); the passage of maternal RNA molecules into the embryo (Bettegowda and Smith 2007; Rassoulzadegan et al. 2006); the potential passage of prion proteins from parent to offspring (Shorter and Lindquist 2005); the biochemical state of the gametes at the time of conception; and the transmission of nutrients, bacteria, or antibodies from maternal circulation to that of the offspring (Boulinier and Staszewski 2008; Grindstaff et al. 2003; Hasselquist and Nilsson 2009). All of these factors can, and do, influence the phenotype of the offspring.

Epigenetics investigates the transmission of phenotypic characteristics in terms of gene expression through mitosis (and potentially meiosis) in the absence of changes in DNA sequence, hence the name epi- (Greek: επί – over, above) genetics (Waddington 1942). The advent of high-throughput techniques such as microarray- and sequencing-based approaches to study the distributions of regulators of gene transcription throughout the genome led to the collective description of the "epigenome", which refers to the epigenetically modified genome. The "epigenotype" refers to mitotically heritable patterns of DNA methylation and modifications to chromatin proteins that package DNA. Henceforth, phenotype is thought to be the result of complex interactions between genotype and current, past, and ancestral environment leading to life-long experience-dependent chromatin plasticity.

This chapter provides an overview of the main components of the epigenome and, using a rodent model of early life social interaction, discusses how epigenetic programming through maternal care subsequently shapes brain development and behavioral function across the life span. Herein, socially directed regulatory processes transfer epigenetic information not only within cells but also between cells and organ systems, as well as across generations. In humans, the epigenome may well function as an interface between the inherited genome and the dynamics imposed by the environment, providing a mechanism for reprogramming gene function in response to changes in lifestyle trajectories, fundamental for adaptive phenotypic plasticity.

11.2 The Dynamic Epigenome: Linking Environment to Genes and Plasticity

Epigenetic events in eukaryotic organisms (plants, insects, reptiles, birds, and mammals) have evolved to provide a more precise and stable control of gene expression and genomic regulation through multiple generations. In eukaryotic cells, the epigenome is encoded in distinct patterns of nuclear organization, global chromatin structure, global and local covalent modification of both histone proteins (regular and variants) (Kadonaga 1998) and DNA (Razin 1998), and the presence of specific macromolecules including small nonprotein-coding RNAs (ncRNAs) termed micro-RNA [other ncRNA include Piwi-interacting RNAs and large intervening non-coding RNAs] (Bergmann and Lane 2003; Chuang and Jones 2007; Saito and Jones 2006). MicroRNA regulates gene expression and cellular fate by controlling chromatin silencing, mRNA stability, or translation, and potentially plays an important role in developmental neuropathology (for review see Mattick et al. 2009). For the purpose of this review, we discuss only DNA and histone modification, considering micro-RNA are regulated by DNA methylation and chromatin structure (Saito and Jones 2006). Unlike the DNA sequence, which is stable and strongly conserved, epigenetic processes can be highly dynamic: chromatin structure and DNA methylation patterns are unique to each type of cell, developmentally regulated, and often induced by exposure to a range of external environmental factors (Dolinoy et al. 2007). Understanding the mechanisms involved in the initiation, maintenance, and heritability of epigenetic states is an important aspect of research in current biology, particularly in the study of phenotypic behavior in humans.

11.2.1 Chromatin Structure, Modifying Enzymes, Histone Code, and Genome Function

In the eukaryotic cell nucleus, chromosomal DNA is packaged into chromatin fibers in repeating protein–DNA complexes called nucleosomes, the basic unit of DNA packaging. Nucleosomes comprise approximately 146 bp of DNA wound 1.8 times around an octamer consisting of two copies each of histone proteins H2A, H2B, H3, and H4 (Kornberg 1974). The attraction between the positively-charged histones and negatively-charged DNA maintains the histone–DNA interaction (Grunstein 1997).

The posttranslational modification of histones, the basic proteins around which DNA is wrapped to form nucleosomes, comprises an epigenetic mechanism related to gene expression. Histone-modifying enzymes are generally not gene specific. Transcription factors or repressors locate and bind to their cognate response elements on the genome (Elf et al. 2007) and concurrently recruit (via protein–protein interactions) specific chromodomain proteins and histone-modifying enzymes to these specific genomic regions. Notably, intracellular signal transduction pathways activated by cell-surface receptors can directly interact with the chromatin structure, linking environmental cues from cell-surface receptors to gene-specific histone posttranslational modification and the level of expression from the underlying genes.

Within the chromatin structure, posttranslational modifications not only occur on the protruding N-terminal tail of histones, but can also affect the histone core and C-terminus [e.g., H3 methylation of lysine 79 residues (H3K79me)] (Tweedie-Cullen et al. 2009). These modifications include acetylation (Wade et al. 1997), poly-ADP-ribosylation, carbonylation (Wondrak et al. 2000), citrullination, biotinylation, formylation, palmitoylation, glycosylation, methylation (Jenuwein 2001), phosphorylation, SUMOylation (Shiio and Eisenman 2003), proline isomerization, and ubiquitination (Shilatifard 2006). The addition or removal of these histone modifications are often regulated together (either positively or negatively), and act in synergy to modulate gene transcription (activation or repression) by altering local chromatin structure and access for transcriptional machinery. Typically, acetylation occurs at lysine residues and all acetylation modifications are associated with transcriptional activation, as are phosphorylation and arginine methylation modifications (Bernstein et al. 2005). The effect of ubiquitination on transcription likewise is dependent on location, with ubiquitination on H2A and H2B associated with transcriptional repression and activation, respectively. In unicellular eukaryotes such as the yeast *Saccharomyces cerevisiae*, histone sumoylation is also associated with transcriptional silencing (Nathan et al. 2006), and H3 proline isomerization with transcriptional activation via negative coupling with H3 methylation of lysine 36 residues (H3K36me) (Nelson et al. 2006). The relationship between regional patterns of histone modifications and locus-specific transcriptional activity provides evidence for the existence of a "histone code" for determining cell-specific gene expression programs (Jenuwein and Allis 2001).

Other chromatin remodeling systems that have been implicated in epigenetic changes include DNA looping, nucleosome sliding (mediated by ATP-dependent chromatin remodeling proteins), and histone substitution (exchange of histones from nucleosome with external histones) (Tsankova et al. 2007). For example, different histone variants, which replace the standard isoforms also play a regulatory role and, in some cases, serve to mark gene activation (Henikoff et al. 2004). The studies discussed in this chapter focus on the functions of H3 and H4 lysine acetylation and methylation (H3/4-KAc/me) with some general considerations concerning gene regulation, activation, and repression during development.

The occurrence of acetylation on histone tails is controlled by the opposing enzymatic activities of histone acetyltransferases [HATs; i.e., CREB-binding protein

(CBP)] and histone deacetylases (HDACs; i.e., the class I HDAC2) (Kuo and Allis 1998). Increased acetylation induces transcription activation – H3 acetylation of lysine 9 residues (H3K9Ac) at the 5′ region of genes is associated with promoter activation – whereas deacetylation usually induces transcription repression. Histone acetylation neutralizes the positive charge of the histone tail and decreases its affinity to negatively charged DNA, generating a more open DNA conformation (euchromatin) (Hong et al. 1993; Sealy and Chalkley 1978). This enables access of transcription factors, regulatory complexes, and RNA polymerase transcription factors to the DNA, and the expression of the corresponding genes is also facilitated. Thus, H3K9Ac is considered as a predominant marker of active gene transcription (Lee et al. 1993; Perry and Chalkley 1982). On the other hand, removal of the acetyl group by HDAC enzymes restores the positive charge to the lysine residue, fostering stronger interactions between histones and DNA (heterochromatin), reducing the accessibility of transcription factors, and the transcription apparatus to their cognate binding sites, resulting in gene silencing (Davie and Chadee 1998).

The amount of methylation on histone tails is controlled by the opposing enzymatic activities of histone methyltransferases (HTMs; i.e., EZH2, G9a, MLL, Suv39H1) (Lachner and Jenuwein 2002; Lachner et al. 2001; Lachner et al. 2003) and histone demethylases (HDMs; i.e., JARID1d, Utx) (Shi et al. 2004; Tsukada et al. 2006). Lysine residues can be mono- (me1), di- (me2), or tri-methylated (me3), and binding of specific proteins that recognize methylated lysine positions can result in different biological outcomes – some specific histone methylation events are associated with gene silencing and some with gene activation depending on the lysine residue (Yan and Boyd 2006). For example, H3 di- or tri-methylation of lysine 4 residues (H3K4me2/3) at the 5′ region of genes is associated with promoter activation, whereas H3 di- or tri-methylation of lysine 9 residues (H3K9me2/3) is associated with Dnmt3a activity, DNA methylation, and repressed gene transcription (Ohm and Baylin 2007). H3 tri-methylation of lysine 27 residues also (H3K27me3), which is catalyzed by the polycomb group (PcG) protein complex, represents transcriptional inactivation. Permissive and repressed intermediate chromatin states provide an additional level of epigenetic regulation (Tsankova et al. 2007).

11.2.2 Genomic Methylation: The Primary Epigenetic Modification

Of DNA methylation, cytosine methylation is the best understood and the most stable epigenetic modification modulating the transcriptional plasticity of mammalian genomes. Recent studies examining whole-genome methylation profiles across the plant and animal kingdoms have revealed both conserved and divergent features of DNA methylation in unicellular eukaryotes to multicellular vertebrates (Feng et al. 2010b; Law and Jacobsen 2010; Zemach et al. 2010). In plants and mammals, the most methylated cytosines are found over repeat elements (Goll and Bestor 2005; Law and Jacobsen 2010; Suzuki and Bird 2008) and loss of this modification is associated with transcriptional reactivation as well as increased mobilization of transposable elements (Slotkin and Martienssen 2007). These observations likely reflect the ancestral role of cytosine methylation in the defense against invasive DNA. Nonrepeat sequences may also be methylated, and methylation of such sequences in the context of gene promoters often correlates with transcriptional silencing in plants (Henderson and Jacobsen 2007) and mammals (Ooi et al. 2009; Suzuki and Bird 2008). Despite similarities in the controlling functions of DNA methylation, the dynamics and deposition of methylation patterns differ in several respects between plants and mammals.

In plant genomes, DNA methylation can occur symmetrically (both strands) at cytosine residues in both 5'-cytosine-phosphodiester-guanine-3' (CpG dinucleotide) and CHG [H = adenine (A), thymine (T) or cytosine (C)] contexts, and also asymmetrically in CHH context, with the latter directed and maintained by RNAs (Law and Jacobsen 2010). Interestingly, in plants, methylation within genes (intragenically) is thought to inhibit cryptic transcription initiation (Zilberman et al. 2007) or suppress recombination or transposon insertion within genes (Zhu 2008).

In mammalian genomes, DNA methylation occurs mostly symmetrically at cytosine residues in the context of CpG dinucleotides in the mammalian genome, to form 5-methylcytosine (5mC) in a cell-specific pattern (Razin and Szyf 1984). However, results from more recent studies suggest that CHH and CHG methylation may be more common than previously appreciated in mammals: in human embryonic stem (ES) cells it accounts for $\sim$25% of all methylated cytosines (Ramsahoye et al. 2000; Lister et al. 2009). In mammals, 5mC patterns are established and maintained during development by the Dnmt1 and Dnmt3 families of DNA methyltransferases, which utilize the final methyl donor produced by one-carbon metabolism, S-adenosylmethionine (also known as SAM, SAMe, ademethione, and adoMet) (Adams et al. 1979). The de novo establishment of DNA methylation is performed by methyltransferases Dnmt3A and Dnmt3B, and modulated by Dnmt3L, which lacks direct catalytic activity (Okano et al. 1999). These enzymes are all expressed in the central nervous system (CNS) and are dynamically regulated during development and differentiation (Feng et al. 2005; Goto et al. 1994). Indeed, Dnmt1 actively methylates CpG dinucleotides within nondividing somatic cells, such as neurons (Okano et al. 1999).

Importantly, global levels of 5mC and gene-specific DNA methylation profiles are dynamic and vary spatially and temporally throughout life, especially during epigenetic remodeling in early development. The Dnmt1 maintenance methyltransferase shows preference hemi-methylated DNA (Bestor and Verdine 1994; Leonhardt and Bestor 1993; Smith 1994) and safeguards the methylome in dividing cells by faithfully copying the methylation pattern from parental to daughter strand during DNA replication (Bestor 1988; Bestor 1992). This process is especially important during embryogenesis, where the methylated maternal and paternal genomes are demethylated upon fertilization (to ensure the totipotency) and specific patterns of methylation are then reestablished progressively commencing in the early postconception period (Okano et al. 1999). Recent work in human cell lines has also shown that dynamic remodeling of epigenetic marks may occur during the cell cycle (Brown and Szyf 2008; Kangaspeska et al. 2008; Metivier et al. 2008).

As previously mentioned, the addition of a methyl group to cytosine nucleotides in DNA does not change the primary DNA sequence per se, but the covalent modification can regulate spatio-temporal gene expression and activity in a mitotically heritable fashion. Through this mechanism, DNA methylation controls cell-specific gene expression, X chromosome inactivation and parental imprinting, cell survival, neuronal migration and maturation in the CNS, and can be modulated by environmental stimuli such as nutrition, drugs, stress, and postnatal care (for review see Weaver 2009). Furthermore, epigenetic regulation through DNA methylation appears to be a critical evolutionary process – the absence of DNA methylation in some eukaryotes such as yeasts *Saccharomyces cerevisiae* and *Schizosaccharomyces pombe*, as well as the flatworm *Caenorhabditis elegans* and fruit fly *Drosophila melanogaster* is associated with the evolutionary loss of DNMT homologues (Goll and Bestor 2005).

11.2.3 Heterochromatin, DNA Methylation, and Gene Silencing

Typically, heterochromatin is associated with hypermethylated DNA and inhibition of transcription (Holliday and Pugh 1975). During early development, for example, repressive heterochromatin is important for X chromosome inactivation (or lyonization) during embryonic development to ensure that females, like males, have one functional copy of the X chromosome in each cell (Orphanides and Reinberg 2002).

DNA methylation of gene promoter regions or enhancer sites inhibits gene expression via two main mechanisms (Bird 2001; Bird and Wolffe 1999; Hashimshony et al. 2003; Kadonaga 1998; Li 2002; Nan et al. 1998). In the direct mechanism, the 5mC marking of CpG-rich promoters (Antequera and Bird 1993; Bird 1996; Gardiner-Garden and Frommer 1987), intragenic, and intergenic regions (Ching et al. 2005; Fazzari and Greally 2004; Khulan et al. 2006) blocks gene expression, thereby establishing a mechanism to direct tissue-specific gene expression – 5mC within transcription factor binding sites displaces the binding of methylation-sensitive transcription factors to their cognate binding sites (Tate and Bird 1993; Watt and Molloy 1988). Here, DNA methylation serves as an epimutation of the transcription factor binding site and repels the transcription factor. DNA methylation within intronic regions may regulate the activity of intragenic micro-RNA involved in regulating RNA splice variation, silencing of chromatin, degradation of mRNA, and blocking translation (Mattick and Makunin 2006). In the indirect mechanism, the methylation sites attract methyl-CpG-binding domain (MBD) containing proteins, such as methyl-CpG-binding protein (MeCP)-2, which are involved in "reading" methylation marks and binding to methylated DNA (Bird 2001; Bird and Wolffe 1999; Hashimshony et al. 2003; Kadonaga 1998; Li 2002; Nan et al. 1998). These MBD proteins affect chromatin condensation by recruiting corepressor proteins such as SIN3A and histone modification enzymes, leading to chromatin compaction and gene silencing (Jones et al. 1998; Ng et al. 1999; Wade et al. 1999; Zhang et al. 1999).

11.2.4   Euchromatin, Active DNA Demethylation, and Gene Activation

Similar to histone modification, DNA methylation is also potentially reversible during development and in somatic tissues (Kersh et al. 2006; Lucarelli et al. 2001) including predominantly postmitotic tissues such as the brain (Feng et al. 2010a; Weaver et al. 2004). Hypomethylated DNA is generally associated with euchromatin and gene activation (Holliday and Pugh 1975).

As discussed previously, in the absence of maintenance and de novo DNA methylation activity, DNA methylation patterns are lost passively during DNA replication in primordial germ cells (Morgan et al. 2005). However, the precise mechanism by which replication-independent (or active) demethylation occurs in the adult mammalian brain remains as a subject of a lively ongoing debate (Ooi and Bestor 2008; Wu and Zhang 2010). One proposed mechanism involves nucleotide excision repair – the removal and replacement of mutations in the DNA and the growth arrest and DNA damage-inducible 45 (Gadd45a) protein has been proposed to promote the DNA repair based mechanism (Barreto et al. 2007; Weiss et al. 1996). In contrast, base excision repair involves the removal of a mutated or chemically altered base and its replacement with the correct base (David and Williams 1998). However, these two mechanisms may not account for the rapid and complete demethylation observed in the paternal genome following fertilization of the embryo (Oswald et al. 2000). The removal of nucleotides would seriously compromise the integrity of the genome, and it is unlikely an excision repair system that would be able to complete genome-wide demethylation and nucleotide replacement within the observed 4-h time frame (Oswald et al. 2000).

Interestingly, some components of the epigenetic machinery long thought to be involved in establishing and maintaining DNA methylation patterns may also be involved in their removal. This should not be unexpected as enzymes often have the potential for bidirectional catalytic activity. A recent publication provides evidence for DNA demethylation induced by MBD3 (Brown et al. 2008), while two other reports propose that DNMT3a and DNMT3b possess deaminase activity and are involved in a dynamic demethylation–methylation pathway that operates during gene transcription (Kangaspeska et al. 2008; Metivier et al. 2008). Prior to these assertions, MBD2b (a shorter isoform of MBD2) was reported to trigger active DNA demethylation by removal of methyl groups directly from the cytosine base and induce gene expression in mammalian cells (Bhattacharya et al. 1999; Cervoni et al. 1999; Cervoni and Szyf 2001; Detich et al. 2002, 2003a, b; Hamm et al. 2008; Ramchandani et al. 1999; Szyf and Bhattacharya 2002a, b). The proposed reaction requires a water molecule and involves the transfer of the methyl group of the cytosine to form methanol (Bhattacharya et al. 1999; Cervoni et al. 1999; Ramchandani et al. 1999). Although the assignment of demethylase activity to MBD2b was contested (Boeke et al. 2000; Ng et al. 1999; Wade et al. 1999), MBD2b levels are inversely correlated with the levels of DNA methylation of certain genes in hepatocytes (Goel et al. 2003) and lymphocytes from lupus patients (Balada et al. 2007), and depletion of MBD2b results in hypermethylation of unmethylated genes in metastatic cancer (Pakneshan et al. 2004; Shukeir et al. 2006). Hence, the ability to epigenetically reprogram differentiated cells is becoming of major medical importance.

More recently, it has been shown that while 5mC constitutes only ~1% of all bases in the mammalian genome, the modified base 5-hydroxymethylcytosine (5hmC) constitutes ~5% of all cytosine species present at CpGs in MspI and TaqαI sites in ES cell DNA and 20% of all cytosine species present at CpGs in the brain, especially in Purkinje neurons (Kriaucionis and Heintz 2009; Tahiliani et al. 2009). Since ES cells are highly proliferative while neurons are postmitotic, the biological functions of 5hmC maybe cell type-specific and may influence chromatin structure and recruit specific factors or may constitute an intermediate component in cytosine demethylation. Herein, 5hmC may (1) displace 5mC-binding proteins (e.g., MeCP2) from methylated DNA (Valinluck et al. 2004); (2) occlude DNMT1 during cell division resulting in passive DNA demethylation (Valinluck and Sowers 2007); (3) be recognized as an aberrant base by DNA repair mechanisms that replace 5hmC with cytosine resulting in active DNA demethylation; or (4) be recognized by transcription factors that recruit and target chromatin-modifying enzymes to specific genomic regions, thus altering chromatin structure and DNA methylation status.

DNMT1-mediated oxidation of cytosine with formaldehyde may generate 5hmC, although this remains to be demonstrated under physiological relevant conditions (Liutkeviciute et al. 2009). Tahiliani et al. (2009) recently reported that the human mixed-lineage leukemia (MLL) fusion protein TET1 – which is an α-ketoglutarate (α-KG) and Fe(II)-dependent dioxygenase – specifically binds 5mC and catalyses the conversion to 5-hydroxymethylcytosine (5hmC) (Tahiliani et al. 2009). Ito et al. (2010) extend these studies by demonstrating that all three murine Tet proteins (Tet1–3) catalyze a similar reaction (Ito et al. 2010). Furthermore, Tet1 was shown to mediate the regulation of Nanog, which is a transcription factor critically involved with self-renewal of undifferentiated ES cells. Ectopic Tet1 expression resulted in increased Nanog promoter 5hmC and increased Nanog expression. Whether 5hmC is further processed to C by an enzyme-catalyzed process or through base excision remains to be determined. Notably, a 5hmC-specific DNA glycosylase activity has been previously reported (Cannon et al. 1988). Alternatively, decreased Tet1 expression in preimplantation embryos was associated with increased methylation of the Nanog promoter, decreased Nanog gene expression, and a bias toward trophectoderm differentiation (Ito et al. 2010). Together, these findings demonstrated a role for Tet1-mediated DNA demethylation during maintenance of pluripotent ES cell self-renewal and specification, including neural differentiation.

In summary, DNA methylation patterns are likely defined by chromatin status, which gates the accessibility of the DNA methylation/demethylation components to the underlying genes. This process may involve transcription factors or repressors that recruit and target chromatin-modifying enzymes to specific genomic regions. The chemical nature of the chromatin modification then defines the methylation status of the underlying genes, either through the facilitation of the DNA demethylation or the recruitment of the DNA methylation machinery (Weaver et al. unpublished). Clearly the exact timing and mechanisms through which a given pattern of chromatin changes from transient effects on gene regulation to more persistent epigenetic programming of gene expression by DNA methylation will be context-dependent (Madhani et al. 2008).

11.2.5   Dsyregulation of the Epigenetic Machinery and Neurodevelopment

Importantly, from a plasticity perspective, loss-of-function mutations in key components of the epigenetic machinery in humans are associated with several developmental and cognitive disorders with implications for risk of later life mental disorders (Jiang et al. 2004). Genetic variants of genes encoding the DNMT enzymes have been identified as risk factors of disease, including cancer (Cebrian et al. 2006; Kelemen et al. 2008; Lee et al. 2005; Montgomery et al. 2004), systemic lupus erythematosus (Park et al. 2004), and a rare autosomal recessive disorder termed ICF (immunodeficiency, centromeric instability, and facial anomalies) syndrome (Hansen et al. 1999), diseases which are characterized by altered DNA methylation patterns. In addition, functional polymorphisms of genes involved in folate metabolism [such as methylenetetrahydrofolate reductase (MTHFR), a regulatory enzyme in folate metabolism] have been shown to alter intracellular SAM levels (Miller et al. 1994; Poirier et al. 2001), decrease global DNA methylation levels in peripheral blood leukocytes (Friso et al. 2005), and to be linked to the increased risk of many serious health conditions (Giovannucci 2004). Thus, genotype is likely to be a further major influence on epigenotype.

The importance of epigenetic mechanisms in neurodevelopmental conditions including mental retardation has been the best characterized by mutations in the X chromosome-linked gene MeCP2 in individuals with Rett syndrome (RTT) (Amir et al. 1999), and mutations in the CBP gene (which has HAT activity) in individuals with Rubinstein–Taybi syndrome (RTS) (Alarcon et al. 2004).

Both MeCP2 and CBP are highly expressed in postmitotic neurons and are involved in regulating neural gene expression (Chen et al. 2003; Martinowich et al. 2003).

Mice with truncated MeCP2 exhibit genome-wide H3 hyperacetylation (H3Ac), neuronal atrophy, increased anxiety, cognitive deficits, and social withdrawal, which can be further exacerbated by forebrain knockout of the brain-derived neurotrophic factor (BDNF) (Shahbazian et al. 2002). Remarkably, many of the physiological, cognitive, and emotional deficits associated with MeCP2 mutant mice are reversed through restoration of the MECP2 gene (Guy et al. 2007), or by ectopic BDNF expression, demonstrating a functional interaction between MeCP2 and BDNF in RTT disease progression (Chang et al. 2006).

Mutations of the CBP HAT domain in several RTS cases are associated with genome-wide histone hypoacetylation and cognitive dysfunction in adulthood (Kalkhoven et al. 2003). The learning and memory deficits are attributed to perturbed neural plasticity (Korzus et al. 2004), however, RTS individuals also exhibit early cognitive dysfunction (Roelfsema and Peters 2007) and display neural dysgenesis, including cortical abnormalities (Sener 1995). Similar to RTS in humans, mice with a heterozygous null mutation of CBP perform poorly in cognitive tasks and show decreased genome-wide histone acetylation (for review see Josselyn 2005). We examined the potential role for CBP in neural precursors born in the subventricular zone of the lateral ventricles of the developing murine cortex, which sequentially generate neurons, astrocytes, and oligodendrocytes (Wang et al. 2010). Herein, we found that phosphorylation of CBP by atypical protein kinase C (aPKC) ζ acts as an epigenetic switch to promote precursor differentiation. Interestingly, this epigenetic mechanism is perturbed in the fetal brains of CBP haploinsufficient mice, which exhibit early behavioral deficits as pups in ultrasound vocalization following maternal separation (Wang et al. 2010). These findings provide a novel mechanism whereby environmental cues, acting through histone modifying enzymes, can regulate stem cell epigenetic status and thereby directly promote differentiation, which regulates neurobehavioral development. This begs the question of whether similar epigenetic mechanisms regulate differentiation in other brain regions, such as in the small number of new neurons that arise from the subgranulare zone of the dentate gyrus within the hippocampus throughout life (Cameron and Gould 1994).

11.3 Experience-Dependent Effects on the Epigenome and Phenotypic Variability in Nature

There are a growing number of examples illustrating the relationship between epigenetic changes and phenotypic variability in divergent eukaryotic species (for review see Weaver 2010). The potential flexibility of the epigenome is a means of responding to changing environmental stimuli, and is especially important for plants, which cannot move in response to unfavorable conditions (Martienssen and Colot 2001). For example, in the flowering plant *Arabidopsis*, the cold-induced acceleration of flowering in different climates (vernalization) is correlated with the rate of epigenetic silencing by H3 tri-methylation of lysine 27 residues (H3K27me3) at the Flowering Locus C (FLC) gene (Shindo et al. 2006).

Another mode of epigenetic inheritance in plants is by paramutation: an epigenetic modification induced by cross-talk between allelic loci (Chandler 2007). The paramutation is inherited by transmitting the RNA transcript from the "paramutating" allele during gametogenesis and by propagating this heritable message to somatic and germ cells of the offspring by an RNA-dependent RNA polymerase (Alleman et al. 2006). Unlike a typical mutation, paramutation results in quantitatively variable phenotypes. Paramutation-like effects suggest the possibility of non-Mendelian heredity comparable to the plant systems, for example, the interallelic transfer of DNA methylation patterns established after heterologous recombination during meiosis (Rassoulzadegan et al. 2002). Currently, the only example of a paramutation mode of epigenetic inheritance in mammals is in transgenic mice carrying a lacZ insertion mutation of the c-kit oncogene, which undergo the zygotic transfer of RNA molecules and inheritance of a white-tail phenotype (Rassoulzadegan et al. 2006).

In social invertebrates, the production of contrasting adult morphologies as well as different reproductive and behavioral systems is critical to their social organization and division of labor (Evans and Wheeler 1999, 2001; Hartfelder and Engels 1998). Recent studies suggest that nutritional effects on epigenetic mechanisms mediate this type of phenotypic plasticity. For example, fertile queens and sterile workers are alternative forms of the adult female honeybee (*Apis mellifera*) that develop from genetically identical larvae following differential feeding with royal jelly – a protein-rich substance secreted from glands on the heads of worker bees. A larva destined to become a queen is fed large quantities of royal jelly inside a specially constructed compartment called a queen cup. The queen is then fed royal honey exclusively for the rest of her life. Findings from recent studies suggest that royal jelly silences Dnmt3, an enzyme involved in genome-wide gene silencing in the newly hatched larvae, with effects on the larval developmental trajectory (Kucharski et al. 2008). Kucharski et al. 2008 showed that Dnmt3 siRNA-treated individuals emerged as queens with fully developed ovaries and a larger abdomen for egg laying, whereas the nontreated control larvae expressing Dnmt3 developed into the default sterile worker variety, due to epigenetic silencing of the genes encoding the queen phenotype. These results suggest that DNA methylation can be differentially altered by nutritional input, and that the flexibility of epigenetic modifications supports shifts in developmental fates, with implications for reproductive and behavioral status. Of course, genome-wide DNA methylation mapping and gene expression profiling in both social and solitary insects would reveal the underlying molecular interactions supporting these complex evolvable biological systems.

Perhaps one of the best illustrations in mammals of how phenotypes can differ dramatically due to epigenetic variability alone is the yellow agouti (A^{vy}) mouse model. These mice have a mutation upstream from the Agouti locus, which involves the de novo retrotransposition of a long terminal repeat (LTR) transposable element (Morgan et al. 1999). This intracisternal A-particle (IAP) transposon provides an alternate promoter for the gene, which drives expression during the development of the hair and causes a yellow fur phenotype. However, this alternate promoter overexpresses the gene in other tissues, leading to the eventual development of obesity and insulin resistance (Morgan et al. 1999). Genetically identical littermates with this IAP transposon have different levels of activity of the alternate promoter, and as a consequence, different degrees of fur discoloration and metabolic consequences. Importantly, the stable interindividual phenotypic variation is associated with the degree of variable histone modification and stochastic 5mC patterns at six CpG dinucleotides within the 5′ LTR of the A^{vy} IAP promoter sequence (Dolinoy et al. 2010). In yellow mice, the A^{vy} IAP promoter LTR is hypomethylated and enriched for H3 and H4 di-acetylation (H3/H4Ac2), which is associated with enhanced A^{vy} IAP promoter activation, leading to yellow fur and susceptibility toward obesity and tumorigenesis. Conversely, in pseudoagouti mice, the A^{vy} IAP promoter LTR is hypermethylated and enriched for H4 tri-methylation of lysine 20 residues (H4K20me3), which is associated with Agouti gene silencing, brown fur, and protection from obesity and cancer in adulthood (Dolinoy et al. 2010).

Variations in parental investment in mammals, such as nutrient supply provided by the parent and behavioral interactions, also affect the development of defensive responses and reproductive strategies in the progeny (Denenberg 1999; Ottinger and Tanabe 1969; Ressler and Anderson 1973). By providing nutrition, the maternal nurturing influences growth and development of offspring health (Morgan et al. 1999). As diet-derived methyl donors and cofactors are necessary for the synthesis of SAM, which serves as the donor of methyl groups for DNA methylation, environmental factors that alter early nutrition and/or SAM synthesis can potentially influence adult metabolism via persistent alterations in DNA methylation (Dolinoy et al. 2006; Waterland et al. 2006a; Waterland and Jirtle 2003; Waterland et al. 2006b; Wolff et al. 1998). In A^{vy} mice, maternal supplementation with methyl donors (Waterland and Jirtle 2003) or the isoflavinoid genistein (Dolinoy et al. 2006) – a phytoestrogen found in soy and present at high levels in infant formula – during gestation can produce offspring with increased methylation of transposable elements in or upstream of the agouti gene, respectively, decreased Agouti gene expression, brown fur, and a reduced risk of lifelong chronic disease.

In the rat, dams fed a diet low in one-carbon donors during pregnancy produce offspring with decreased DNA methylation and increased association of H3K9Ac at promoter regions of specific genes, including the glucocorticoid receptor (GR) exon 1_{10} and peroxisome proliferator-activated receptor-alpha (PPARα), and increased mRNA expression in the liver of juvenile (Lillycrop et al. 2005) and adult offspring (Lillycrop et al. 2007). These epigenetic changes and reduced DNMT1 expression were largely prevented by maternal folic acid supplementation during pregnancy (Lillycrop et al. 2005, 2007, 2008) as well as by increasing folic acid intake during the juvenile–pubertal period (Burdge et al. 2009). Together with the A^{vy} mice findings, these data suggest that early life nutrition has the potential to influence epigenetic programming in the brain not only during early development but also in adult life, thereby modulating health throughout life.

From an evolutionary perspective, the effects of nutrient restriction may be in response to adaptive programs that sense the organisms' nutritional state in gestation, which results in tissue-specific chromatin remodeling (Ke et al. 2006; MacLennan et al. 2004; Sinclair et al. 2007). Indeed, the availability of dietary methionine and folate alter the parent-of-origin effects on the methylation status of imprinted genes [including insulin-like growth factor (IGF)-2] (Luedi et al. 2005; Waterland et al. 2006b) that mediate many of the actions of growth hormone on somatic growth and tissue maintenance (Feinberg 2007). Support of this phenomenon is evidenced by recent studies in nonhuman primates that show maternal nutrient deprivation during pregnancy produce organ- and gestational age-dependent perturbations in global DNA methylation levels in the kidney and forebrain of the developing fetus (Unterberger et al. 2009).

In humans, it has long been proposed (Hales and Barker 1992) that poor fetal and infant growth; and the subsequent development of disease later in life emerge from nutritional programming early in life (Wells 2003). Epidemiological data reveal that cardiovascular and diabetes mortality in children can be influenced by the nutritional status of their parents and grandparents (Kaati et al. 2002). However, the most comprehensive study to date of adaptive transgenerational epigenetic effects in mammals is that of the maternally transmitted responses to stress in the rat. In particular, differential maternal behavior in the rat alters the epigenetic status of the promoter of the hippocampal GR, which is associated with stable individual differences on stress responsivity and cognitive and emotional development in the offspring.

11.4   Natural Variations of Maternal Care in the Rat and Phenotypic Variability in the Adult Offspring

Natural variations in maternal care in humans and nonhuman primates are also observed in rodents and similarly are associated with divergent behavioral phenotypes in the offspring. In the rat, naturally occurring variations in the frequency of maternal pup licking/grooming and arched-back nursing (LG-ABN) are associated with stable interindividual differences on stress responsiveness, emotionality, cognitive performance, and reproductive behavior in the adult offspring (Caldji et al. 1998; Francis et al. 1999; Liu et al. 1997; Myers et al. 1989; Stern 1997). In adulthood, the female offspring of mothers that exhibit increased levels of pup LG-ABN (i.e., High LG-ABN mothers) over the first week of life are themselves high in maternal LG-ABN behavior toward their pups and likewise, the offspring of Low LG-ABN mothers are low in maternal LG-ABN behavior toward their pups (Francis et al. 1999). Neonatal cross-fostering as well as postweaning environmental enrichment and impoverishment can reverse behavioral differences between female High and Low LG-ABN offspring on measures of maternal behavior and anxiety (Champagne and Meaney 2007). Furthermore, gestational stress during the third trimester reduces LG-ABN behavior in High LG-ABN mothers and the adult offspring resemble those of Low LG-ABN mothers on measures of anxiety and maternal behaviors, an effect which is sustained through the second and third litter (Champagne and Meaney 2006). These findings suggest that individual differences in stress reactivity and maternal care are transmitted across generations through a behavioral mode of transmission linked to variations in maternal behavior, which serves to enhance the capacity for defensive responses in the progeny toward increased sensitivity to future (stressful) environments.

11.4.1   Hypothalamic–Pituitary–Adrenal and Behavioral Responses to Stress

The relationship between early life environment and health in the adult offspring is mediated by maternal influences on the development of neuroendocrine systems that underlie hypothalamic–pituitary–adrenal (HPA) and behavioral responses to stress (Francis and Meaney 1999; Heim et al. 2000; Nemeroff 1996; Repetti et al. 2002; Seckl and Meaney 1993; Sroufe 1997). Exposure to different levels of maternal LG-ABN during the postnatal period is associated with HPA blunting and changes in forebrain GR expression levels that persist into adulthood (Francis et al. 1999; Liu et al. 1997). The magnitude of the HPA response to stress is a function of the neural stimulation of hypothalamic corticotropin-releasing factor (CRF) release. This activates the pituitary–adrenal system as well as modulatory influences, as evidenced by glucocorticoid (GC) negative feedback in the hippo-campus that inhibits CRF synthesis and release, dampening HPA responses to stress (De Kloet et al. 1998). GCs bind to GR to mediate the peripheral stress response and feedback to the CNS to modulate further activation of the HPA response (Herman et al. 2003).

The adult offspring of High LG-ABN mothers show increased hippocampal GR mRNA expression, enhanced feedback sensitivity to GCs, decreased hypothalamic CRF mRNA expression, and consequently more modest ACTH and cortisol stress responsivity, and reduced fearful behavior under conditions of stress in comparison with adult animals reared by Low LG-ABN dams (Caldji et al. 1998; Francis et al. 1999; Liu et al. 1997; Weaver et al. 2004, 2006, 2007). Interestingly, removing the difference in hippocampal GR levels erases the effects of early experience on HPA responses to stress in adulthood (Meaney et al. 1989), demonstrating that the difference in hippocampal GR expression serves as a mechanism for the effects of early experience on the development of individual differences in HPA responses to stress (Meaney 2001). Likewise, impairments to HPA axis regulation and an increase in anxiety-related behavior were observed in mice with forebrain-specific disruption of the GR gene and loss of hippocampal GR expression (Boyle et al. 2006). Furthermore, the adult offspring of the gestationally stressed High LG-ABN mothers have reduced hippocampal GR protein expression (Weaver et al. unpub-lished data) and resemble those of low LG-ABN mothers on behavioral measures of anxiety and maternal behavior (Champagne and Meaney 2006).

11.4.2   Maternal Effects and the Emerging Importance of the Epigenome

The observations so far suggest that the developing rodent forebrain is vulnerable to tactile stimulation provided by the mother during the first week of life and that different frequencies of LG-ABN presented during this period help to program neurodevelopment with long-lasting consequences on hippocampal GR function and HPA responses to stress. Cross-fostering paradigms show direct effects of maternal care on the behavioral and neuroendocrine responses to stress, and there-fore, support an epigenetic mechanism (Francis et al. 1999; Liu et al. 1997). In accordance with this hypothesis, we found differences in 5mC patterns and chromatin

H3K9Ac status in the exon 1_7 promoter, an upstream regulatory region that regulates the expression of the coding regions of the GR gene (McCormick et al. 2000) in the hippocampus of the offspring of High and Low LG-ABN mothers (Weaver et al. 2004). These group differences emerge over the first week of life, remain stable into adulthood, and are reversed by cross-fostering (Weaver et al. 2004). More specifically, our data suggest that an epimutation within the transcription factor nerve growth factor-inducible protein-A (NGFI-A) response element in the GR exon 1_7 promoter alters NGFI-A binding and might explain the sustained effect of maternal care on hippocampal GR expression and HPA responses to stress (Weaver et al. 2007).

The ability of maternal behavior to affect several behavioral phenotypes in the offspring, including maternal care, provides a mechanism by which acquired and stable behavioral traits can be propagated across generations through epigenetic modifications of DNA and chromatin structure. Support of this idea is evidenced by the increased hypothalamic CRF and GR exon 1_7 promoter methylation, decreased central CRF and GR expression, and increased HPA responsivity in adult mice born to gestationally stressed dams (Mueller and Bale 2008). On the other hand, brief ($\leq$15 min) periods of handling of daily for the first weeks of life (which increases maternal LG-ABN behavior) is associated with increased repressor neuron-restrictive silencer factor (NRSF) and decreased hypothalamic CRF promoter expression in the adult offspring (Korosi et al. 2010). Within the CRF promoter is a NRSF response element (Seth and Majzoub 2001). Increased NRSF binding and recruitment of additional repressor complexes to the CRF promoter might explain the sustained effect of handling on hypothalamic CRF expression (Zheng et al. 2009).

Together with our findings, these data suggest that the enzymes required for DNA methylation are involved in programming of neuroendocrine function and behavior, and may also contribute to the timing and sensitivity of the neonate to maternal adversity during pregnancy and lactation.

11.4.3 From Maternal Care to Chromatin Plasticity and Beyond

We propose that maternal behavior stimulates a signaling pathway that activates specific transcription factors, directing the epigenetic machinery (chromatin and DNA modifying enzymes) to exact targets within the genome. Our in vivo and in vitro studies suggest that maternal LG-ABN in early life elicits a thyroid hormone-dependent increase in serotonin (5-HT) activity at 5-HT$_7$ receptors, subsequent activation of cAMP and cAMP-dependent protein kinase A (PKA) accompanied by the recruitment of the transcription factor NGFI-A. NGFI-A, in turn, recruits CBP (which has HAT activity) (Chawla et al. 1998; Meaney et al. 1987, 2000; Weaver et al. 2007; Yu et al. 2004) and the demethylating enzyme MBD2b (Carvin et al. 2003) to the GR exon 1_7 promoter (McCormick et al. 2000). Our data suggest that CBP activity increases H3K9Ac, opening the chromatin structure enabling the binding of both NGFI-A and MBD2b proteins simultaneously to the same GR exon 1_7 promoter sequence (Weaver et al. unpublished data). MBD2b demethylates the NGFI-A response element, allowing stable binding of NGFI-A to its cognate binding site resulting in an increase in levels of hippocampal GR expression in the neonatal offspring. NGFI-A discriminates between the methylated and unmethylated GR exon 1_7 promoters and selectively activates the unmethylated sequences. Therefore, the different methylation states of the GR exon 1_7 promoter from the offspring of High and Low LG-ABN results in different levels of hippocampal GR expression in the adult offspring. These data chart a course through which maternal behavior results in epigenetic modification of a specific gene in the brain. Interestingly, although MBD2-deficient mice are viable, the postpartum MBD2-null mothers were significantly slower at retrieving pups to their nests in comparison with the wild-type dams (Hendrich et al. 2001). This suggests that MBD2 might also have an important role in the behavioral transmission of epigenetic modifications across generations by the mother. Indeed, we have previously shown that this behavioral transmission is associated with cytosine methylation of the estrogen receptor (ER)-α 1b promoter and ER-α expression in the medial preoptic (MPOA) area of female offspring (Champagne et al. 2003, 2006). Notably, maternal care influences the maternal behavior of female offspring, an effect that also appears to be related to epigenetic regulation of endocrine function, providing a mechanism for transgenerational inheritance of maternal behavior from mother to offspring. As environmental stressors influence the nature of maternal behavior, maternal care remains a key mediator of epigenetic programming of neurodevelopment, and in turn, the expression of biological defense systems that respond to environmental adversity.

Similar processes at comparable epigenetic labile regions could explain why the adult offspring of High and Low LG-ABN dams exhibit wide spread differences in hippocampal gene expression and cognitive function (Weaver et al. 2006). For example, the adult offspring of Low LG-ABN mothers show enhanced binding of MECP2 to the BDNF promoter in the hippocampus (Weaver et al. unpublished data), decreased hippocampal BDNF mRNA and protein expression, reduced hippocampal neuronal survival, reduced hippocampal synaptogenesis, and synaptic plasticity (Bredy et al. 2003a; Liu et al. 2000; Weaver et al. 2002). Consequently, these offspring perform worse in tests of spatial learning and object recognition by comparison with adult animals reared by High LG-ABN dams (Bredy et al. 2003b; Liu et al. 2000). This is consistent with recent studies demonstrating that exposure of infant rats to stressed caretakers that predominately displayed abusive behaviors (e.g., dragging and rough handling) produces offspring with increased BDNF IV promoter methylation and decreased in forebrain BDNF mRNA expression throughout life, with evidence of transgenerational inheritance of these traits in the abused female offspring (Roth et al. 2009). Central infusion of the DNA methylation inhibitor zeburaline increases forebrain BDNF mRNA expression in the abused offspring to levels comparable with the nonabused offspring. Interestingly, the effect of maternal care on cognitive function in the offspring of Low LG-ABN mothers is largely reversed with peripubertal exposure to an enriched environment (Bredy et al. 2003b, 2004; Champagne et al. 2008), implying that epigenetic labile regions in the rat brain remain environmentally responsive well beyond the perinatal period.

11.4.4   Evidence of Epigenetic Reprogramming in the Adult Brain

Although the majority of epigenetic programming is thought to occur early in postnatal life, it is possible to reverse these patterns through social experience, diet, or pharmacological intervention (Fischer et al. 2007; Weaver et al. 2004, 2005). The potential for epigenetic programs to be reversed has several important implications, especially for interventions aimed at improving behavioral outcomes and cognitive performance in children born into adversity (Olds et al. 1998, 2004a, b).

Animal models suggest that there is the potential for phenotypic plasticity in response to social experience during adolescence and adulthood. In rodents, social isolation during the postweaning period is associated with decreased forebrain expression of 5-HT receptor subtypes and increased anxiety-like responses, and is attenuated by antidepressant treatment (Bibancos et al. 2007; Heritch et al. 1990). Similarly, adult rodents exposed to a single stressful agonistic behavioral encounter (social defeat) show prolonged increased CRF expression and HPA responses to stress (Buwalda et al. 1999; Cooper and Huhman 2007). Social avoidance behavior that was induced by chronic social defeat stress given in adulthood coincided with demethylation of the CRF gene and increased hypothalamic CRF mRNA transcript expression (Evan et al. 2010). Conversely, juvenile environmental enrichment in rats is associated with increased hippocampal NGFI-A and GR expression (Olsson et al. 1994), reduced basal coticosterone levels, and a reduced HPA response to stress (Belz et al. 2003). Long-term stress in the adult has been shown to result in hippocampal cell loss (Anderton 1997), promoting the notion that stress in early life might also alter hippocampal neuron structure and function permanently (Kerr et al. 1991; Sapolsky 1985). Remarkably, environmental enrichment increases hippocampal H3 and H4 acetylation and enhances cognitive performance in juvenile rodents that have selective loss of hippocampal neurons (Fischer et al. 2007).

We therefore examined the effects of pharmacological intervention on brain gene expression and physiological and behavioral responses to stress within the context of tactile stimulation in early life. Central infusion of the HDAC inhibitor (HDACi) trichostatin A (TSA) in the adult offspring of Low LG-ABN mothers increased the H3K9Ac, cytosine demethylation, NGFI-A binding, and GR exon 1_7 promoter activation and reduced the HPA responses and anxiety-related behavior to levels comparable with those observed in the offspring of High LG-ABN dams (Weaver et al. 2004, 2006). Conversely, chronic central infusion of adult offspring of High or Low LG-ABN mothers with the dietary amino acid L-methionine, the precursor of SAM (Cantoni 1975; Mudd and Cantoni 1958) and inhibitor of demethylation (Pascale et al. 1991), increased the DNA methylation within the NGFI-A-binding site. This resulted in reduced NGFI-A binding to the exon 1_7 promoter selectively in

the offspring of High LG-ABN dams, removing group differences in both hippocampal GR expression and HPA responses to stress (Weaver et al. 2005). The idea
that DNA methylation patterns remain dynamic in adulthood is supported by recent
work in rats receiving hippocampal-dependent contextual fear conditioning training
(Miller et al. 2008; Miller and Sweatt 2007). Herein, TSA likely targets the class I
HDAC2, as HDAC2 deficiency in mice results in increased synapse number and
memory facilitation, similar to HDACi treatment (Guan et al. 2009). Together, these
data suggest that the machinery required for de novo DNA methylation or demethylation remains present and responsive to cellular signaling cascades in the mature
mammalian brain. Indeed, gene expression profiling of hippocampal tissue from the
adult offspring of High and Low LG-ABN mothers reveal specific effects on the
hippocampal transcriptome (Weaver et al. 2006).

11.5 Interindividual Differences in Human Behavior and Health

Studies in humans suggest that the forebrain GR function is complicit in the regulation
of the HPA axis and the development of affective disorders (DeRijk and Sternberg
1997; Holsboer 2000; Invitti et al. 1999). This raises the question of whether epigenetic modification in response to early environmental conditions can explain the
effects of early infant adversity on adult health in humans (for detailed review see
Weaver 2009). Interestingly, during their lifetime, monozygotic twins increasingly
differ in their epigenotype (lifelong drift) (Fraga et al. 2005), which might explain the
frequent discordance of neuropsychiatric disorders such as schizophrenia and bipolar
disorder (Kato et al. 2005). Although higher epigenetic discordance in fraternal
(dizygotic) twins can result from differences in DNA sequence, recent in silico single
nucleotide polymorphism (SNP) analyses together with animal studies favor epigenomic differences in the zygotes (Kaminsky et al. 2009). A recent review by Schlinzig
et al. (2009) found that global DNA methylation levels in cord white blood cells
are higher in newborns delivered by Caesarean section (CS) than those delivered by
normal vaginal delivery. Although it is currently unknown how gene expression is
affected in this case, individuals born by CS have been reported to face an increased
risk for common diseases later in life (Cardwell et al. 2008; Hakansson and Kallen
2003). These studies raise the possibility that suboptimal epigenetic modifications
arise over time resulting in late onset mental pathologies.

Indeed, aberrant gene transcription resulting from altered epigenetic regulation
is associated with cognitive defects in several progressive pathologies including
Alzheimer's disease (AD), schizophrenia, and depression. Increased expression
of presenilin 1 (PS1), a member of the γ-secretase complex, correlates with PS1
promoter hypomethylation in postmortem brain samples from AD patients, and
with increased β-amyloid formation in vitro (Scarpa et al. 2003; Wang et al. 2008).
Down regulation of reelin, a glycoprotein involved in neuronal migration during
development and cognitive functions in adults, and of the glutamate decarboxylase

that catalyzes GABA synthesis (GAD_{67}), are associated with promoter hyper-methylation in postmortem samples of schizophrenic patients (Abdolmaleky et al. 2005; Guidotti et al. 2000; Impagnatiello et al. 1998).

Consistent with this hypothesis, ribosomal RNA (rRNA) promoter methylation (Brown and Szyf 2007, 2008) was shown to be increased in suicide victims who were victims of abuse during childhood compared with controls (McGowan et al. 2008), suggesting a reduced capacity for protein synthesis in suicide brains (Brown and Szyf 2007, 2008). Protein synthesis has long been known to be required for associative learning to consolidate into long-term memory (Agranoff et al. 1967), which involves epigenetic regulation (Korzus et al. 2004), and a decline in cognitive plasticity is commonly observed with age (Kadar et al. 1990). More recently, it was found that the expression levels of DNMT enzymes are altered in suicide brains and specific genes are aberrantly silenced by DNA methylation (Poulter et al. 2008). For example, the GABA-A $\alpha 1$ receptor subunit (Poulter et al. 2008) and BDNF exon IV (Keller et al. 2010) promoter regions are both hypermethylated and their gene expression reduced in the forebrains of depressed patients who committed suicide in comparison with controls, further suggesting a link between mental disease and abnormal methylation. These findings suggest that a shift in the steady-state balance between DNA methylating and demethylating machinery might influence specific neural pathways and account for interindividual differences in emotional reactivity and mental health in humans.

The effects of tactile stimulation through mother–infant interactions on interindividual differences in cognitive development and stress responses in rodents is supported by work in humans (Feldman et al. 2002) and nonhuman primates (Harlow and Zimmermann 1959). This raises the question of whether comparable epigenetic labile regions to the GR exon 1_7 promoter exist in the human genome. Alignment of splice sites reveals that the distally located exon 1F promoter of human type II GR (hGR, OMIM +138040; NR3C1) shows high homology to the GR exon 1_7 promoter in the rat, and contains an NGFI-A-binding site (Turner and Muller 2005). Interestingly, studies in healthy human subjects show that CpG methylation patterns of conserved transcription factor binding sites on the NR3C1 exon 1F promoter are both stochastic and unique to the individual (Turner et al. 2008). Furthermore, neonatal methylation at the $5'$ CpG dinucleotide within the NGFI-A-binding site on the NR3C1 exon 1F promoter has been suggested as an early epigenetic marker of maternal mood and risk of altered HPA function in infants 3 months of age (Oberlander et al. 2008). Although future studies are required to examine the functional consequence of the methylated $5'$ CpG dinucleotide, these findings are consistent with our studies in the neonate and adult offspring of Low LG-ABN mothers that show hypermethylation of the $5'$ CpG dinucleotide within the NGFI-A-binding site on the exon 1_7 promoter, decreased GR expression and increased HPA responsivity (Weaver et al. 2004). In support of this paradigm, a recent study shows that the NGFI-A-binding sites on the NR3C1 exon 1F promoter are hypermethylated in the hippocampus of suicide victims with a history of childhood abuse and mRNA transcript expression from the exon 1F promoter is decreased by comparison to controls (victims of sudden, accidental death with no history of abuse) (McGowan et al. 2009), suggesting that the transmission of vulnerability for depression from parent to offspring could occur through the epigenetic modification of genomic regions that are implicated in the regulation of stress responses.

11.6 Concluding Remarks

The dynamic interdependence of an individual's genome, lifestyle, and health later in life has lead to the realization that the epigenome is essentially the study of gene–environment interactions. Sensory input during early development plays an important role in brain development with long-term consequences on brain functioning in adulthood. The studies presented in this chapter provide support for the idea that mother–offspring interactions early in life enhance the capacity for defensive responses in the progeny by programming emotional, cognitive, and endocrine systems toward increased sensitivity to adversity, and that these programs can be transmitted across generations via an epigenetic mode of inheritance involving maternal behavior, which in turn is responsive to changes in environmental stimuli (biotic, physical, and social). However, epigenetic reprogramming of distinct patterns of gene expression can take place at several points throughout life in response to developmental, physiological, psychological, pathological, and/or environmental cues.

These findings are restricted to the study of a single promoter in only one gene in one brain region; at this time, these results might be best thought of as a proof of principle. The degree to which this mechanism generalizes to environmental programming in other systems remains to be determined, and may well reveal an alternative mechanism for programming of the epigenome. The challenge will be to find comparable epigenetic labile regions. Genome-wide methodologies (epigenomics, metabolomics, proteomics, transcriptomics, etc.) of epigenetic changes assessing different regions and cell types in the brain are necessary. The examination of genotype–epigenotype–environment interactions from a developmental perspective has broad ranging implications for our understanding social, physiological, and pathological processes and their interrelations. Accordingly, we are only beginning to understand the mechanisms whereby early life experience suppresses or enhances expression of adaptive phenotypic behaviors throughout life.

11.7 Competing Interests Statement

The author declares that he has no competing financial interests.

Acknowlegments I would like to thank Dr. Shelley E. Brown for her helpful comments and numerous constructive suggestions throughout the preparation of this manuscript.

References

Abdolmaleky HM, Cheng KH, Russo A, Smith CL, Faraone SV, Wilcox M, Shafa R, Glatt SJ, Nguyen G, Ponte JF et al (2005) Hypermethylation of the reelin (RELN) promoter in the brain of schizophrenic patients: a preliminary report. Am J Med Genet B Neuropsychiatr Genet 134B: 60–66

Adams RL, McKay EL, Craig LM, Burdon RH (1979) Mouse DNA methylase: methylation of native DNA. Biochim Biophys Acta 561:345–357

Agranoff BW, Davis RE, Casola L, Lim R (1967) Actinomycin D blocks formation of memory of shock-avoidance in goldfish. Science 158:1600–1601

Alarcon JM, Malleret G, Touzani K, Vronskaya S, Ishii S, Kandel ER, Barco A (2004) Chromatin acetylation, memory, and LTP are impaired in CBP+/- mice: a model for the cognitive deficit in Rubinstein-Taybi syndrome and its amelioration. Neuron 42:947–959

Alleman M, Sidorenko L, McGinnis K, Seshadri V, Dorweiler JE, White J, Sikkink K, Chandler VL (2006) An RNA-dependent RNA polymerase is required for paramutation in maize. Nature 442:295–298

Amir RE, Van den Veyver IB, Wan M, Tran CQ, Francke U, Zoghbi HY (1999) Rett syndrome is caused by mutations in X-linked MECP2, encoding methyl-CpG-binding protein 2. Nat Genet 23:185–188

Anderton BH (1997) Changes in the ageing brain in health and disease. Philos Trans R Soc Lond B Biol Sci 352:1781–1792

Antequera F, Bird A (1993) CpG islands. EXS 64:169–185

Baccarelli A, Bollati V (2009) Epigenetics and environmental chemicals. Curr Opin Pediatr 21: 243–251

Balada E, Ordi-Ros J, Serrano-Acedo S, Martinez-Lostao L, Vilardell-Tarres M (2007) Transcript overexpression of the MBD2 and MBD4 genes in CD4+ T cells from systemic lupus erythematosus patients. J Leukoc Biol 81:1609–1616

Barker DJ, Eriksson JG, Forsen T, Osmond C (2002) Fetal origins of adult disease: strength of effects and biological basis. Int J Epidemiol 31:1235–1239

Barreto G, Schäfer A, Marhold J, Stach D, Swaminathan SK, Handa V, Döderlein G, Maltry N, Wu W, Lyko F, Niehrs C (2007) Gadd45a promotes epigenetic gene activation by repair-mediated DNA demethylation. Nature 445:671–675

Belz EE, Kennell JS, Czambel RK, Rubin RT, Rhodes ME (2003) Environmental enrichment lowers stress-responsive hormones in singly housed male and female rats. Pharmacol Biochem Behav 76:481–486

Bergmann A, Lane ME (2003) HIDden targets of microRNAs for growth control. Trends Biochem Sci 28:461–463

Bernstein BE, Kamal M, Lindblad-Toh K, Bekiranov S, Bailey DK, Huebert DJ, McMahon S, Karlsson EK, Kulbokas EJ 3rd, Gingeras TR et al (2005) Genomic maps and comparative analysis of histone modifications in human and mouse. Cell 120:169–181

Bestor T (1988) Structure of mammalian DNA methyltransferase as deduced from the inferred amino acid sequence and direct studies of the protein. Biochem Soc Trans 16:944–947

Bestor TH (1992) Activation of mammalian DNA methyltransferase by cleavage of a Zn binding regulatory domain. EMBO J 11:2611–2617

Bestor TH, Verdine GL (1994) DNA methyltransferases. Curr Opin Cell Biol 6:380–389

Bettegowda A, Smith GW (2007) Mechanisms of maternal mRNA regulation: implications for mammalian early embryonic development. Front Biosci 12:3713–3726

Bhattacharya SK, Ramchandani S, Cervoni N, Szyf M (1999) A mammalian protein with specific demethylase activity for mCpG DNA. Nature 397:579–583

Bibancos T, Jardim DL, Aneas I, Chiavegatto S (2007) Social isolation and expression of serotonergic neurotransmission-related genes in several brain areas of male mice. Genes Brain Behav 6:529–539

Bird AP (1996) The relationship of DNA methylation to cancer. Cancer Surv 28:87–101

Bird A (2001) Molecular biology. Methylation talk between histones and DNA. Science 294: 2113–2115

Bird AP, Wolffe AP (1999) Methylation-induced repression–belts, braces, and chromatin. Cell 99:451–454

Boeke J, Ammerpohl O, Kegel S, Moehren U, Renkawitz R (2000) The minimal repression domain of MBD2b overlaps with the methyl-CpG-binding domain and binds directly to Sin3A. J Biol Chem 275:34963–34967

Boulinier T, Staszewski V (2008) Maternal transfer of antibodies: raising immuno-ecology issues. Trends Ecol Evol 23:282–288

Boyle MP, Kolber BJ, Vogt SK, Wozniak DF, Muglia LJ (2006) Forebrain glucocorticoid receptors modulate anxiety-associated locomotor activation and adrenal responsiveness. J Neurosci 26:1971–1978

Bradshaw AD (1965) Evolutionary significance of phenotypic plasticity in plants. Adv Genet 13: 115–155

Bredy TW, Grant RJ, Champagne DL, Meaney MJ (2003a) Maternal care influences neuronal survival in the hippocampus of the rat. Eur J Neurosci 18:2903–2909

Bredy TW, Humpartzoomian RA, Cain DP, Meaney MJ (2003b) Partial reversal of the effect of maternal care on cognitive function through environmental enrichment. Neuroscience 118: 571–576

Bredy TW, Zhang TY, Grant RJ, Diorio J, Meaney MJ (2004) Peripubertal environmental enrichment reverses the effects of maternal care on hippocampal development and glutamate receptor subunit expression. Eur J Neurosci 20:1355–1362

Brown SE, Szyf M (2007) Epigenetic programming of the rRNA promoter by MBD3. Mol Cell Biol 27:4938–4952

Brown SE, Szyf M (2008) Dynamic epigenetic states of ribosomal RNA promoters during the cell cycle. Cell Cycle 7:382–390

Brown SE, Suderman MJ, Hallett M, Szyf M (2008) DNA demethylation induced by the methyl-CpG-binding domain protein MBD3. Gene 420:99–106

Burdge GC, Lillycrop KA, Phillips ES, Slater-Jefferies JL, Jackson AA, Hanson MA (2009) Folic acid supplementation during the juvenile-pubertal period in rats modifies the phenotype and epigenotype induced by prenatal nutrition. J Nutr 139:1054–1060

Buwalda B, de Boer SF, Schmidt ED, Felszeghy K, Nyakas C, Sgoifo A, Van der Vegt BJ, Tilders FJ, Bohus B, Koolhaas JM (1999) Long-lasting deficient dexamethasone suppression of hypothalamic-pituitary-adrenocortical activation following peripheral CRF challenge in socially defeated rats. J Neuroendocrinol 11:513–520

Caldji C, Tannenbaum B, Sharma S, Francis D, Plotsky PM, Meaney MJ (1998) Maternal care during infancy regulates the development of neural systems mediating the expression of fearfulness in the rat. Proc Natl Acad Sci USA 95:5335–5340

Cameron HA, Gould E (1994) Adult neurogenesis is regulated by adrenal steroids in the dentate gyrus. Neuroscience 61:203–209

Canetti L, Bachar E, Galili-Weisstub E, De-Nour AK, Shalev AY (1997) Parental bonding and mental health in adolescence. Adolescence 32:381–394

Cannon SV, Cummings A, Teebor GW (1988) 5-Hydroxymethylcytosine DNA glycosylase activity in mammalian tissue. Biochem Biophys Res Comm 151:1173–1179

Cantoni GL (1975) Biological methylation: selected aspects. Annu Rev Biochem 44:435–451

Cardwell CR, Stene LC, Joner G, Cinek O, Svensson J, Goldacre MJ, Parslow RC, Pozzilli P, Brigis G, Stoyanov D et al (2008) Caesarean section is associated with an increased risk of childhood-onset type 1 diabetes mellitus: a meta-analysis of observational studies. Diabetologia 51:726–735

Carvin CD, Parr RD, Kladde MP (2003) Site-selective in vivo targeting of cytosine-5 DNA methylation by zinc-finger proteins. Nucleic Acids Res 31:6493–6501

Cebrian A, Pharoah PD, Ahmed S, Ropero S, Fraga MF, Smith PL, Conroy D, Luben R, Perkins B, Easton DF et al (2006) Genetic variants in epigenetic genes and breast cancer risk. Carcinogenesis 27:1661–1669

Cervoni N, Szyf M (2001) Demethylase activity is directed by histone acetylation. J Biol Chem 276:40778–40787

Cervoni N, Bhattacharya S, Szyf M (1999) DNA demethylase is a processive enzyme. J Biol Chem 274:8363–8366

Champagne FA, Meaney MJ (2006) Stress during gestation alters postpartum maternal care and the development of the offspring in a rodent model. Biol Psychiatry 59:1227–1235

Champagne FA, Meaney MJ (2007) Transgenerational effects of social environment on variations in maternal care and behavioral response to novelty. Behav Neurosci 121:1353–1363

Champagne FA, Weaver IC, Diorio J, Sharma S, Meaney MJ (2003) Natural variations in maternal care are associated with estrogen receptor alpha expression and estrogen sensitivity in the medial preoptic area. Endocrinology 144:4720–4724

Champagne FA, Weaver IC, Diorio J, Dymov S, Szyf M, Meaney MJ (2006) Maternal care associated with methylation of the estrogen receptor-alpha1b promoter and estrogen receptor-alpha expression in the medial preoptic area of female offspring. Endocrinology 147: 2909–2915

Champagne DL, Bagot RC, van Hasselt F, Ramakers G, Meaney MJ, de Kloet ER, Joels M, Krugers H (2008) Maternal care and hippocampal plasticity: evidence for experience-dependent structural plasticity, altered synaptic functioning, and differential responsiveness to glucocorticoids and stress. J Neurosci 28:6037–6045

Chandler VL (2007) Paramutation: from maize to mice. Cell 128:641–645

Chang Q, Khare G, Dani V, Nelson S, Jaenisch R (2006) The disease progression of Mecp2 mutant mice is affected by the level of BDNF expression. Neuron 49:341–348

Chawla S, Hardingham GE, Quinn DR, Bading H (1998) CBP: a signal-regulated transcriptional coactivator controlled by nuclear calcium and CaM kinase IV. Science 281:1505–1509

Chen WG, Chang Q, Lin Y, Meissner A, West AE, Griffith EC, Jaenisch R, Greenberg ME (2003) Derepression of BDNF transcription involves calcium-dependent phosphorylation of MeCP2. Science 302:885–889

Ching TT, Maunakea AK, Jun P, Hong C, Zardo G, Pinkel D, Albertson DG, Fridlyand J, Mao JH, Shchors K et al (2005) Epigenome analyses using BAC microarrays identify evolutionary conservation of tissue-specific methylation of SHANK3. Nat Genet 37:645–651

Chong S, Whitelaw E (2004) Epigenetic germline inheritance. Curr Opin Genet Dev 14:692–696

Chuang JC, Jones PA (2007) Epigenetics and microRNAs. Pediatr Res 61:24R–29R

Coe CL, Lubach GR (2005) Prenatal origins of individual variation in behavior and immunity. Neurosci Biobehav Rev 29:39–49

Cooper MA, Huhman KL (2007) Corticotropin-releasing factor receptors in the dorsal raphe nucleus modulate social behavior in Syrian hamsters. Psychopharmacology (Berl) 194: 297–307

David SS, Williams SD (1998) Chemistry of glycosylases and endonucleases involved in base-excision repair. Chem Rev 98:1221–1262

Davie JR, Chadee DN (1998) Regulation and regulatory parameters of histone modifications. J Cell Biochem Suppl 30–31:203–213

De Kloet ER, Vreugdenhil E, Oitzl MS, Joels M (1998) Brain corticosteroid receptor balance in health and disease. Endocr Rev 19:269–301

Dempfle A, Scherag A, Hein R, Beckmann L, Chang-Claude J, Schafer H (2008) Gene-environment interactions for complex traits: definitions, methodological requirements and challenges. Eur J Hum Genet 16:1164–1172

Denenberg VH (1999) Commentary: is maternal stimulation the mediator of the handling effect in infancy? Dev Psychobiol 34:1–3

DeRijk R, Sternberg EM (1997) Corticosteroid resistance and disease. Ann Med 29:79–82

Detich N, Theberge J, Szyf M (2002) Promoter-specific activation and demethylation by MBD2/demethylase. J Biol Chem 277:35791–35794

Detich N, Bovenzi V, Szyf M (2003a) Valproate induces replication-independent active DNA demethylation. J Biol Chem 278:27586–27592

Detich N, Hamm S, Just G, Knox JD, Szyf M (2003b) The methyl donor S-Adenosylmethionine inhibits active demethylation of DNA: a candidate novel mechanism for the pharmacological effects of S-Adenosylmethionine. J Biol Chem 278:20812–20820

Dolinoy DC, Weidman JR, Waterland RA, Jirtle RL (2006) Maternal genistein alters coat color and protects Avy mouse offspring from obesity by modifying the fetal epigenome. Environ Health Perspect 114:567–572

Dolinoy DC, Weidman JR, Jirtle RL (2007) Epigenetic gene regulation: linking early developmental environment to adult disease. Reprod Toxicol 23:297–307

Dolinoy DC, Weinhouse C, Jones T, Rozek LS, Jirtle RL (2010) Variable histone modifications at the A(vy) metastable epiallele. Epigenetics 5:637–644

Elf J, Li GW, Xie XS (2007) Probing transcription factor dynamics at the single-molecule level in a living cell. Science 316:1191–1194

Elliott E, Ezra-Nevo G, Regev L, Neufeld-Cohen A, Chen A (2010) Resilience to social stress coincides with functional DNA methylation of the Crf gene in adult mice. Nat Neurosci 13:1351–3

Evans JD, Wheeler DE (1999) Differential gene expression between developing queens and workers in the honey bee, *Apis mellifera*. Proc Natl Acad Sci USA 96:5575–5580

Evans JD, Wheeler DE (2001) Expression profiles during honeybee caste determination. Genome Biol 2, RESEARCH0001

Fazzari MJ, Greally JM (2004) Epigenomics: beyond CpG islands. Nat Rev Genet 5:446–455

Feinberg AP (2007) An epigenetic approach to cancer etiology. Cancer J 13:70–74

Feldman R, Eidelman AI, Sirota L, Weller A (2002) Comparison of skin-to-skin (kangaroo) and traditional care: parenting outcomes and preterm infant development. Pediatrics 110:16–26

Feng J, Chang H, Li E, Fan G (2005) Dynamic expression of de novo DNA methyltransferases Dnmt3a and Dnmt3b in the central nervous system. J Neurosci Res 79:734–746

Feng J, Zhou Y, Campbell SL, Le T, Li E, Sweatt JD, Silva AJ, Fan G (2010a) Dnmt1 and Dnmt3a maintain DNA methylation and regulate synaptic function in adult forebrain neurons. Nat Neurosci 13:423–430

Feng S, Cokus SJ, Zhang X, Chen PY, Bostick M, Goll MG, Hetzel J, Jain J, Strauss SH, Halpern ME et al (2010b) Conservation and divergence of methylation patterning in plants and animals. Proc Natl Acad Sci USA 107:8689–8694

Fischer A, Sananbenesi F, Wang X, Dobbin M, Tsai LH (2007) Recovery of learning and memory is associated with chromatin remodelling. Nature 447:178–182

Fowden AL, Giussani DA, Forhead AJ (2006) Intrauterine programming of physiological systems: causes and consequences. Physiology (Bethesda) 21:29–37

Fraga MF, Ballestar E, Paz MF, Ropero S, Setien F, Ballestar ML, Heine-Suner D, Cigudosa JC, Urioste M, Benitez J et al (2005) Epigenetic differences arise during the lifetime of monozygotic twins. Proc Natl Acad Sci USA 102:10604–10609

Francis DD, Meaney MJ (1999) Maternal care and the development of stress responses. Curr Opin Neurobiol 9:128–134

Francis D, Diorio J, Liu D, Meaney MJ (1999) Nongenomic transmission across generations of maternal behavior and stress responses in the rat. Science 286:1155–1158

Gardiner-Garden M, Frommer M (1987) CpG islands in vertebrate genomes. J Mol Biol 196: 261–282

Giovannucci E (2004) Alcohol, one-carbon metabolism, and colorectal cancer: recent insights from molecular studies. J Nutr 134:2475S–2481S

Gluckman PD, Hanson MA, Cooper C, Thornburg KL (2008) Effect of in utero and early-life conditions on adult health and disease. N Engl J Med 359:61–73

Goel A, Mathupala SP, Pedersen PL (2003) Glucose metabolism in cancer. Evidence that demethylation events play a role in activating type II hexokinase gene expression. J Biol Chem 278:15333–15340

Goll MG, Bestor TH (2005) Eukaryotic cytosine methyltransferases. Annu Rev Biochem 74: 481–514

Goto K, Numata M, Komura JI, Ono T, Bestor TH, Kondo H (1994) Expression of DNA methyltransferase gene in mature and immature neurons as well as proliferating cells in mice. Differentiation 56:39–44

Grindstaff JL, Brodie ED 3rd, Ketterson ED (2003) Immune function across generations: integrating mechanism and evolutionary process in maternal antibody transmission. Proc Biol Sci 270:2309–2319

Grunstein M (1997) Histone acetylation in chromatin structure and transcription. Nature 389: 349–352

Guan JS, Haggarty SJ, Giacometti E, Dannenberg JH, Joseph N, Gao J, Nieland TJ, Zhou Y, Wang X, Mazitschek R et al (2009) HDAC2 negatively regulates memory formation and synaptic plasticity. Nature 459:55–60

Guidotti A, Auta J, Davis JM, Di-Giorgi-Gerevini V, Dwivedi Y, Grayson DR, Impagnatiello F, Pandey G, Pesold C, Sharma R et al (2000) Decrease in reelin and glutamic acid decarboxylase67 (GAD67) expression in schizophrenia and bipolar disorder: a postmortem brain study. Arch Gen Psychiatry 57:1061–1069

Guy J, Gan J, Selfridge J, Cobb S, Bird A (2007) Reversal of neurological defects in a mouse model of Rett syndrome. Science 315:1143–7

Hakansson S, Kallen K (2003) Caesarean section increases the risk of hospital care in childhood for asthma and gastroenteritis. Clin Exp Allergy 33:757–764

Hales CN, Barker DJ (1992) Type 2 (non-insulin-dependent) diabetes mellitus: the thrifty phenotype hypothesis. Diabetologia 35:595–601

Hamm S, Just G, Lacoste N, Moitessier N, Szyf M, Mamer O (2008) On the mechanism of demethylation of 5-methylcytosine in DNA. Bioorg Med Chem Lett 18:1046–1049

Hansen RS, Wijmenga C, Luo P, Stanek AM, Canfield TK, Weemaes CM, Gartler SM (1999) The DNMT3B DNA methyltransferase gene is mutated in the ICF immunodeficiency syndrome. Proc Natl Acad Sci USA 96:14412–14417

Harlow HF, Zimmermann RR (1959) Affectional responses in the infant monkey; orphaned baby monkeys develop a strong and persistent attachment to inanimate surrogate mothers. Science 130:421–432

Hartfelder K, Engels W (1998) Social insect polymorphism: hormonal regulation of plasticity in development and reproduction in the honeybee. Curr Top Dev Biol 40:45–77

Hashimshony T, Zhang J, Keshet I, Bustin M, Cedar H (2003) The role of DNA methylation in setting up chromatin structure during development. Nat Genet 34:187–192

Hasselquist D, Nilsson JA (2009) Maternal transfer of antibodies in vertebrates: trans-generational effects on offspring immunity. Philos Trans R Soc Lond B Biol Sci 364:51–60

Heim C, Newport DJ, Heit S, Graham YP, Wilcox M, Bonsall R, Miller AH, Nemeroff CB (2000) Pituitary-adrenal and autonomic responses to stress in women after sexual and physical abuse in childhood. JAMA 284:592–597

Henderson IR, Jacobsen SE (2007) Epigenetic inheritance in plants. Nature 447:418–424

Hendrich B, Guy J, Ramsahoye B, Wilson VA, Bird A (2001) Closely related proteins MBD2 and MBD3 play distinctive but interacting roles in mouse development. Genes Dev 15:710–723

Henikoff S, Furuyama T, Ahmad K (2004) Histone variants, nucleosome assembly and epigenetic inheritance. Trends Genet 20:320–326

Heritch AJ, Henderson K, Westfall TC (1990) Effects of social isolation on brain catecholamines and forced swimming in rats: prevention by antidepressant treatment. J Psychiatr Res 24: 251–258

Herman JP, Figueiredo H, Mueller NK, Ulrich-Lai Y, Ostrander MM, Choi DC, Cullinan WE (2003) Central mechanisms of stress integration: hierarchical circuitry controlling hypothalamo-pituitary-adrenocortical responsiveness. Front Neuroendocrinol 24:151–180

Holliday R, Pugh JE (1975) DNA modification mechanisms and gene activity during development. Science 187:226–232

Holsboer F (2000) The corticosteroid receptor hypothesis of depression. Neuropsychopharmacology 23:477–501

Hong L, Schroth GP, Matthews HR, Yau P, Bradbury EM (1993) Studies of the DNA binding properties of histone H4 amino terminus. Thermal denaturation studies reveal that acetylation markedly reduces the binding constant of the H4 "tail" to DNA. J Biol Chem 268:305–314

Huizink AC, Mulder EJ, Buitelaar JK (2004) Prenatal stress and risk for psychopathology: specific effects or induction of general susceptibility? Psychol Bull 130:115–142

Impagnatiello F, Guidotti AR, Pesold C, Dwivedi Y, Caruncho H, Pisu MG, Uzunov DP, Smalheiser NR, Davis JM, Pandey GN et al (1998) A decrease of reelin expression as a putative vulnerability factor in schizophrenia. Proc Natl Acad Sci USA 95:15718–15723

Invitti C, Redaelli G, Baldi G, Cavagnini F (1999) Glucocorticoid receptors in anorexia nervosa and Cushing's disease. Biol Psychiatry 45:1467–1471

Ishibe N, Kelsey KT (1997) Genetic susceptibility to environmental and occupational cancers. Canc Causes Contr 8:504–513

Ito S, D'Alessio AC, Taranova OV, Hong K, Sowers LC, Zhang Y (2010) Role of Tet proteins in 5mC to 5hmC conversion, ES-cell self-renewal and inner cell mass specification. Nature 466:1129–1133

Jenuwein T (2001) Re-SET-ting heterochromatin by histone methyltransferases. Trends Cell Biol 11:266–273

Jenuwein T, Allis CD (2001) Translating the histone code. Science 293:1074–1080

Jiang YH, Bressler J, Beaudet AL (2004) Epigenetics and human disease. Annu Rev Genomics Hum Genet 5:479–510

Jones PL, Veenstra GJ, Wade PA, Vermaak D, Kass SU, Landsberger N, Strouboulis J, Wolffe AP (1998) Methylated DNA and MeCP2 recruit histone deacetylase to repress transcription. Nat Genet 19:187–191

Josselyn SA (2005) What's right with my mouse model? New insights into the molecular and cellular basis of cognition from mouse models of Rubinstein-Taybi Syndrome. Learn Mem 12:80–83

Kaati G, Bygren LO, Edvinsson S (2002) Cardiovascular and diabetes mortality determined by nutrition during parents' and grandparents' slow growth period. Eur J Hum Genet 10:682–688

Kadar T, Silbermann M, Brandeis R, Levy A (1990) Age-related structural changes in the rat hippocampus: correlation with working memory deficiency. Brain Res 512:113–120

Kadonaga JT (1998) Eukaryotic transcription: an interlaced network of transcription factors and chromatin-modifying machines. Cell 92:307–313

Kalkhoven E, Roelfsema JH, Teunissen H, den Boer A, Ariyurek Y, Zantema A, Breuning MH, Hennekam RC, Peters DJ (2003) Loss of CBP acetyltransferase activity by PHD finger mutations in Rubinstein-Taybi syndrome. Hum Mol Genet 12:441–450

Kaminsky ZA, Tang T, Wang SC, Ptak C, Oh GH, Wong AH, Feldcamp LA, Virtanen C, Halfvarson J, Tysk C et al (2009) DNA methylation profiles in monozygotic and dizygotic twins. Nat Genet 41:240–245

Kangaspeska S, Stride B, Metivier R, Polycarpou-Schwarz M, Ibberson D, Carmouche RP, Benes V, Gannon F, Reid G (2008) Transient cyclical methylation of promoter DNA. Nature 452:112–115

Kato T, Iwamoto K, Kakiuchi C, Kuratomi G, Okazaki Y (2005) Genetic or epigenetic difference causing discordance between monozygotic twins as a clue to molecular basis of mental disorders. Mol Psychiatry 10:622–630

Ke X, Lei Q, James SJ, Kelleher SL, Melnyk S, Jernigan S, Yu X, Wang L, Callaway CW, Gill G et al (2006) Uteroplacental insufficiency affects epigenetic determinants of chromatin structure in brains of neonatal and juvenile IUGR rats. Physiol Genomics 25:16–28

Kelemen LE, Sellers TA, Schildkraut JM, Cunningham JM, Vierkant RA, Pankratz VS, Fredericksen ZS, Gadre MK, Rider DN, Liebow M et al (2008) Genetic variation in the one-carbon transfer pathway and ovarian cancer risk. Cancer Res 68:2498–2506

Keller S, Sarchiapone M, Zarrilli F, Videtic A, Ferraro A, Carli V, Sacchetti S, Lembo F, Angiolillo A, Jovanovic N et al (2010) Increased BDNF promoter methylation in the Wernicke area of suicide subjects. Arch Gen Psychiatry 67:258–267

Kerr DS, Campbell LW, Applegate MD, Brodish A, Landfield PW (1991) Chronic stress-induced acceleration of electrophysiologic and morphometric biomarkers of hippocampal aging. J Neurosci 11:1316–1324

Kersh EN, Fitzpatrick DR, Murali-Krishna K, Shires J, Speck SH, Boss JM, Ahmed R (2006) Rapid demethylation of the IFN-gamma gene occurs in memory but not naive CD8 T cells. J Immunol 176:4083–4093

Khulan B, Thompson RF, Ye K, Fazzari MJ, Suzuki M, Stasiek E, Figueroa ME, Glass JL, Chen Q, Montagna C et al (2006) Comparative isoschizomer profiling of cytosine methylation: the HELP assay. Genome Res 16:1046–1055

Kornberg RD (1974) Chromatin structure: a repeating unit of histones and DNA. Science 184: 868–871

Korosi A, Shanabrough M, McClelland S, Liu ZW, Borok E, Gao XB, Horvath TL, Baram TZ (2010) Early-life experience reduces excitation to stress-responsive hypothalamic neurons and reprograms the expression of corticotropin-releasing hormone. J Neurosci 30:703–713

Korzus E, Rosenfeld MG, Mayford M (2004) CBP histone acetyltransferase activity is a critical component of memory consolidation. Neuron 42:961–972

Kraft P, Hunter D (2005) Integrating epidemiology and genetic association: the challenge of gene-environment interaction. Philos Trans R Soc Lond B Biol Sci 360:1609–1616

Kriaucionis S, Heintz N (2009) The nuclear DNA base 5-hydroxymethylcytosine is present in Purkinje neurons and the brain. Science 324:929–930

Kucharski R, Maleszka J, Foret S, Maleszka R (2008) Nutritional control of reproductive status in honeybees via DNA methylation. Science 319:1827–1830

Kuo MH, Allis CD (1998) Roles of histone acetyltransferases and deacetylases in gene regulation. Bioessays 20:615–626

Lachner M, Jenuwein T (2002) The many faces of histone lysine methylation. Curr Opin Cell Biol 14:286–298

Lachner M, O'Carroll D, Rea S, Mechtler K, Jenuwein T (2001) Methylation of histone H3 lysine 9 creates a binding site for HP1 proteins. Nature 410:116–120

Lachner M, O'Sullivan RJ, Jenuwein T (2003) An epigenetic road map for histone lysine methylation. J Cell Sci 116:2117–2124

Law JA, Jacobsen SE (2010) Establishing, maintaining and modifying DNA methylation patterns in plants and animals. Nat Rev Genet 11:204–220

Lee DY, Hayes JJ, Pruss D, Wolffe AP (1993) A positive role for histone acetylation in transcription factor access to nucleosomal DNA. Cell 72:73–84

Lee SJ, Jeon HS, Jang JS, Park SH, Lee GY, Lee BH, Kim CH, Kang YM, Lee WK, Kam S et al (2005) DNMT3B polymorphisms and risk of primary lung cancer. Carcinogenesis 26:403–409

Leonhardt H, Bestor TH (1993) Structure, function and regulation of mammalian DNA methyl-transferase. EXS 64:109–119

Li E (2002) Chromatin modification and epigenetic reprogramming in mammalian development. Nat Rev Genet 3:662–673

Lillycrop KA, Phillips ES, Jackson AA, Hanson MA, Burdge GC (2005) Dietary protein restriction of pregnant rats induces and folic acid supplementation prevents epigenetic modification of hepatic gene expression in the offspring. J Nutr 135:1382–1386

Lillycrop KA, Slater-Jefferies JL, Hanson MA, Godfrey KM, Jackson AA, Burdge GC (2007) Induction of altered epigenetic regulation of the hepatic glucocorticoid receptor in the offspring of rats fed a protein-restricted diet during pregnancy suggests that reduced DNA methyltransferase-1 expression is involved in impaired DNA methylation and changes in histone modifications. Br J Nutr 97:1064–1073

Lillycrop KA, Phillips ES, Torrens C, Hanson MA, Jackson AA, Burdge GC (2008) Feeding pregnant rats a protein-restricted diet persistently alters the methylation of specific cytosines in the hepatic PPAR alpha promoter of the offspring. Br J Nutr 100:278–282

Lister R, Pelizzola M, Dowen RH, Hawkins RD, Hon G, Tonti-Filippini J, Nery JR, Lee L, Ye Z, Ngo QM, Edsall L, Antosiewicz-Bourget J, Stewart R, Ruotti V, Millar AH, Thomson JA,

Ren B, Ecker JR (2009) Human DNA methylomes at base resolution show widespread epigenomic differences. Nature 462(7271):315–22

Liu D, Diorio J, Tannenbaum B, Caldji C, Francis D, Freedman A, Sharma S, Pearson D, Plotsky PM, Meaney MJ (1997) Maternal care, hippocampal glucocorticoid receptors, and hypotha-lamic- pituitary-adrenal responses to stress [see comments]. Science 277:1659–1662

Liu D, Diorio J, Day JC, Francis DD, Meaney MJ (2000) Maternal care, hippocampal synapto-genesis and cognitive development in rats. Nat Neurosci 3:799–806

Liutkeviciute Z, Lukinavicius G, Masevicius V, Daujotyte D, Klimasauskas S (2009) Cytosine-5-methyltransferases add aldehydes to DNA. Nat Chem Biol 5:400–402

London SJ, Romieu I (2009) Gene by environment interaction in asthma. Annu Rev Public Health 30:55–80

Lucarelli M, Fuso A, Strom R, Scarpa S (2001) The dynamics of myogenin site-specific demeth-ylation is strongly correlated with its expression and with muscle differentiation. J Biol Chem 276:7500–7506

Luedi PP, Hartemink AJ, Jirtle RL (2005) Genome-wide prediction of imprinted murine genes. Genome Res 15:875–884

MacLennan NK, James SJ, Melnyk S, Piroozi A, Jernigan S, Hsu JL, Janke SM, Pham TD, Lane RH (2004) Uteroplacental insufficiency alters DNA methylation, one-carbon metabolism, and histone acetylation in IUGR rats. Physiol Genomics 18:43–50

Madhani HD, Francis NJ, Kingston RE, Kornberg RD, Moazed D, Narlikar GJ, Panning B, Struhl K (2008) Epigenomics: a roadmap, but to where? Science 322:43–44

Martienssen RA, Colot V (2001) DNA methylation and epigenetic inheritance in plants and filamentous fungi. Science 293:1070–1074

Martinowich K, Hattori D, Wu H, Fouse S, He F, Hu Y, Fan G, Sun YE (2003) DNA methylation-related chromatin remodeling in activity-dependent BDNF gene regulation. Science 302:890–893

Mattick JS, Makunin IV (2006) Non-coding RNA. Hum Mol Genet 15(Spec No 1):R17–R29

Mattick JS, Amaral PP, Dinger ME, Mercer TR, Mehler MF (2009) RNA regulation of epigenetic processes. Bioessays 31:51–59

McCormick JA, Lyons V, Jacobson MD, Noble J, Diorio J, Nyirenda M, Weaver S, Ester W, Yau JL, Meaney MJ et al (2000) 5′-heterogeneity of glucocorticoid receptor messenger RNA is tissue specific: differential regulation of variant transcripts by early-life events. Mol Endocri-nol 14:506–517

McEwen BS (2004) Protection and damage from acute and chronic stress: allostasis and allostatic overload and relevance to the pathophysiology of psychiatric disorders. Ann NY Acad Sci 1032:1–7

McGowan PO, Sasaki A, Huang TC, Unterberger A, Suderman M, Ernst C, Meaney MJ, Turecki G, Szyf M (2008) Promoter-wide hypermethylation of the ribosomal RNA gene promoter in the suicide brain. PLoS ONE 3:e2085

McGowan PO, Sasaki A, D'Alessio AC, Dymov S, Labonte B, Szyf M, Turecki G, Meaney MJ (2009) Epigenetic regulation of the glucocorticoid receptor in human brain associates with childhood abuse. Nat Neurosci 12:342–348

Meaney MJ (2001) Maternal care, gene expression, and the transmission of individual differences in stress reactivity across generations. Annu Rev Neurosci 24:1161–1192

Meaney MJ, Aitken DH, Sapolsky RM (1987) Thyroid hormones influence the development of hippocampal glucocorticoid receptors in the rat: a mechanism for the effects of postnatal handling on the development of the adrenocortical stress response. Neuroendocrinology 45:278–283

Meaney MJ, Aitken DH, Viau V, Sharma S, Sarrieau A (1989) Neonatal handling alters adreno-cortical negative feedback sensitivity and hippocampal type II glucocorticoid receptor binding in the rat. Neuroendocrinology 50:597–604

Meaney MJ, Diorio J, Francis D, Weaver S, Yau J, Chapman K, Seckl JR (2000) Postnatal handling increases the expression of cAMP-inducible transcription factors in the rat hippo-campus: the effects of thyroid hormones and serotonin. J Neurosci 20:3926–3935

Metivier R, Gallais R, Tiffoche C, Le Peron C, Jurkowska RZ, Carmouche RP, Ibberson D, Barath P, Demay F, Reid G et al (2008) Cyclical DNA methylation of a transcriptionally active promoter. Nature 452:45–50

Miller CA, Sweatt JD (2007) Covalent modification of DNA regulates memory formation. Neuron 53:857–869

Miller JW, Nadeau MR, Smith J, Smith D, Selhub J (1994) Folate-deficiency-induced homocysteinaemia in rats: disruption of S-adenosylmethionine's co-ordinate regulation of homocysteine metabolism. Biochem J 298(Pt 2):415–419

Miller CA, Campbell SL, Sweatt JD (2008) DNA methylation and histone acetylation work in concert to regulate memory formation and synaptic plasticity. Neurobiol Learn Mem 89:599–603

Montgomery KG, Liu MC, Eccles DM, Campbell IG (2004) The DNMT3B C–>T promoter polymorphism and risk of breast cancer in a British population: a case-control study. Breast Cancer Res 6:R390–R394

Morgan HD, Sutherland HG, Martin DI, Whitelaw E (1999) Epigenetic inheritance at the agouti locus in the mouse. Nat Genet 23:314–318

Morgan HD, Santos F, Green K, Dean W, Reik W (2005) Epigenetic reprogramming in mammals. Hum Mol Genet 14:R47–R58

Mousseau TA, Fox CW (1998) The adaptive significance of maternal effects. Trends Ecol Evol 13:403–407

Mudd SH, Cantoni GL (1958) Activation of methionine for transmethylation III. The methionine-activating enzyme of Bakers' yeast. J Biol Chem 231:481–492

Mueller BR, Bale TL (2008) Sex-specific programming of offspring emotionality after stress early in pregnancy. J Neurosci 28:9055–9065

Myers MM, Brunelli SA, Shair HN, Squire JM, Hofer MA (1989) Relationships between maternal behavior of SHR and WKY dams and adult blood pressures of cross-fostered F1 pups. Dev Psychobiol 22:55–67

Nan X, Ng HH, Johnson CA, Laherty CD, Turner BM, Eisenman RN, Bird A (1998) Transcriptional repression by the methyl-CpG-binding protein MeCP2 involves a histone deacetylase complex. Nature 393:386–389

Nathan D, Ingvarsdottir K, Sterner DE, Bylebyl GR, Dokmanovic M, Dorsey JA, Whelan KA, Krsmanovic M, Lane WS, Meluh PB et al (2006) Histone sumoylation is a negative regulator in *Saccharomyces cerevisiae* and shows dynamic interplay with positive-acting histone modifications. Genes Dev 20:966–976

Nelson CJ, Santos-Rosa H, Kouzarides T (2006) Proline isomerization of histone H3 regulates lysine methylation and gene expression. Cell 126:905–916

Nemeroff CB (1996) The corticotropin-releasing factor (CRF) hypothesis of depression: new findings and new directions. Mol Psychiatry 1:336–342

Ng HH, Zhang Y, Hendrich B, Johnson CA, Turner BM, Erdjument-Bromage H, Tempst P, Reinberg D, Bird A (1999) MBD2 is a transcriptional repressor belonging to the MeCP1 histone deacetylase complex. Nat Genet 23:58–61

Oberlander TF, Weinberg J, Papsdorf M, Grunau R, Misri S, Devlin AM (2008) Prenatal exposure to maternal depression, neonatal methylation of human glucocorticoid receptor gene (NR3C1) and infant cortisol stress responses. Epigenetics 3:97–106

Ohm JE, Baylin SB (2007) Stem cell chromatin patterns: an instructive mechanism for DNA hypermethylation? Cell Cycle 6:1040–1043

Okano M, Bell DW, Haber DA, Li E (1999) DNA methyltransferases Dnmt3a and Dnmt3b are essential for de novo methylation and mammalian development. Cell 99:247–257

Olds D, Henderson CR Jr, Cole R, Eckenrode J, Kitzman H, Luckey D, Pettitt L, Sidora K, Morris P, Powers J (1998) Long-term effects of nurse home visitation on children's criminal and antisocial behavior: 15-year follow-up of a randomized controlled trial. JAMA 280:1238–1244

Olds DL, Kitzman H, Cole R, Robinson J, Sidora K, Luckey DW, Henderson CR Jr, Hanks C, Bondy J, Holmberg J (2004a) Effects of nurse home-visiting on maternal life course and child development: age 6 follow-up results of a randomized trial. Pediatrics 114:1550–1559

Olds DL, Robinson J, Pettitt L, Luckey DW, Holmberg J, Ng RK, Isacks K, Sheff K, Henderson CR Jr (2004b) Effects of home visits by paraprofessionals and by nurses: age 4 follow-up results of a randomized trial. Pediatrics 114:1560–1568

Oli MK, Dobson FS (2003) The relative importance of life-history variables to population growth rate in mammals: Cole's prediction revisited. Am Nat 161:422–440

Olsson T, Mohammed AH, Donaldson LF, Henriksson BG, Seckl JR (1994) Glucocorticoid receptor and NGFI-A gene expression are induced in the hippocampus after environmental enrichment in adult rats. Brain Res Mol Brain Res 23:349–353

Ooi SK, Bestor TH (2008) The colorful history of active DNA demethylation. Cell 133:1145–1148

Ooi SK, O'Donnell AH, Bestor TH (2009) Mammalian cytosine methylation at a glance. J Cell Sci 122:2787–2791

Orphanides G, Reinberg D (2002) A unified theory of gene expression. Cell 108:439–451

Oswald J, Engemann S, Lane N, Mayer W, Olek A, Fundele R, Dean W, Reik W, Walter J (2000) Active demethylation of the paternal genome in the mouse zygote. Curr Biol 10:475–478

Ottinger DR, Tanabe G (1969) Maternal food restriction: effects on offspring behavior and development. Dev Psychobiol 2:7–9

Pakneshan P, Tetu B, Rabbani SA (2004) Demethylation of urokinase promoter as a prognostic marker in patients with breast carcinoma. Clin Cancer Res 10:3035–3041

Park BL, Kim LH, Shin HD, Park YW, Uhm WS, Bae SC (2004) Association analyses of DNA methyltransferase-1 (DNMT1) polymorphisms with systemic lupus erythematosus. J Hum Genet 49:642–646

Pascale RM, Simile MM, Satta G, Seddaiu MA, Daino L, Pinna G, Vinci MA, Gaspa L, Feo F (1991) Comparative effects of L-methionine, S-adenosyl-L-methionine and 5'-methylthioadenosine on the growth of preneoplastic lesions and DNA methylation in rat liver during the early stages of hepatocarcinogenesis. Anticancer Res 11:1617–1624

Perry M, Chalkley R (1982) Histone acetylation increases the solubility of chromatin and occurs sequentially over most of the chromatin. A novel model for the biological role of histone acetylation. J Biol Chem 257:7336–7347

Poirier LA, Wise CK, Delongchamp RR, Sinha R (2001) Blood determinations of S-adenosylmethionine, S-adenosylhomocysteine, and homocysteine: correlations with diet. Cancer Epidemiol Biomark Prev 10:649–655

Poulter MO, Du L, Weaver IC, Palkovits M, Faludi G, Merali Z, Szyf M, Anisman H (2008) GABA(A) receptor promoter hypermethylation in suicide brain: implications for the involvement of epigenetic processes. Biol Psychiatry 64:645–652

Ramchandani S, Bhattacharya SK, Cervoni N, Szyf M (1999) DNA methylation is a reversible biological signal. Proc Natl Acad Sci USA 96:6107–6112

Ramsahoye BH, Biniszkiewicz D, Lyko F, Clark V, Bird AP, Jaenisch R (2000) Non-CpG methylation is prevalent in embryonic stem cells and may be mediated by DNA methyltransferase 3a. Proc Natl Acad Sci USA 97:5237–42

Rassoulzadegan M, Magliano M, Cuzin F (2002) Transvection effects involving DNA methylation during meiosis in the mouse. EMBO J 21:440–450

Rassoulzadegan M, Grandjean V, Gounon P, Vincent S, Gillot I, Cuzin F (2006) RNA-mediated non-mendelian inheritance of an epigenetic change in the mouse. Nature 441:469–474

Razin A (1998) CpG methylation, chromatin structure and gene silencing-a three-way connection. EMBO J 17:4905–4908

Razin A, Szyf M (1984) DNA methylation patterns. Formation and function. Biochim Biophys Acta 782:331–342

Repetti RL, Taylor SE, Seeman TE (2002) Risky families: family social environments and the mental and physical health of offspring. Psychol Bull 128:330–366

Ressler RH, Anderson LT (1973) Avoidance conditioning in mice as a function of their mothers' exposure to shock. Dev Psychobiol 6:105–111

Robinson GE, Fernald RD, Clayton DF (2008) Genes and social behavior. Science 322:896–900

Roelfsema JH, Peters DJ (2007) Rubinstein-Taybi syndrome: clinical and molecular overview. Expert Rev Mol Med 9:1–16

Roff D (2002) Life-history evolution. Sinauer Associates, Sunderland, MA

Roth TL, Lubin FD, Funk AJ, Sweatt JD (2009) Lasting epigenetic influence of early-life adversity on the BDNF gene. Biol Psychiatry 65:760–769

Saccheri I, Hanski I (2006) Natural selection and population dynamics. Trends Ecol Evol 21: 341–347

Saito Y, Jones PA (2006) Epigenetic activation of tumor suppressor microRNAs in human cancer cells. Cell Cycle 5:2220–2222

Sapolsky RM (1985) Glucocorticoid toxicity in the hippocampus: temporal aspects of neuronal vulnerability. Brain Res 359:300–305

Scarpa S, Fuso A, D'Anselmi F, Cavallaro RA (2003) Presenilin 1 gene silencing by S-adeno-sylmethionine: a treatment for Alzheimer disease? FEBS Lett 541:145–148

Schlinzig T, Johansson S, Gunnar A, Ekstrom TJ, Norman M (2009) Epigenetic modulation at birth - altered DNA-methylation in white blood cells after Caesarean section. Acta Paediatr 98:1096–1099

Sealy L, Chalkley R (1978) DNA associated with hyperacetylated histone is preferentially digested by DNase I. Nucleic Acids Res 5:1863–1876

Seckl JR, Meaney MJ (1993) Early life events and later development of ischaemic heart disease. Lancet 342:1236

Sener RN (1995) Rubinstein-Taybi syndrome: cranial MR imaging findings. Comput Med Imaging Graph 19:417–418

Seth KA, Majzoub JA (2001) Repressor element silencing transcription factor/neuron-restrictive silencing factor (REST/NRSF) can act as an enhancer as well as a repressor of corticotropin-releasing hormone gene transcription. J Biol Chem 276:13917–13923

Shahbazian M, Young J, Yuva-Paylor L, Spencer C, Antalffy B, Noebels J, Armstrong D, Paylor R, Zoghbi H (2002) Mice with truncated MeCP2 recapitulate many Rett syndrome features and display hyperacetylation of histone H3. Neuron 35:243–254

Shi Y, Lan F, Matson C, Mulligan P, Whetstine JR, Cole PA, Casero RA (2004) Histone demethylation mediated by the nuclear amine oxidase homolog LSD1. Cell 119:941–953

Shiio Y, Eisenman RN (2003) Histone sumoylation is associated with transcriptional repression. Proc Natl Acad Sci USA 100:13225–13230

Shilatifard A (2006) Chromatin modifications by methylation and ubiquitination: implications in the regulation of gene expression. Annu Rev Biochem 75:243–269

Shindo C, Lister C, Crevillen P, Nordborg M, Dean C (2006) Variation in the epigenetic silencing of FLC contributes to natural variation in Arabidopsis vernalization response. Genes Dev 20: 3079–3083

Shorter J, Lindquist S (2005) Prions as adaptive conduits of memory and inheritance. Nat Rev Genet 6:435–450

Shukeir N, Pakneshan P, Chen G, Szyf M, Rabbani SA (2006) Alteration of the methylation status of tumor-promoting genes decreases prostate cancer cell invasiveness and tumorigenesis in vitro and in vivo. Cancer Res 66:9202–9210

Sinclair KD, Allegrucci C, Singh R, Gardner DS, Sebastian S, Bispham J, Thurston A, Huntley JF, Rees WD, Maloney CA et al (2007) DNA methylation, insulin resistance, and blood pressure in offspring determined by maternal periconceptional B vitamin and methionine status. Proc Natl Acad Sci USA 104:19351–19356

Slotkin RK, Martienssen R (2007) Transposable elements and the epigenetic regulation of the genome. Nat Rev Genet 8:272–285

Smith SS (1994) Biological implications of the mechanism of action of human DNA (cytosine-5) methyltransferase. Prog Nucleic Acid Res Mol Biol 49:65–111

Sroufe LA (1997) Psychopathology as an outcome of development. Dev Psychopathol 9:251–268

Stern JM (1997) Offspring-induced nurturance: animal-human parallels. Dev Psychobiol 31: 19–37

Suzuki MM, Bird A (2008) DNA methylation landscapes: provocative insights from epigenomics. Nat Rev Genet 9:465–476

Szyf M, Bhattacharya SK (2002a) Extracting DNA demethylase activity from mammalian cells. Methods Mol Biol 200:163–176

Szyf M, Bhattacharya SK (2002b) Measuring DNA demethylase activity in vitro. Methods Mol Biol 200:155–161

Tahiliani M, Koh KP, Shen Y, Pastor WA, Bandukwala H, Brudno Y, Agarwal S, Iyer LM, Liu DR, Aravind L et al (2009) Conversion of 5-methylcytosine to 5-hydroxymethylcytosine in mammalian DNA by MLL partner TET1. Science 324:930–935

Tate PH, Bird AP (1993) Effects of DNA methylation on DNA-binding proteins and gene expression. Curr Opin Genet Dev 3:226–231

Tsankova N, Renthal W, Kumar A, Nestler EJ (2007) Epigenetic regulation in psychiatric disorders. Nat Rev Neurosci 8:355–367

Tsukada Y, Fang J, Erdjument-Bromage H, Warren ME, Borchers CH, Tempst P, Zhang Y (2006) Histone demethylation by a family of JmjC domain-containing proteins. Nature 439:811–816

Turner JD, Muller CP (2005) Structure of the glucocorticoid receptor (NR3C1) gene 5' untranslated region: identification, and tissue distribution of multiple new human exon 1. J Mol Endocrinol 35:283–292

Turner JD, Pelascini LP, Macedo JA, Muller CP (2008) Highly individual methylation patterns of alternative glucocorticoid receptor promoters suggest individualized epigenetic regulatory mechanisms. Nucleic Acids Res 36:7207–7218

Tweedie-Cullen RY, Reck JM, Mansuy IM (2009) Comprehensive mapping of post-translational modifications on synaptic, nuclear, and histone proteins in the adult mouse brain. J Proteome Res 8:4966–4982

Unterberger A, Szyf M, Nathanielsz PW, Cox LA (2009) Organ and gestational age effects of maternal nutrient restriction on global methylation in fetal baboons. J Med Primatol 38: 219–227

Valinluck V, Sowers LC (2007) Endogenous cytosine damage products alter the site selectivity of human DNA maintenance methyltransferase DNMT1. Cancer Res 67:946–950

Valinluck V, Tsai HH, Rogstad DK, Burdzy A, Bird A, Sowers LC (2004) Oxidative damage to methyl-CpG sequences inhibits the binding of the methyl-CpG binding domain (MBD) of methyl-CpG binding protein 2 (MeCP2). Nucleic Acids Res 32:4100–4108

Waddington CH (1942) Epigenotype. Endeavour 1:18–21

Wade PA, Pruss D, Wolffe AP (1997) Histone acetylation: chromatin in action. Trends Biochem Sci 22:128–132

Wade PA, Gegonne A, Jones PL, Ballestar E, Aubry F, Wolffe AP (1999) Mi-2 complex couples DNA methylation to chromatin remodelling and histone deacetylation. Nat Genet 23:62–66

Wang SC, Oelze B, Schumacher A (2008) Age-specific epigenetic drift in late-onset Alzheimer's disease. PLoS ONE 3:e2698

Wang J, Weaver IC, Gauthier-Fisher A, Wang H, He L, Yeomans J, Wondisford F, Kaplan DR, Miller FD (2010) CBP histone acetyltransferase activity regulates embryonic neural differentiation in the normal and Rubinstein-Taybi syndrome brain. Dev Cell 18:114–125

Waterland RA, Jirtle RL (2003) Transposable elements: targets for early nutritional effects on epigenetic gene regulation. Mol Cell Biol 23:5293–5300

Waterland RA, Dolinoy DC, Lin JR, Smith CA, Shi X, Tahiliani KG (2006a) Maternal methyl supplements increase offspring DNA methylation at Axin Fused. Genesis 44:401–406

Waterland RA, Lin JR, Smith CA, Jirtle RL (2006b) Post-weaning diet affects genomic imprinting at the insulin-like growth factor 2 (Igf2) locus. Hum Mol Genet 15:705–716

Watt F, Molloy PL (1988) Cytosine methylation prevents binding to DNA of a HeLa cell transcription factor required for optimal expression of the adenovirus major late promoter. Genes Dev 2:1136–1143

Weaver ICG (2009) Life at the interface between a dynamic environment and a fixed genome: epigenetic programming of stress responses by maternal behavior. In: D Janigro (ed)

Mammalian brain development, contemporary neuroscience. Humana Press, a part of Springer Science + Business Media, LLC, pp 17–39

Weaver IC (2010) Epigenetic programming of stress responses and trans-generational inheritance through natural variations in maternal care: a role for DNA methylation in experience-dependent (re)programming of defensive responses. In: Lajtha A (ed) Genomics, proteomics and the nervous system. Springer US. Biomedical and Life Sciences, Heidelberg

Weaver IC, Grant RJ, Meaney MJ (2002) Maternal behavior regulates long-term hippocampal expression of BAX and apoptosis in the offspring. J Neurochem 82:998–1002

Weaver IC, Cervoni N, Champagne FA, D'Alessio AC, Sharma S, Seckl JR, Dymov S, Szyf M, Meaney MJ (2004) Epigenetic programming by maternal behavior. Nat Neurosci 7:847–854

Weaver IC, Champagne FA, Brown SE, Dymov S, Sharma S, Meaney MJ, Szyf M (2005) Reversal of maternal programming of stress responses in adult offspring through methyl supplementation: altering epigenetic marking later in life. J Neurosci 25:11045–11054

Weaver IC, Meaney MJ, Szyf M (2006) Maternal care effects on the hippocampal transcriptome and anxiety-mediated behaviors in the offspring that are reversible in adulthood. Proc Natl Acad Sci USA 103:3480–3485

Weaver IC, D'Alessio AC, Brown SE, Hellstrom IC, Dymov S, Sharma S, Szyf M, Meaney MJ (2007) The transcription factor nerve growth factor-inducible protein a mediates epigenetic programming: altering epigenetic marks by immediate-early genes. J Neurosci 27:1756–1768

Weiss A, Keshet I, Razin A, Cedar H (1996) DNA demethylation in vitro: involvement of RNA. Cell 86:709–718

Wells JC (2003) The thrifty phenotype hypothesis: thrifty offspring or thrifty mother? J Theor Biol 221:143–161

West-Eberhard MJ (2005) Developmental plasticity and the origin of species differences. Proc Natl Acad Sci USA 102(Suppl 1):6543–6549

Wolff GL, Kodell RL, Moore SR, Cooney CA (1998) Maternal epigenetics and methyl supplements affect agouti gene expression in Avy/a mice. FASEB J 12:949–957

Wondrak GT, Cervantes-Laurean D, Jacobson EL, Jacobson MK (2000) Histone carbonylation in vivo and in vitro. Biochem J 351(Pt 3):769–777

Wu SC, Zhang Y (2010) Active DNA demethylation: many roads lead to Rome. Nat Rev Mol Cell Biol 11:607–620

Yu J, de Belle I, Liang H, Adamson ED (2004) Coactivating factors p300 and CBP are transcriptionally crossregulated by Egr1 in prostate cells, leading to divergent responses. Mol Cell 15: 83–94

Yan C, Boyd DD (2006) Histone H3 acetylation and H3 K4 methylation define distinct chromatin regions permissive for transgene expression. Molecular and cellular biology 26:6357–6371

Zemach A, McDaniel IE, Silva P, Zilberman D (2010) Genome-wide evolutionary analysis of eukaryotic DNA methylation. Science 328:916–919

Zhang Y, Ng HH, Erdjument-Bromage H, Tempst P, Bird A, Reinberg D (1999) Analysis of the NuRD subunits reveals a histone deacetylase core complex and a connection with DNA methylation. Genes Dev 13:1924–1935

Zheng D, Zhao K, Mehler MF (2009) Profiling RE1/REST-mediated histone modifications in the human genome. Genome Biol 10:R9

Zhu JK (2008) Epigenome sequencing comes of age. Cell 133:395–397

Zilberman D, Gehring M, Tran RK, Ballinger T, Henikoff S (2007) Genome-wide analysis of *Arabidopsis thaliana* DNA methylation uncovers an interdependence between methylation and transcription. Nat Genet 39:61–69

Chapter 12
Histone Deacetylase Inhibitors: A Novel Therapeutic Approach for Cognitive Disorders

Viviane Labrie

Abstract Epigenetic mechanisms have a central role in regulating gene expression and are capable of influencing complex cognitive functions. In particular, acetylation of histone proteins is an epigenetic modification involved in mediating synaptic plasticity, learning, and memory. Emerging evidence indicates that increased histone acetylation through the inhibition of histone deacetylases (HDACs) can facilitate the formation of long-term memories in preclinical studies. Moreover, HDAC inhibitors have been reported to ameliorate cognitive deficits in animal models relevant to neurodegenerative and neurodevelopmental disorders. HDAC inhibitors have also been found to enhance the extinction of learned behaviors, including drug-seeking behaviors. Consequently, HDAC inhibition may be a useful approach in the treatment of a wide range of disorders characterized by cognitive dysfunction. Future HDAC-based pharmacotherapies will benefit from a greater understanding of different HDAC isoforms and the molecular pathways specifically involved in inducing cognitive enhancement.

Keywords Drug addiction · Histone deacetylase (HDAC) inhibitors · Memory · Neurodegenerative disorders · Neurodevelopmental disorders · Synaptic plasticity

12.1 Introduction

Epigenetics, a cellular mechanism once considered to be stable after development, has now been found to be a dynamic process that occurs in fully differentiated, postmitotic cells of the central nervous system in response to environmental signals (Borrelli et al. 2008; Graff and Mansuy 2008; Feinberg 2007). Epigenetic mechanisms regulate the structure of the chromatin through posttranslational modifications

V. Labrie
Krembil Family Epigenetics Laboratory, Centre for Addiction and Mental Health, 250 College St, Toronto, ON, M5G 1X5, Canada
e-mail: Viviane_Labrie@camh.net

A. Petronis and J. Mill (eds.), *Brain, Behavior and Epigenetics*,
Epigenetics and Human Health, DOI 10.1007/978-3-642-17426-1_12,
© Springer-Verlag Berlin Heidelberg 2011

of histone proteins and covalent DNA modifications. Alterations in chromatin structure changes the accessibility of DNA to regulatory proteins, resulting in changes in gene transcription. Changes in gene expression and subsequent protein synthesis affect synaptic function and morphology, which is essential for many cognitive processes, including learning and memory (Costa-Mattioli et al. 2009; Loebrich and Nedivi 2009). In this manner, epigenetic mechanisms act as a means of translating external stimuli into modifications of gene expression and neural activity that affect cognitive function and behavioral outcome.

One of the most extensively studied cognitive processes is memory formation. Recent studies have demonstrated that chromatin modifications, especially histone acetylation, are involved in synaptic plasticity and memory formation (Fischer et al. 2007; Levenson et al. 2004; Korzus et al. 2004; Guan et al. 2002). In general, histone acetylation is associated with transcriptional activation and is regulated by the balance between histone acetyltransferases (HAT) and histone deacetylases (HDAC). Increased histone acetylation has been shown to facilitate learning behaviors (Guan et al. 2009; Fischer et al. 2007; Levenson et al. 2004). This has led a number of researchers to investigate the potential of HDAC inhibitors to improve memory, particularly in diseases characterized by cognitive impairments. Nonselective HDAC inhibitors have demonstrated ameliorative effects in preclinical models relevant to Alzheimer's disease, Huntington's disease, Rubinstein–Taybi syndrome, and other cognitive disorders (Fischer et al. 2007; Kilgore et al. 2010; Ferrante et al. 2003; Alarcón et al. 2004; Korzus et al. 2004). HDAC inhibitors have also been found to augment extinction, a learned adaptive response capable of benefiting treatments for persistent maladaptive behaviors observed in many psychiatric illnesses and drug addiction (Lattal et al. 2007; Bredy and Barad 2008). These promising therapeutic effects have stimulated considerable interest in determining the HDAC isoforms, gene targets, and molecular pathways involved in mediating cognitive improvement. Consequently, the development and analysis of HDAC inhibitors is a rapidly expanding field. This chapter reviews recent insights about the contributions of chromatin acetylation to physiological and pathological cognitive functioning, and the application of HDAC inhibitors for the treatment of neurodegenerative, neurodevelopmental, and psychiatric disorders.

12.2   Histone Modifications

Histone proteins are components of the chromatin architecture that function to compress genomic DNA within the nucleus and are intimately involved in regulating gene expression by controlling access and signaling to the transcriptional machinery (for review, see Kouzarides 2007; Berger 2007). Complexes of DNA and histones form the nucleosome, the basic unit of the chromatin, in which 146 base pairs of DNA is wrapped around an octamer of core histone proteins: H2A, H2B, H3, and H4. Histones are small, conserved, and highly basic proteins composed of a globular domain and an amino-terminal tail that protrudes from the surface of the nucleosome. Histone tails are the site of numerous posttranslation modifications, including acetylation, phosphorylation, methylation, sumoylation, ubiquitination, and ADP-ribosylation. Patterns of histone modifications have been proposed to encode information, since these modifications affect chromatin structure and correspond to differing degrees of transcriptional activation or repression. These patterns are often referred to as the "histone code" (Strahl and Allis 2000) and can be altered in response to external stimuli (Borrelli et al. 2008; Graff and Mansuy 2008).

Acetylation of histones has been correlated with active gene expression (for review, see MacDonald and Howe 2009; Choi and Howe 2009). Histone acetylation occurs at lysine residues on histone tails and neutralizes existing positive charges, which weaken the histone–DNA interaction. This relaxes the chromatin structure and allows transcription factors to interact with their target DNA. The steady-state levels of histone acetylation are determined by the balance between the activity of HATs and HDACs. HAT enzymes catalyze the addition of acetyl groups to lysine residues within histones, thereby facilitating gene transcription. Removal of acetyl groups is the responsibility of HDACs. Elevated HDAC activity shifts the chromatin to a more condensed conformation, repressing gene expression. Interestingly, recent gene-array findings suggest that the effect of HDAC activity on gene expression is not global. Less than 20% of genes demonstrate an altered expression level in response to HDAC inhibition *in vitro* (Li and Li 2006; Iacomino et al. 2001; Tabuchi et al. 2006; Glaser et al. 2003; Chiba et al. 2004) and *in vivo* (Shafaati et al. 2009; Bosetti et al. 2005; Covington et al. 2009).

The superfamily of HDACs is divided into four main classes: I, II, III, and IV (for review, see Kazantsev and Thompson 2008; Carey and La Thangue 2006). Class I and II are the most well studied in the nervous system and contain Zn^{2+}-dependent active sites. Class I HDACs consist of HDAC1, HDAC2, and HDAC3, which are ubiquitously expressed and HDAC8, which is primarily restricted to smooth muscle cells. Class I HDACs are predominately localized in the nucleus. Class II HDACs are further divided into two subgroups: class IIa (HDAC4, HDAC5, HDAC7, and HDAC9) and class IIb (HDAC6 and HDAC10). Class II enzymes share considerable structural and sequence homology, and can shuttle between the cytoplasm and nucleus. Class III HDACs, known as the sirtuins (SIRT1–7), require nicotinamide adenine dinucleotide (NAD^+) for their enzymatic activity. Class IV is represented by a single member, HDAC11, which is principally located in the nucleus of cells.

With the exception of HDAC8, all HDAC isoforms exist in large multisubunit complexes and associate with other proteins or HDACs for optimal enzymatic activity (Balasubramanian et al. 2009). For example, HDAC4, HDAC5, and HDAC7 are unable to deacetylate histones in isolation and require interaction with HDAC3 to be active (Fischle et al. 2002). Also, in the cell, HDAC3 is complexed with NCOR/SMRT, which improves HDAC3 deacetylation activity (Guenther et al. 2001). HDAC1 and HDAC2 are associated with mSin3, NuRD, and CoREST in the cell, forming complexes that are recruited to gene promoters by DNA binding proteins, which may contribute to gene-specific transcriptional regulation (Laherty et al. 1997; Zhang et al. 1999; Wen et al. 2000). Thus, the diversity of isoforms, multiprotein complexes, and cofactors makes development of selective HDAC inhibitors a formidable challenge.

12.3 HDAC Inhibitors

The development of new HDAC inhibitors is currently undergoing a period of sudden growth in the pharmaceutical industry due to the potential application of these compounds as anticancer therapies and the emerging possibility that HDAC inhibitors may be useful in treating neurological and psychiatric illnesses. HDAC inhibitors can be classified into four major categories based on chemical structure (1) the short-chain fatty acids, such as sodium butyrate, valproate, and phenylbutyrate; (2) the hyroxamic acids, such as trichostatin A (TSA) and suberoylanilide hydroxamic acid (SAHA); (3) the benzamides, such as MS-275, 4b, and 106; and (4) the cyclic peptides, including apicidin and depsipeptide (Thomas 2009; Ma et al. 2009). In cancer, HDAC inhibitors can suppress tumor cell proliferation, induce cell differentiation, and upregulate crucial genes associated with anticancer effects (Carey and La Thangue 2006; Carew et al. 2008). As a consequence, various HDAC inhibitors have entered phase I and II clinical trials for cancer treatment, and have so far demonstrated promising antitumor activity for several types of cancers (Ma et al. 2009). However, the goal of reversing or impeding pathophysiological processes in disorders of the central nervous system is fundamentally different than the objectives of anticancer therapies. Harnessing the therapeutic potential of HDAC inhibitors for neurological and psychiatric disorders requires stable and bioavailable compounds capable of crossing the blood–brain barrier to reach diseased brain tissues. Some of the most commonly investigated HDAC inhibitors in the central nervous system include sodium butyrate, valproate, phenylbutyrate, TSA, and SAHA. These compounds are predominately broad-spectrum inhibitors, targeting many HDAC isoforms in both class I and II. Valproate affects only class I HDAC isoforms, however, valproate is also known to have many additional targets, and so the contribution of HDAC inhibition to the therapeutic effects of this drug is unclear. Certain HDAC inhibitors, such as SAHA and sodium butyrate display greater potencies in inhibiting class I HDACs than class II enzymes (Kilgore et al. 2010). Indeed, SAHA displays a high affinity for class I HDACs, with effective concentrations in the low nanomolar range (Kilgore et al. 2010; Khan et al. 2008).

The design of class- and isoform-specific HDAC inhibitors has been highly difficult due to the evolutionarily conserved architecture of HDAC active sites. However, attempts to improve selectivity by exploiting subtle differences in active site components, including the capping group, linker region, and metal-binding domains, have had some success (Bieliauskas and Pflum 2008). Selective compounds targeting exclusively HDAC1 or HDAC8 in the class I category and HDAC4 or HDAC6 in the class II category have been developed (Perez-Balado et al. 2007; Kozikowski et al. 2008; Krennhrubec et al. 2007; Bieliauskas and Pflum 2008).

Certain compounds are specific for a limited number of HDAC isoforms, such as SHI-1:2 inhibitors, which demonstrate an intrinsic activity against HDAC1 and HDAC2 that is at least a 100-fold greater than for other HDACs (Methot et al. 2008). Furthermore, a family of pimelic diphenylamide HDAC inhibitors demonstrating class I specificity with no class II activity have been created (Chou et al. 2008). These compounds also show a more than 15-fold selectivity for HDAC3 in comparison with HDAC1 and HDAC2 (Chou et al. 2008). Other compounds selective for class I or class II HDAC enzymes have been generated (Hamblett et al. 2007; Jones et al. 2008; Ontoria et al. 2009; Bieliauskas and Pflum 2008). As these compounds have just emerged, reports on their effects in the central nervous system are very limited. However, these compounds will be important in determining the roles of individual HDACs in physiological and disease processes in the brain. In addition, isoform- and class-selective HDAC inhibitors may more effectively targeting the pathophysiological disturbances involved in cognitive disorders.

An important caveat in interpreting all studies using HDAC inhibitors is that modifications of the epigenetic histone code may not be the exclusive or even primary mechanism underlying the effects of HDAC inhibitors. It is becoming increasingly apparent that HDAC enzymes not only target histones, but also regulate the acetylation of a variety of nonhistone proteins (Glozak et al. 2005; Lin et al. 2006; Carey and La Thangue 2006). This includes transcription factors, signal transduction mediators, cytoskeletal proteins, and several metabolic enzymes (Glozak et al. 2005; Lin et al. 2006; Carey and La Thangue 2006). Although histones are the most thoroughly studied substrate of HDACs, lysine residues on many nonhistone proteins are deacetylated by HDACs. Consequently, HDAC enzymes are more accurately considered as "lysine deacetylases". Changes in the acetylation of nonhistone proteins can potentially influence stability, localization, protein dimerization, and binding activity of these proteins and may be an additional method by which HDACs mediate transcriptional regulation (Caron et al. 2005; Levy et al. 2004; Gronroos et al. 2002; Wang et al. 2001). Therefore, the behavioral effects of HDAC inhibitors may be due to alterations in the acetylation of a diverse number of intracellular targets.

Another key point concerning the effects of HDAC inhibition is that patterns of histone acetylation are intricately linked to other epigenetic modifications. Indeed, extensive cross-talk occurs between different histone modifications and DNA methylation (Kouzarides 2007; Latham and Dent 2007). This involves multiple feed-forward and feed-back mechanisms within- and between-nucleosomes, allowing epigenetic modifications to act in concert (Kouzarides 2007; Latham and Dent 2007). For example, methylated DNA, a genomic sequence with a transcriptionally repressive epigenetic mark, can recruit methyl-binding proteins (MBDs), such as methyl-CpG-binding protein 2 (MeCP2) (Meehan et al. 1992; Hendrich and Bird 1998). MBDs associate with histone methyltransferases (HMTs) and HDACs that methylate and deacetylate histones, respectively, further silencing gene expression (Jones et al. 1998; Fuks et al. 2003). In addition, class I HDAC inhibitors valproate and MS-275 have been found to induce histone acetylation and lower DNA methylation in the frontal cortex of mice with hypermethylated DNA (Dong et al. 2007).

Similarly, the pan-HDAC inhibitor TSA has been shown to induce global and gene-specific DNA demethylation in human cancer cells (Ou et al. 2007). Thus, histone acetylation is unlikely to be the only epigenetic modification altered by HDAC inhibitors. Also, due to the complexity of the interactions, classification of epigenetic mechanisms as gene activating or suppressing is likely an oversimplification.

12.4   Regulation of Histone Acetylation in Learning and Memory

Histone acetylation has been implicated in many complex behaviors, particularly learning and memory. Memory is described as an array of processes employed by the brain for the long-term storage of information. The formation of long-term memories entails lasting changes in gene expression. Indeed, studies have demonstrated that the establishment of long-term memories requires the engagement of many signal pathways, changes in gene transcription, and de novo protein synthesis (Costa-Mattioli et al. 2009; Loebrich and Nedivi 2009).

Memory formation has been found to induce increases in histone acetylation in the hippocampus. The hippocampus is a brain region of particular importance to the formation and retrieval of memories (Kim and Fanselow 1992; Szapiro et al. 2002). In rodents, learning and memory can be investigated using a number of well-established hippocampus-dependent tests, including spatial mazes, contextual fear conditioning, and novel object recognition. In contextual fear conditioning, animals learn to associate a novel context with an aversive stimulus, and a single training session is sufficient to induce the formation of long-term memories. Animals exposed to a contextual fear conditioning paradigm demonstrated a significant increase in histone acetylation (Levenson et al. 2004). The increase in acetylation was transient and found at 1 h, but not 24 h after training, and only in histone H3, but not H4 (Levenson et al. 2004). The solely transient and H3-specific change in acetylation observed may be the result of using pan-specific antibodies that probe multiple acetylation sites. However, the finding that memory consolidation correlates with increased histone acetylation has been reproduced in a number of other learning paradigms using rodents (Fischer et al. 2007; Vecsey et al. 2007; Fontan-Lozano et al. 2008; Levenson et al. 2004) and invertebrates (Federman et al. 2009). Interestingly, transient elevations in histone acetylation associated with memory formation were found to be mediated by N-methyl-D-aspartate (NMDA) receptor-dependent synaptic transmission and the mitogen-activated protein kinase (MAPK) signaling cascade (Levenson et al. 2004). NMDA receptor activation and MAPK signaling are cellular processes critically involved in the formation of long-term memories in the hippocampus (Atkins et al. 1998).

Consistent with the idea that histone acetylation has a functional role in learning and memory, mice with a disruption in HAT activity display memory impairments. CREB-binding protein (CBP) is an enzyme involved in recruiting other components of the transcriptional machinery and contains endogenous HAT activity

(Bannister and Kouzarides 1996). Several genetically-modified mice with impaired CBP function have been developed (Alarcón et al. 2004; Wood et al. 2005, 2006; Oike et al. 1999). These models consistently demonstrate that abnormal CBP function leads to deficits in a number of memory tests, including novel object recognition, spatial memory, and contextual and cued fear conditioning (Alarcón et al. 2004; Wood et al. 2005, 2006; Oike et al. 1999). However, it is possible that memory abnormalities in CBP transgenic animals are not only the result of altered HAT activity, since CBP interacts with multiple transcriptional regulators (Janknecht 2002). To address this, mice expressing a CBP transgene with an inactivated HAT domain (CBP^{HAT}) were generated (Korzus et al. 2004). Expression of CBP^{HAT} was spatially restricted to forebrain neurons and temporally restricted using the tetracycline system, thereby avoiding potential developmental abnormalities. CBP^{HAT} expression in adult mice decreased histone acetylation and produced impairments in spatial and recognition memory that could be normalized by transgene suppression. In support of these findings, studies examining other HAT enzymes, E1A-binding protein (p300), and p300/CBP-associated factor (PCAF) have also shown a role for these HATs in memory processes (Oliveira et al. 2007; Maurice et al. 2008). Transgenic mice expressing an inhibitory truncated version of p300 that lacks HAT activity were demonstrated to have deficits in long-term recognition and contextual fear memory (Oliveira et al. 2007). These studies indicate that HAT activity contributes to memory formation, and the role of HAT in learning and memory may be mediated through histone acetylation. However, like HDACs, HATs are also known to target several nonhistone proteins. HAT-induced acetylation of transcription factors, such as p53, GATA-1, and Myo-D, has been shown to alter their DNA binding affinity and enhance transcription (Boyes et al. 1998; Gu and Roeder 1997; Polesskaya et al. 2000).

Histone acetylation may also facilitate synaptic plasticity. Synaptic plasticity refers to the ability of synapses to undergo activity-dependent changes in strength. At a cellular level, memory formation is dependent on synaptic plasticity (Bliss and Collingridge 1993; Costa-Mattioli et al. 2009). In *Aplysia*, histone acetylation was found to be differentially regulated by opposing forms of synaptic plasticity (Guan et al. 2002). The sensorimotor synapse of *Aplysia* demonstrates two major forms of long-term synaptic plasticity: long-term facilitation (LTF), which is a lasting enhancement in synaptic transmission, and long-term depression (LTD), which is a persistent decrease in synaptic transmission. LTF was accompanied by an increase in binding of the HAT CBP to the CAAT/enhancer-binding protein (C/EBP) gene promoter with a concurrent increase in histone H3 and H4 acetylation at the same promoter (Guan et al. 2002). In contrast, LTD led to a decrease in histone acetylation at the C/EBP promoter that was mediated at least in part by HDAC5 (Guan et al. 2002). Changes in histone acetylation have also been observed during the induction of synaptic plasticity in mammalian systems. Long-term potentiation (LTP) reflects an increase in synaptic transmission in response to high-frequency stimulation. LTP requires the activation of NMDA receptors and engages the MAPK signaling cascade (Kauer et al. 1988; Kelleher et al. 2004). Activation of NMDA receptors in the hippocampus was shown to increase histone H3 acetylation and this effect was blocked by inhibition of MAPK signaling (Levenson et al. 2004). MAPK activation in the hippocampus also augmented histone H3 acetylation (Levenson et al. 2004). The MAPK signaling pathway may promote histone acetylation through CBP HAT activity, as the MAPK cascade is known to lead to the phosphorylation and activation of CREB, which recruits CBP for subsequent transcriptional activation (Impey et al. 2002). Genetically-manipulated mice with deficient CBP function demonstrate impaired synaptic plasticity in the late-phase of LTP (L-LTP), which is known to require gene transcription (Alarcón et al. 2004). Administration of the HDAC inhibitor SAHA to hippocampal slices of CBP-deficient mice significantly improved L-LTP (Alarcón et al. 2004). Therefore, these studies indicate that histone acetylation may be involved in the synaptoplastic processes underlying memory formation.

12.5 Modulation of Learning and Memory by HDAC Inhibitors

Since memory formation is associated with an increase in histone acetylation and can be disrupted by reduced HAT activity, it may follow that compounds that increase histone acetylation effectively enhance memory formation. To test this directly, a number of studies have investigated the effects of HDAC inhibitors on long-term memory formation in normal animals. Systemic administration of an HDAC inhibitor, such as TSA, sodium butyrate, valproate, or SAHA, improved long-term memory in tests of contextual fear conditioning (Levenson et al. 2004; Fischer et al. 2007; Guan et al. 2009; Bredy and Barad 2008), cued fear conditioning (Bredy and Barad 2008), spatial learning in a water maze (Fischer et al. 2007), eyeblink conditioning (Fontan-Lozano et al. 2008), and object recognition (Fontan-Lozano et al. 2008) in normal rodents. Direct infusion of TSA into the hippocampus or amygdala has also been found to enhance fear-associated memories (Vecsey et al. 2007; Yeh et al. 2004). Some studies did not observe a memory improvement in wild-type animals following HDAC inhibitor administration in certain behavioral tasks (Kilgore et al. 2010; Vecsey et al. 2007). However, the degree of memory enhancement observed is likely determined by the properties of the HDAC inhibitor investigated (for example, the binding affinity and HDAC isotype selectivity) and by the dosing strategy, learning procedure, genetic background, and age of the animals employed.

Supporting the facilitatory effects of HDAC inhibitors on memory formation, these compounds have been demonstrated to augment synaptic plasticity and synaptogenesis. In the normal rodent hippocampus, induction of LTP was significantly enhanced by HDAC inhibition, using TSA, sodium butyrate, or SAHA (Levenson et al. 2004; Alarcón et al. 2004). In addition, LTP induced in the amygdala was increased by TSA (Yeh et al. 2004). Recently, chronic administration of SAHA in wild-type mice was found to enhance dendritic spine density and synapse numbers (Guan et al. 2009), which are cellular processes known to contribute to synaptic plasticity and memory formation (Yang et al. 2009; Bourne and Harris 2010).

HDAC inhibitors have also been shown to transform a learning event that would not normally result in long-term memory into an event that is remembered long-term. Mice exposed to a novel object for a short period of time will not remember this object after 24 h (Stefanko et al. 2009; Fontan-Lozano et al. 2008). However, mice treated with an HDAC inhibitor such as sodium butyrate or TSA displayed a lasting memory for the object that persisted after 24 h and 7 days (Stefanko et al. 2009; Fontan-Lozano et al. 2008). Similarly, in invertebrates, a weak training protocol that is insufficient to establish lasting memories was shown to potentiate long-term memory in animals treated with sodium butyrate or TSA (Federman et al. 2009). Administration of TSA to sensorimotor neurons of *Aplysia* resulted in a switch from short- to long-term facilitation of synaptic transmission (Guan et al. 2002). In mouse hippocampal slices, early-LTP (E-LTP), which does not require transcription or translation, was transformed into a transcription-dependent long-lasting form of LTP (Vecsey et al. 2007). Furthermore, HDAC inhibition decreased the threshold for learning-induced changes in histone acetylation and expression of memory-associated genes. Mice treated with sodium butyrate or TSA displayed a greater increase in histone H3 acetylation in the hippocampus and perirhinal cortex after exposure to an object recognition task (Fontan-Lozano et al. 2008) and contextual fear conditioning paradigm (Vecsey et al. 2007). In addition, HDAC inhibitors increased the expression of genes specifically associated with learning and memory following a learning task (Fontan-Lozano et al. 2008; Vecsey et al. 2007). This is consistent with studies demonstrating that HDAC inhibitors do not act globally, but can regulate a smaller subset of genes in the brain (Bosetti et al. 2005; Covington et al. 2009). Overall, these findings indicate that HDAC inhibitors can generate long-term memories under conditions that are typically insufficient to induce lasting memories, and that these facilitatory effects may be mediated by changes in histone acetylation and transcription of genes involved in memory formation.

Recently, HDAC inhibitors have been demonstrated to improve the extinction of memories. Extinction is regarded as a distinct form of learning that acts to suppress, but not erase, previously established memories (Davis et al. 2006). Like other forms of learning, extinction has been shown to depend on an intricate regulatory network of signaling cascades, gene transcription, and protein synthesis (Davis et al. 2006). Extinction of conditioned fear has been associated with changes in histone acetylation (Bredy et al. 2007). Following extinction, the promoter region of brain-derived neurotrophic factor (BDNF), a gene implicated in memory and synaptic plasticity, was found to have altered histone H3 and H4 acetylation in the prefrontal cortex of mice (Bredy et al. 2007). Moreover, systemic or intrahippocampal administration of sodium butyrate, TSA, or valproate in normal mice was found to enhance the extinction of contextual and cued fear (Lattal et al. 2007; Bredy and Barad 2008). Valproate was shown to improve the effects of a weak extinction protocol and induced similar changes in histone H4 acetylation in the BDNF promoter region as a strong extinction protocol (Bredy et al. 2007). Thus, in addition to having therapeutic potential for diseases involving impaired memory, these results suggest that HDAC inhibitors may be useful in treating diseases characterized by persistent maladaptive memories, such as posttraumatic stress disorder and drug addiction.

12.6   HDAC Inhibitors as a Potential Treatment for Cognitive Disorders

Since HDAC inhibitors benefit memory processes in normal mice, several studies have investigated the potential of these compounds in ameliorating cognitive symptoms in disease models. Cognitive dysfunction is a central component of many neurological and psychiatric illnesses, and often includes disturbances in learning and memory. Consequently, the capacity of HDAC inhibitors to improve learning and memory has been examined in several animal models of cognitive impairment, including models of neurodegenerative diseases, neurodevelopmental disorders, and drug addiction.

12.6.1   Neurodegenerative Diseases: Recovering Lost Memories

Marked neuronal atrophy accompanied by a progressive decline in memory is a prominent characteristic of neurodegenerative disorders such as Alzheimer's disease (Heese and Akatsu 2006). Several mouse models with extensive neurodegeneration have been developed and recent studies have begun to explore the potential of HDAC inhibitors to improve memory formation in these models (Eriksen and Janus 2007). In CK-p25 transgenic mice, postnatal induction of p25, a protein implicated in various neurodegenerative diseases, specifically in the forebrain resulted in cyclin-dependent kinase 5 (Cdk5) hyperactivation (Fischer et al. 2005). This led to deficits in spatial and associative fear memory, along with severe synaptic and neuronal loss in forebrain structures such as the hippocampus (Fischer et al. 2005). Chronic administration of the HDAC inhibitor sodium butyrate prior to a learning task was shown to effectively enhance associative and spatial memory, and also increased synaptic connectivity (Fischer et al. 2007). Furthermore, the possibility that HDAC inhibitors may reestablish access to memories that had become lost or inaccessible as a result of neurodegenerative processes was also investigated using the CK-p25 transgenic mice (Fischer et al. 2007). Mice were initially trained in fear conditioning and spatial learning procedures. Following a rest period to allow long-term memory consolidation, induction of p25 was initiated, causing brain atrophy and neuronal loss. After p25 induction, animals were given chronic injections of sodium butyrate or vehicle, and then fear-associated and spatial memories were assessed. Remarkably, chronic HDAC inhibitor administration led to the recovery of memories that would otherwise be inaccessible. Thus, HDAC inhibitors were found to improve memory formation and restored the capacity for memory recall in a mouse model of neurodegeneration. Interestingly, the permissive effects of HDAC inhibitors on memory in CK-p25 transgenic mice were mimicked by environmental enrichment (Fischer et al. 2007). Environmental enrichment, a combination of exercise and cognitive training, is a well known but poorly understood means of enhancing memory in rodents and humans. It has been reported to delay the onset and development of memory deficits and neuropathologies associated with Alzheimer's disease (Berardi et al. 2007; Lazarov et al. 2005; Jankowsky et al. 2005). CK-p25 mice subjected to environmental enrichment demonstrated a similar increase in histone acetylation and in memory formation and retrieval as mice treated with an HDAC inhibitor (Fischer et al. 2007). This suggests that environmental enrichment and HDAC inhibitors may facilitate memories through a similar mechanism that could involve histone acetylation.

HDAC inhibitors have been tested in other mouse models relevant to Alzheimer's disease. The accumulation of neurotoxic amyloid plaques and neurofibrillary tangles in the brain are neuropathological hallmarks of Alzheimer's disease. Genetic mutations in amyloid precursor protein (APP) and presenilin-1 (PS1) have been implicated in plaque formation in early-onset cases of Alzheimer's disease (Selkoe 2001). Overexpression of human APP and PS1 mutations in mice induced amyloidosis and prominent cognitive deficits (Jankowsky et al. 2004; Savonenko et al. 2005). HDAC inhibitors, including valproate, sodium butyrate, and SAHA, were shown to reverse impairments in contextual fear memory in mice expressing mutant APP and PS1 transgenes (Kilgore et al. 2010). In addition, treatment with an HDAC inhibitor allowed the newly formed memories to remain stable, as the memories continued to be present after 2 weeks (Kilgore et al. 2010). Nicotinamide, a competitive inhibitor of class III HDACs, was also found to prevent impairments in spatial memory, object recognition, and fear conditioning in genetically-modified mice that develop both amyloid plaques and neurofibrillary tangles (Green et al. 2008). In these mice, nicotinamide reduced intracellular aggregates of a specific phospho-species of tau associated with microtubule depolymerization and neurofibrillary tangles (Green et al. 2008). Finally, in mice treated with kainic acid, a neurotoxic agent that induces hippocampal neurodegeneration and cognitive impairments, HDAC inhibitors sodium butyrate and TSA were found to restore short- and long-term memory in an object recognition task (Fontan-Lozano et al. 2008). Thus, these animal models indicate that HDAC inhibitors may be suitable for treating cognitive dysfunction in Alzheimer's disease. However, the mechanisms underlying Alzheimer's disease are far more complex than those reproduced in these animal models, and evidence has argued that Alzheimer's disease is associated with an increase and decrease in histone acetylation (Cao and Sudhof 2001; Marambaud et al. 2003; Kim et al. 2004, 2007; Rouaux et al. 2003; Saura et al. 2004). Conceivably, both types of changes in histone acetylation co-occur in Alzheimer's disease, and vary depending on brain structure, cell type, and genomic region. Consequently, it remains to be determined whether HDAC inhibitors will indeed provide therapeutic benefits to Alzheimer's patients.

Alterations in histone acetylation have also been implicated in Huntington's disease (HD), a neurodegenerative disorder characterized by cognitive impairments, mood disturbances, and motor deficits (Sadri-Vakili and Cha 2006). HD is caused by a CAG repeat expansion in the coding region of the *huntingtin* gene, producing mutant huntingtin protein with a lengthened polyglutamine tract (Sadri-Vakili and Cha 2006). The polyglutamine extension was found to directly bind and inhibit the activity of the HAT domain of CBP and PCAF (Steffan et al. 2001). This inhibitory interaction was demonstrated to lead to a reduction in histone H3 and H4 acetylation in cultured *Drosophila* cells that was reversed by administration of sodium butyrate, TSA, or SAHA (Steffan et al. 2001). In mouse models of HD, treatment with HDAC inhibitors, such as phenylbutyrate, sodium butyrate, 4b, and SAHA, have been shown to attenuate neuronal atrophy, increase motor function, and extend survival (Ferrante et al. 2003; Hockly et al. 2003; Thomas et al. 2008; Gardian et al. 2005). This was accompanied by an increase in the acetylation of histones and nonhistone proteins associated with neurotoxicity and HD pathology (Ferrante et al. 2003; Hockly et al. 2003; Gardian et al. 2005; Sadri-Vakili et al. 2007; Dompierre et al. 2007). The effects of HDAC inhibitors on cognitive performance in animal models of HD have not been reported, likely due to the confounding effects of motor deficits in these models. However, clinical trials investigating the efficacy and safety of the HDAC inhibitor phenylbutyrate as a treatment for HD have been initiated (study ID: R01NS45242), and will shed light on the capacity of these compounds to improve the cognitive symptoms of HD.

12.6.2   Neurodevelopmental Disorders

Rubinstein-Taybi syndrome (RTS) is a rare developmental disease that is characterized by mental retardation and skeletal abnormalities (Hallam and Bourtchouladze 2006). RTS is caused by mutations in the gene encoding CBP (Petrij et al. 1995; Blough et al. 2000). Recent evidence indicates that RTS symptoms are also caused by mutations in the gene encoding p300 (Roelfsema et al. 2005; Bartholdi et al. 2007). As mentioned earlier, CBP and p300 have HAT activity and function as transcriptional coactivators that recruit other components of the transcriptional machinery. Mouse models with deficient CBP or p300 display cognitive and physiological deficits associated with RTS (Alarcón et al. 2004; Korzus et al. 2004; Wood et al. 2005; Oliveira et al. 2007). Memory impairments induced by a CBP deficiency were demonstrated to be reversed by systemic or intraventricular injections of the HDAC inhibitors TSA and SAHA (Alarcón et al. 2004; Korzus et al. 2004). In addition, HDAC inhibition ameliorated synaptic plasticity in CBP-deficient mice, as SAHA reversed impaired L-LTP (Alarcón et al. 2004). At the molecular level, reduced HAT activity and histone acetylation in CBP transgenic mice was increased by HDAC inhibitors (Alarcón et al. 2004; Korzus et al. 2004). Thus, HDAC inhibitors constitute a promising therapeutic approach for the cognitive features of RTS.

Fragile X syndrome (FXS) is a common heritable disease in which patients exhibit a wide range of neurological disturbances, including cognitive deficits, autism, seizures, peripheral neuropathy, and abnormal autonomic function (Garber et al. 2008). FXS is caused by an expanded repeat of CGG trinucleotides at the 5' end of the fragile X mental retardation 1 (*FMR1*) gene (Verkerk et al. 1991; Pieretti et al. 1991). The trinucleotide expansions cause an increase in DNA methylation at the *FMR1* gene promoter, reducing the translational of the fragile X mental retardation protein (FMRP) (Pieretti et al. 1991; Godler et al. 2010). FMRP is a selective RNA-binding protein that regulates mRNA transport to neuronal dendrites and local translation, affecting synaptic plasticity and neuronal maturation (Weiler et al. 1997). Treatment of lymphoblastoid cells from FXS patients with demethylating agents such as 5-aza-2-deoxycytidine reactivated *FMR1* gene expression and restored normal levels of *FMR1* mRNA and protein (Chiurazzi et al. 1998). Administration of the HDAC inhibitors 4-phenylbutyrate, sodium butyrate, or TSA in combination with 5-aza-2-deoxycytidine was far more effective, indicating a synergistic effect between histone hyperacetylation and DNA demethylation (Chiurazzi et al. 1998). Accordingly, subsequent studies demonstrated that DNA methylation is tightly coupled to histone acetylation and histone methylation at the *FMR1* gene (Coffee et al. 2002; Tabolacci et al. 2008). Recently, inhibitors of class III HDACs, nicotinamide and splitomicin, were shown to induce *FMR1* gene reactivation and the acetylation of histones at the 5' end of the *FMR1* gene in cells derived from FXS patients (Biacsi et al. 2008). These findings support the need for further investigation about the ability of HDAC inhibitors to improve the symptoms of FXS.

12.6.3 Drug Addiction

Exposure therapy is one of the most effective forms of psychotherapy and is commonly used to treat anxiety syndromes and substance abuse (Hofmann 2007; Marlatt 1990). Exposure therapy is based on the concept of extinction. For drug addictions, treatment involves prolonged and repeated exposures to drug-associated environmental cues without access to the substance of abuse. Consequently, this form of treatment allows patients to diminish conditioned responses elicited by the drug-associated cues (Heather and Bradley 1990; O'Brien et al. 1990). Recent evidence indicates that pharmacotherapies capable of enhancing extinction in rodents have the potential to improve the effectiveness of exposure therapy in humans (Davis et al. 2006; Norberg et al. 2008).

Drug-seeking behaviors in mice can be measured using the conditioned place paradigm (CPP). In this task, animals learn to pair the effects of an addictive substance with a distinct environment. Extinction is induced by repetitive exposures to the drug-associated context without reinforcement. Extinction of cocaine-seeking behaviors measured in the CPP was enhanced by treatments with the HDAC inhibitor sodium butyrate (Malvaez et al. 2009). Reinstatement of drug-seeking behaviors after the extinction sessions can be induced by administering a drug prime. Sodium butyrate was found to significantly attenuate the reinstatement of cocaine-seeking behaviors (Malvaez et al. 2009). Thus, HDAC inhibition enhanced the rate of extinction and its persistence, suggesting that HDAC inhibitors may facilitate the effects of exposure therapy for substance abuse disorders in the clinic.

12.7 Mechanisms by Which HDAC Inhibitors Facilitate Cognitive Function

One of the major open questions that arise from studies investigating the therapeutic utility of HDAC inhibitors is: What are the mechanisms by which HDAC inhibitors enhance cognitive function and synaptic plasticity? To address this question, Guan et al. (2009) recently performed a series of experiments investigating the HDAC family members specifically involved in memory formation. Initially, SAHA, an HDAC inhibitor that primarily targets class I HDACs (HDAC1, HDAC2, and HDAC3 in the brain) and HDAC6, was confirmed to enhance memory formation in normal mice. The possibility that SAHA induces memory improvements by reducing HDAC6 activity was eliminated by demonstrating that a selective HDAC6 inhibitor, WT-161, did not increase memory in normal mice. The contributions of HDAC1 and HDAC2 to memory formation were investigated using genetic knock-out or overexpression mouse models. HDAC2 overexpression was found to decrease dendritic spine density, synapse number, and synaptic plasticity. More-over, elevated HDAC2 levels attenuated memory formation in behavioral measures of contextual and cued fear conditioning, spatial long-term memory, and spatial working memory. In contrast, overexpression of HDAC1 did not alter memory or synaptic function. Genetic inactivation of HDAC2 was found to increase synapto-genesis, synaptic plasticity, context- and tone-associated memories, and spatial working memory. If HDAC inhibitors induce memory enhancements via HDAC2, then it would be expected that HDAC inhibition would readily reverse the learning impairments in mice overexpressing HDAC2, but have no effect in mice lacking HDAC2 activity. Indeed, SAHA enhanced associative fear memories and completely abrogated the decrease in spine density and synapse abnormalities in HDAC2-overexpressing mice. Conversely, SAHA did not affect associative fear memory, spine density, synapse numbers, or synaptic plasticity in HDAC2 knockout animals. This suggests that HDAC2 is the major target of SAHA in facilitating memory formation. Further studies are necessary to determine whether these effects are reproduced using other HDAC inhibitors. Importantly, mice lacking HDAC2 did not display gross changes in neuronal morphology or behavioral deficits, indicating that HDAC2 may be safely targeted without causing obvious disruptions in neuronal physiology and brain function. Thus, selective HDAC2 inhibitors may be a suitable treatment for cognitive disorders.

HDAC2 has been proposed to mediate changes in memory formation and synaptic function by binding to the regulatory element of memory-associated genes and suppressing their expression (Guan et al. 2009). HDAC2 was found to be enriched at the promoter regions of *BDNF*, *CBP*, cAMP responsive element binding protein 1 (*Crebl*), early growth response factor 1 (*Egr1*), FBJ osteosarcoma oncogene (*Fos*), neuritin 1 (*Nrn1*), neurexin 3 (*Nrxn3*), and NMDA receptor subunits (Guan et al. 2009). All these genes are implicated in synaptic plasticity and remodeling or regulated by neuronal activity (Loebrich and Nedivi 2009). In addition, HDAC1 was demonstrated to be more enriched at the promoter region of activity regulated cytoskeletal-associated protein (*Arc*), a gene associated with learning and memory processes (Guan et al. 2009). This indicates that although HDAC2 appears to be the principal isoform negatively regulating memory formation, HDAC1 may also provide important contributions. Interestingly, S-nitrosylation of HDAC2 has been found to release HDAC2 from the promoter of *Egr1*, a memory-associated gene (Nott et al. 2008). S-nitrosylation is induced by nitric oxide, a free radical molecule that can be synthesized in response to neuronal activation (Nott et al. 2008). Reduced HDAC2 activity following S-nitrosylation or in HDAC2 knockout mice was correlated with an increase in the acetylation of histones in synaptic plasticity genes, such as *BDNF*, *Egr1*, *Fos*, and the NMDA receptor subunit *GLUR1* (Guan et al. 2009; Nott et al. 2008). Accordingly, the expression of these genes was also elevated (Guan et al. 2009; Nott et al. 2008). Thus, HDAC inhibitors may improve memory formation by decreasing the activity of HDAC2 (and other pertinent isoforms), resulting in an increase in histone acetylation and a subsequent elevation in the transcription of genes involved in synaptic plasticity and synaptogenesis.

HDAC inhibitors have also been reported to enhance memory formation and synaptic plasticity through CREB- and CBP-dependent transcriptional activation (Vecsey et al. 2007). Genetic elimination of CREB function was shown to attenuate the enhancement in contextual fear memory and hippocampal LTP induced by the HDAC inhibitor TSA. Transgenic mice carrying a version of CBP lacking the CREB-binding domain were found to be resistant to the facilitatory effects of TSA on hippocampal LTP. Furthermore, HDAC inhibitors were shown to augment the expression of CREB-targeted genes after a contextual fear conditioning procedure. This suggests that in order for HDAC inhibitors to improve memory, simply inducing a histone hyperacetylated state is not sufficient and activation of the CREB and CBP transcriptional complex may also be required.

Other nonhistone targets have been implicated in the memory enhancement elicited by HDAC inhibitors. Nuclear actor-kappa-B (NF-κB) is a transcription factor that positively regulates the expression of genes and influences synaptic plasticity, learning, and memory (Hoffmann et al. 2006; Romano et al. 2006). Acetylation of the p65 subunit (RelA) of the NF-κB complex enhances its DNA binding affinity and transcriptional activity (Chen et al. 2002). p65 acetylation was found to be transiently increased in the rodent amygdala following associative fear learning (Yeh et al. 2004). Treatment with the HDAC inhibitors TSA or sodium butyrate prior to the learning task was shown to significantly prolong the expression of p65 and increase its DNA binding affinity (Yeh et al. 2004). Eliminating p65 accessibility using a decoy κB DNA segment attenuated the TSA-induced improvement in associative fear conditioning (Yeh et al. 2004). Furthermore, many other transcription factors and nonhistone proteins are regulated by changes in acetylation, including p53, FOXO1, p300, Hsp90, and tubulin (Glozak et al. 2005; Lin et al. 2006). Consequently, acetylation of nonhistone substrates likely contributes to the mechanism by which HDAC inhibitors mediate memory improvements.

12.8   Conclusions and Future Directions

To date, pan-HDAC inhibitors have demonstrated a capacity to improve memory formation in a wide diversity of models relevant to neurodegenerative and neurodevelopmental diseases (Fischer et al. 2007; Kilgore et al. 2010; Ferrante et al. 2003; Alarcón et al. 2004; Korzus et al. 2004). HDAC inhibitors have also been shown to facilitate the extinction of persistent and maladaptive behaviors (Lattal et al. 2007; Bredy and Barad 2008), indicating that HDAC inhibitors may enhance the effects of exposure therapy used to treat anxiety syndromes and addiction. HDAC inhibitors therefore demonstrate promising effects for the treatment of many cognitive disorders involving deficits in learning and memory. However, there remain many open questions critical to our understanding of the effects of HDAC inhibitors on complex cognitive functions in the brain. First, determining the effects of HDAC inhibitors on different cell types and structures of brain will be necessary to better predict the consequences of HDAC inhibition. Indeed, evidence demonstrates that expression patterns of many HDAC isoforms is different among brain regions (Broide et al. 2007), suggesting that the outcome of distinct HDAC inhibitors may vary depending on the targeted isoforms. Second, we are still far from understanding the signaling cascades and gene expression changes that are necessary and sufficient to mediate the cognitive improvements induced by HDAC inhibitors. Third, how are HDAC inhibitors capable of exerting transcriptional control on a select subset of genes? A recent high-resolution mass spectrometry study identified 3,600 lysine acetylation sites on 1,750 proteins and found that HDAC inhibitors only upregulated about 10% of all acetylation sites (Choudhary et al. 2009). Moreover, understanding the relative contributions of histone and nonhistone proteins will be central to determining the mechanisms mediating the effects of HDAC inhibitors. Finally, knowledge of the HDAC isoforms involved in eliciting the cognitive improvements will lead to the development of selective HDAC-based therapies. In this regard, genetic animal models targeting specific HDAC isoforms indicate that HDAC2 inhibitors may be particularly useful in treating cognitive dysfunction (Guan et al. 2009). Currently, the development of isoform- and class-selective HDAC inhibitors is undergoing a rapid expansion. Investigations of these selective HDAC inhibitors will uncover the role of HDAC subtypes in normal physiology and disease, and will facilitate rational drug design based on pathophysiological insight. In addition, improving selectivity will likely limit the number of untoward side effects in the clinical setting. Thus, selective HDAC inhibitors represent a fundamentally novel approach for treating cognitive disorders that may deliver symptomatic improvements with fewer adverse effects.

Acknowledgments V.L. is supported by a Canadian Institutes of Health (CIHR) fellowship.

References

Alarcón JM et al (2004) Chromatin acetylation, memory, and LTP are impaired in CBP+/- mice: a model for the cognitive deficit in Rubinstein-Taybi syndrome and its amelioration. Neuron 42:947–959

Atkins CM, Selcher JC, Petraitis JJ, Trzaskos JM, Sweatt JD (1998) The MAPK cascade is required for mammalian associative learning. Nat Neurosci 1:602–609

Balasubramanian S, Verner E, Buggy JJ (2009) Isoform-specific histone deacetylase inhibitors: the next step? Cancer Lett 280:211–221

Bannister AJ, Kouzarides T (1996) The CBP co-activator is a histone acetyltransferase. Nature 384:641–643

Bartholdi D et al (2007) Genetic heterogeneity in Rubinstein-Taybi syndrome: delineation of the phenotype of the first patients carrying mutations in EP300. J Med Genet 44:327–333

Berardi N, Braschi C, Capsoni S, Cattaneo A, Maffei L (2007) Environmental enrichment delays the onset of memory deficits and reduces neuropathological hallmarks in a mouse model of Alzheimer-like neurodegeneration. J Alzheimers Dis 11:359–370

Berger SL (2007) The complex language of chromatin regulation during transcription. Nature 447:407–412

Biacsi R, Kumari D, Usdin K (2008) SIRT1 inhibition alleviates gene silencing in Fragile X mental retardation syndrome. PLoS Genet 4:e1000017

Bieliauskas AV, Pflum MK (2008) Isoform-selective histone deacetylase inhibitors. Chem Soc Rev 37:1402–1413

Bliss TV, Collingridge GL (1993) A synaptic model of memory: long-term potentiation in the hippocampus. Nature 361:31–39

Blough RI et al (2000) Variation in microdeletions of the cyclic AMP-responsive element-binding protein gene at chromosome band 16p13.3 in the Rubinstein-Taybi syndrome. Am J Med Genet 90:29–34

Borrelli E, Nestler EJ, Allis CD, Sassone-Corsi P (2008) Decoding the epigenetic language of neuronal plasticity. Neuron 60:961–974

Bosetti F, Bell JM, Manickam P (2005) Microarray analysis of rat brain gene expression after chronic administration of sodium valproate. Brain Res Bull 65:331–338

Bourne JN, Harris KM (2010) Coordination of size and number of excitatory and inhibitory synapses results in a balanced structural plasticity along mature hippocampal CA1 dendrites during LTP. Hippocampus

Boyes J, Byfield P, Nakatani Y, Ogryzko V (1998) Regulation of activity of the transcription factor GATA-1 by acetylation. Nature 396:594–598

Bredy TW, Barad M (2008) The histone deacetylase inhibitor valproic acid enhances acquisition, extinction, and reconsolidation of conditioned fear. Learn Mem 15:39–45

Bredy TW, Wu H, Crego C, Zellhoefer J, Sun YE, Barad M (2007) Histone modifications around individual BDNF gene promoters in prefrontal cortex are associated with extinction of conditioned fear. Learn Mem 14:268–276

Broide RS, Redwine JM, Aftahi N, Young W, Bloom FE, Winrow CJ (2007) Distribution of histone deacetylases 1-11 in the rat brain. J Mol Neurosci 31:47–58

Cao X, Sudhof TC (2001) A transcriptionally [correction of transcriptively] active complex of APP with Fe65 and histone acetyltransferase Tip60. Science 293:115–120

Carew JS, Giles FJ, Nawrocki ST (2008) Histone deacetylase inhibitors: mechanisms of cell death and promise in combination cancer therapy. Cancer Lett 269:7–17

Carey N, La Thangue NB (2006) Histone deacetylase inhibitors: gathering pace. Curr Opin Pharmacol 6:369–375

Caron C, Boyault C, Khochbin S (2005) Regulatory cross-talk between lysine acetylation and ubiquitination: role in the control of protein stability. Bioessays 27:408–415

Chen LF, Mu Y, Greene WC (2002) Acetylation of RelA at discrete sites regulates distinct nuclear functions of NF-kappaB. EMBO J 21:6539–6548

Chiba T et al (2004) Identification of genes up-regulated by histone deacetylase inhibition with cDNA microarray and exploration of epigenetic alterations on hepatoma cells. J Hepatol 41:436–445

Chiurazzi P, Pomponi MG, Willemsen R, Oostra BA, Neri G (1998) In vitro reactivation of the FMR1 gene involved in fragile X syndrome. Hum Mol Genet 7:109–113

Choi JK, Howe LJ (2009) Histone acetylation: truth of consequences? Biochem Cell Biol 87: 139–150

Chou CJ, Herman D, Gottesfeld JM (2008) Pimelic diphenylamide 106 is a slow, tight-binding inhibitor of class I histone deacetylases. J Biol Chem 283:35402–35409

Choudhary C et al (2009) Lysine acetylation targets protein complexes and co-regulates major cellular functions. Science 325:834–840

Coffee B, Zhang F, Ceman S, Warren ST, Reines D (2002) Histone modifications depict an aberrantly heterochromatinized FMR1 gene in fragile x syndrome. Am J Hum Genet 71: 923–932

Costa-Mattioli M, Sossin WS, Klann E, Sonenberg N (2009) Translational control of long-lasting synaptic plasticity and memory. Neuron 61:10–26

Covington HE 3rd et al (2009) Antidepressant actions of histone deacetylase inhibitors. J Neurosci 29:11451–11460

Davis M, Ressler K, Rothbaum BO, Richardson R (2006) Effects of D-cycloserine on extinction: translation from preclinical to clinical work. Biol Psychiatry 60:369–375

Dompierre JP et al (2007) Histone deacetylase 6 inhibition compensates for the transport deficit in Huntington's disease by increasing tubulin acetylation. J Neurosci 27:3571–3583

Dong E, Guidotti A, Grayson DR, Costa E (2007) Histone hyperacetylation induces demethylation of reelin and 67-kDa glutamic acid decarboxylase promoters. Proc Natl Acad Sci USA 104:4676–4681

Eriksen JL, Janus CG (2007) Plaques, tangles, and memory loss in mouse models of neurodegeneration. Behav Genet 37:79–100

Federman N, Fustinana MS, Romano A (2009) Histone acetylation is recruited in consolidation as a molecular feature of stronger memories. Learn Mem 16:600–606

Feinberg AP (2007) Phenotypic plasticity and the epigenetics of human disease. Nature 447: 433–440

Ferrante RJ et al (2003) Histone deacetylase inhibition by sodium butyrate chemotherapy ameliorates the neurodegenerative phenotype in Huntington's disease mice. J Neurosci 23: 9418–9427

Fischer A, Sananbenesi F, Pang PT, Lu B, Tsai LH (2005) Opposing roles of transient and prolonged expression of p25 in synaptic plasticity and hippocampus-dependent memory. Neuron 48:825–838

Fischer A, Sananbenesi F, Wang X, Dobbin M, Tsai LH (2007) Recovery of learning and memory is associated with chromatin remodelling. Nature 447:178–182

Fischle W et al (2002) Enzymatic activity associated with class II HDACs is dependent on a multiprotein complex containing HDAC3 and SMRT/N-CoR. Mol Cell 9:45–57

Fontan-Lozano A, Romero-Granados R, Troncoso J, Munera A, Delgado-Garcia JM, Carrion AM (2008) Histone deacetylase inhibitors improve learning consolidation in young and in KA-induced-neurodegeneration and SAMP-8-mutant mice. Mol Cell Neurosci 39:193–201

Fuks F, Hurd PJ, Wolf D, Nan X, Bird AP, Kouzarides T (2003) The methyl-CpG-binding protein MeCP2 links DNA methylation to histone methylation. J Biol Chem 278:4035–4040

Garber KB, Visootsak J, Warren ST (2008) Fragile X syndrome. Eur J Hum Genet 16:666–672

Gardian G et al (2005) Neuroprotective effects of phenylbutyrate in the N171-82Q transgenic mouse model of Huntington's disease. J Biol Chem 280:556–563

Glaser KB, Staver MJ, Waring JF, Stender J, Ulrich RG, Davidsen SK (2003) Gene expression profiling of multiple histone deacetylase (HDAC) inhibitors: defining a common gene set produced by HDAC inhibition in T24 and MDA carcinoma cell lines. Mol Cancer Ther 2: 151–163

Glozak MA, Sengupta N, Zhang X, Seto E (2005) Acetylation and deacetylation of non-histone proteins. Gene 363:15–23

Godler DE et al (2010) Methylation of novel markers of fragile X alleles is inversely correlated with FMRP expression and FMR1 activation ratio. Hum Mol Genet 19(8):1618–1632

Graff J, Mansuy IM (2008) Epigenetic codes in cognition and behaviour. Behav Brain Res 192:70–87

Green KN et al (2008) Nicotinamide restores cognition in Alzheimer's disease transgenic mice via a mechanism involving sirtuin inhibition and selective reduction of Thr231-phosphotau. J Neurosci 28:11500–11510

Gronroos E, Hellman U, Heldin CH, Ericsson J (2002) Control of Smad7 stability by competition between acetylation and ubiquitination. Mol Cell 10:483–493

Gu W, Roeder RG (1997) Activation of p53 sequence-specific DNA binding by acetylation of the p53 C-terminal domain. Cell 90:595–606

Guan Z et al (2002) Integration of long-term-memory-related synaptic plasticity involves bidirectional regulation of gene expression and chromatin structure. Cell 111:483–493

Guan JS et al (2009) HDAC2 negatively regulates memory formation and synaptic plasticity. Nature 459:55–60

Guenther MG, Barak O, Lazar MA (2001) The SMRT and N-CoR corepressors are activating cofactors for histone deacetylase 3. Mol Cell Biol 21:6091–6101

Hallam TM, Bourtchouladze R (2006) Rubinstein-Taybi syndrome: molecular findings and therapeutic approaches to improve cognitive dysfunction. Cell Mol Life Sci 63:1725–1735

Hamblett CL et al (2007) The discovery of 6-amino nicotinamides as potent and selective histone deacetylase inhibitors. Bioorg Med Chem Lett 17:5300–5309

Heather N, Bradley BP (1990) Cue exposure as a practical treatment for addictive disorders: why are we waiting? Addict Behav 15:335–337

Heese K, Akatsu H (2006) Alzheimer's disease–an interactive perspective. Curr Alzheimer Res 3: 109–121

Hendrich B, Bird A (1998) Identification and characterization of a family of mammalian methyl-CpG binding proteins. Mol Cell Biol 18:6538–6547

Hockly E et al (2003) Suberoylanilide hydroxamic acid, a histone deacetylase inhibitor, ameliorates motor deficits in a mouse model of Huntington's disease. Proc Natl Acad Sci USA 100:2041–2046

Hoffmann A, Natoli G, Ghosh G (2006) Transcriptional regulation via the NF-kappaB signaling module. Oncogene 25:6706–6716

Hofmann SG (2007) Enhancing exposure-based therapy from a translational research perspective. Behav Res Ther 45:1987–2001

Iacomino G, Tecce MF, Grimaldi C, Tosto M, Russo GL (2001) Transcriptional response of a human colon adenocarcinoma cell line to sodium butyrate. Biochem Biophys Res Commun 285:1280–1289

Impey S et al (2002) Phosphorylation of CBP mediates transcriptional activation by neural activity and CaM kinase IV. Neuron 34:235–244

Janknecht R (2002) The versatile functions of the transcriptional coactivators p300 and CBP and their roles in disease. Histol Histopathol 17:657–668

Jankowsky JL et al (2004) Mutant presenilins specifically elevate the levels of the 42 residue beta-amyloid peptide in vivo: evidence for augmentation of a 42-specific gamma secretase. Hum Mol Genet 13:159–170

Jankowsky JL et al (2005) Environmental enrichment mitigates cognitive deficits in a mouse model of Alzheimer's disease. J Neurosci 25:5217–5224

Jones PL et al (1998) Methylated DNA and MeCP2 recruit histone deacetylase to repress transcription. Nat Genet 19:187–191

Jones P et al (2008) 2-Trifluoroacetylthiophenes, a novel series of potent and selective class II histone deacetylase inhibitors. Bioorg Med Chem Lett 18:3456–3461

Kauer JA, Malenka RC, Nicoll RA (1988) NMDA application potentiates synaptic transmission in the hippocampus. Nature 334:250–252

Kazantsev AG, Thompson LM (2008) Therapeutic application of histone deacetylase inhibitors for central nervous system disorders. Nat Rev Drug Discov 7:854–868

Kelleher RJ III, Govindarajan A, Jung HY, Kang H, Tonegawa S (2004) Translational control by MAPK signaling in long-term synaptic plasticity and memory. Cell 116:467–479

Khan N et al (2008) Determination of the class and isoform selectivity of small-molecule histone deacetylase inhibitors. Biochem J 409:581–589

Kilgore M et al (2010) Inhibitors of class 1 histone deacetylases reverse contextual memory deficits in a mouse model of Alzheimer's disease. Neuropsychopharmacology 35:870–880

Kim JJ, Fanselow MS (1992) Modality-specific retrograde amnesia of fear. Science 256:675–677

Kim HS et al (2004) Inhibition of histone deacetylation enhances the neurotoxicity induced by the C-terminal fragments of amyloid precursor protein. J Neurosci Res 75:117–124

Kim D et al (2007) SIRT1 deacetylase protects against neurodegeneration in models for Alzheimer's disease and amyotrophic lateral sclerosis. EMBO J 26:3169–3179

Korzus E, Rosenfeld MG, Mayford M (2004) CBP histone acetyltransferase activity is a critical component of memory consolidation. Neuron 42:961–972

Kouzarides T (2007) Chromatin modifications and their function. Cell 128:693–705

Kozikowski AP, Tapadar S, Luchini DN, Kim KH, Billadeau DD (2008) Use of the nitrile oxide cycloaddition (NOC) reaction for molecular probe generation: a new class of enzyme selective histone deacetylase inhibitors (HDACIs) showing picomolar activity at HDAC6. J Med Chem 51:4370–4373

Krennhrubec K, Marshall BL, Hedglin M, Verdin E, Ulrich SM (2007) Design and evaluation of 'Linkerless' hydroxamic acids as selective HDAC8 inhibitors. Bioorg Med Chem Lett 17:2874–2878

Laherty CD, Yang WM, Sun JM, Davie JR, Seto E, Eisenman RN (1997) Histone deacetylases associated with the mSin3 corepressor mediate mad transcriptional repression. Cell 89: 349–356

Latham JA, Dent SY (2007) Cross-regulation of histone modifications. Nat Struct Mol Biol 14: 1017–1024

Lattal KM, Barrett RM, Wood MA (2007) Systemic or intrahippocampal delivery of histone deacetylase inhibitors facilitates fear extinction. Behav Neurosci 121:1125–1131

Lazarov O et al (2005) Environmental enrichment reduces Abeta levels and amyloid deposition in transgenic mice. Cell 120:701–713

Levenson JM, O'Riordan KJ, Brown KD, Trinh MA, Molfese DL, Sweatt JD (2004) Regulation of histone acetylation during memory formation in the hippocampus. J Biol Chem 279: 40545–40559

Levy L et al (2004) Acetylation of beta-catenin by p300 regulates beta-catenin-Tcf4 interaction. Mol Cell Biol 24:3404–3414

Li RW, Li C (2006) Butyrate induces profound changes in gene expression related to multiple signal pathways in bovine kidney epithelial cells. BMC Genomics 7:234

Lin HY, Chen CS, Lin SP, Weng JR, Chen CS (2006) Targeting histone deacetylase in cancer therapy. Med Res Rev 26:397–413

Loebrich S, Nedivi E (2009) The function of activity-regulated genes in the nervous system. Physiol Rev 89:1079–1103

Ma X, Ezzeldin HH, Diasio RB (2009) Histone deacetylase inhibitors: current status and overview of recent clinical trials. Drugs 69:1911–1934

MacDonald VE, Howe LJ (2009) Histone acetylation: where to go and how to get there. Epigenetics 4:139–143

Malvaez M, Barrett RM, Wood MA, Sanchis-Segura C (2009) Epigenetic mechanisms underlying extinction of memory and drug-seeking behavior. Mamm Genome 20:612–623

Marambaud P et al (2003) A CBP binding transcriptional repressor produced by the PS1/epsilon-cleavage of N-cadherin is inhibited by PS1 FAD mutations. Cell 114:635–645

Marlatt GA (1990) Cue exposure and relapse prevention in the treatment of addictive behaviors. Addict Behav 15:395–399

Maurice T et al (2008) Altered memory capacities and response to stress in p300/CBP-associated factor (PCAF) histone acetylase knockout mice. Neuropsychopharmacology 33:1584–1602

Meehan RR, Lewis JD, Bird AP (1992) Characterization of MeCP2, a vertebrate DNA binding protein with affinity for methylated DNA. Nucleic Acids Res 20:5085–5092

Methot JL et al (2008) Exploration of the internal cavity of histone deacetylase (HDAC) with selective HDAC1/HDAC2 inhibitors (SHI-1:2). Bioorg Med Chem Lett 18:973–978

Norberg MM, Krystal JH, Tolin DF (2008) A meta-analysis of D-cycloserine and the facilitation of fear extinction and exposure therapy. Biol Psychiatry 63:1118–1126

Nott A, Watson PM, Robinson JD, Crepaldi L, Riccio A (2008) S-Nitrosylation of histone deacetylase 2 induces chromatin remodelling in neurons. Nature 455:411–415

O'Brien CP, Childress AR, McLellan T, Ehrman R (1990) Integrating systemic cue exposure with standard treatment in recovering drug dependent patients. Addict Behav 15:355–365

Oike Y et al (1999) Truncated CBP protein leads to classical Rubinstein-Taybi syndrome phenotypes in mice: implications for a dominant-negative mechanism. Hum Mol Genet 8:387–396

Oliveira AM, Wood MA, McDonough CB, Abel T (2007) Transgenic mice expressing an inhibitory truncated form of p300 exhibit long-term memory deficits. Learn Mem 14:564–572

Ontoria JM et al (2009) Identification of novel, selective, and stable inhibitors of class II histone deacetylases. Validation studies of the inhibition of the enzymatic activity of HDAC4 by small molecules as a novel approach for cancer therapy. J Med Chem 52:6782–6789

Ou JN et al (2007) Histone deacetylase inhibitor Trichostatin A induces global and gene-specific DNA demethylation in human cancer cell lines. Biochem Pharmacol 73:1297–1307

Perez-Balado C et al (2007) Bispyridinium dienes: histone deacetylase inhibitors with selective activities. J Med Chem 50:2497–2505

Petrij F et al (1995) Rubinstein-Taybi syndrome caused by mutations in the transcriptional co-activator CBP. Nature 376:348–351

Pieretti M et al (1991) Absence of expression of the FMR-1 gene in fragile X syndrome. Cell 66:817–822

Polesskaya A et al (2000) CREB-binding protein/p300 activates MyoD by acetylation. J Biol Chem 275:34359–34364

Roelfsema JH et al (2005) Genetic heterogeneity in Rubinstein-Taybi syndrome: mutations in both the CBP and EP300 genes cause disease. Am J Hum Genet 76:572–580

Romano A, Freudenthal R, Merlo E, Routtenberg A (2006) Evolutionarily-conserved role of the NF-kappaB transcription factor in neural plasticity and memory. Eur J Neurosci 24:1507–1516

Rouaux C, Jokic N, Mbebi C, Boutillier S, Loeffler JP, Boutillier AL (2003) Critical loss of CBP/p300 histone acetylase activity by caspase-6 during neurodegeneration. EMBO J 22: 6537–6549

Sadri-Vakili G, Cha JH (2006) Mechanisms of disease: histone modifications in Huntington's disease. Nat Clin Pract Neurol 2:330–338

Sadri-Vakili G et al (2007) Histones associated with downregulated genes are hypo-acetylated in Huntington's disease models. Hum Mol Genet 16:1293–1306

Saura CA et al (2004) Loss of presenilin function causes impairments of memory and synaptic plasticity followed by age-dependent neurodegeneration. Neuron 42:23–36

Savonenko A et al (2005) Episodic-like memory deficits in the APPswe/PS1dE9 mouse model of Alzheimer's disease: relationships to beta-amyloid deposition and neurotransmitter abnormalities. Neurobiol Dis 18:602–617

Selkoe DJ (2001) Alzheimer's disease: genes, proteins, and therapy. Physiol Rev 81:741–766

Shafaati M, O'Driscoll R, Bjorkhem I, Meaney S (2009) Transcriptional regulation of cholesterol 24-hydroxylase by histone deacetylase inhibitors. Biochem Biophys Res Commun 378:689–694

Stefanko DP, Barrett RM, Ly AR, Reolon GK, Wood MA (2009) Modulation of long-term memory for object recognition via HDAC inhibition. Proc Natl Acad Sci USA 106:9447–9452

Steffan JS et al (2001) Histone deacetylase inhibitors arrest polyglutamine-dependent neurodegeneration in Drosophila. Nature 413:739–743

Strahl BD, Allis CD (2000) The language of covalent histone modifications. Nature 403:41–45

Szapiro G et al (2002) Molecular mechanisms of memory retrieval. Neurochem Res 27:1491–1498

Tabolacci E et al (2008) Modest reactivation of the mutant FMR1 gene by valproic acid is accompanied by histone modifications but not DNA demethylation. Pharmacogenet Genomics 18:738–741

Tabuchi Y, Takasaki I, Doi T, Ishii Y, Sakai H, Kondo T (2006) Genetic networks responsive to sodium butyrate in colonic epithelial cells. FEBS Lett 580:3035–3041

Thomas EA (2009) Focal nature of neurological disorders necessitates isotype-selective histone deacetylase (HDAC) inhibitors. Mol Neurobiol 40:33–45

Thomas EA et al (2008) The HDAC inhibitor 4b ameliorates the disease phenotype and transcriptional abnormalities in Huntington's disease transgenic mice. Proc Natl Acad Sci USA 105: 15564–15569

Vecsey CG et al (2007) Histone deacetylase inhibitors enhance memory and synaptic plasticity via CREB:CBP-dependent transcriptional activation. J Neurosci 27:6128–6140

Verkerk AJ et al (1991) Identification of a gene (FMR-1) containing a CGG repeat coincident with a breakpoint cluster region exhibiting length variation in fragile X syndrome. Cell 65:905–914

Wang C et al (2001) Direct acetylation of the estrogen receptor alpha hinge region by p300 regulates transactivation and hormone sensitivity. J Biol Chem 276:18375–18383

Weiler IJ et al (1997) Fragile X mental retardation protein is translated near synapses in response to neurotransmitter activation. Proc Natl Acad Sci USA 94:5395–5400

Wen YD et al (2000) The histone deacetylase-3 complex contains nuclear receptor corepressors. Proc Natl Acad Sci USA 97:7202–7207

Wood MA et al (2005) Transgenic mice expressing a truncated form of CREB-binding protein (CBP) exhibit deficits in hippocampal synaptic plasticity and memory storage. Learn Mem 12: 111–119

Wood MA, Attner MA, Oliveira AM, Brindle PK, Abel T (2006) A transcription factor-binding domain of the coactivator CBP is essential for long-term memory and the expression of specific target genes. Learn Mem 13:609–617

Yang G, Pan F, Gan WB (2009) Stably maintained dendritic spines are associated with lifelong memories. Nature 462:920–924

Yeh SH, Lin CH, Gean PW (2004) Acetylation of nuclear factor-kappaB in rat amygdala improves long-term but not short-term retention of fear memory. Mol Pharmacol 65:1286–1292

Zhang Y, Ng HH, Erdjument-Bromage H, Tempst P, Bird A, Reinberg D (1999) Analysis of the NuRD subunits reveals a histone deacetylase core complex and a connection with DNA methylation. Genes Dev 13:1924–1935

Chapter 13
Epigenetic Mechanisms of Memory Consolidation

Marcel A. Estevez and Ted Abel

Abstract The requirement of gene transcription for memory consolidation has been established for several decades, but not until recently has it been recognized that epigenetic mechanisms play a role in the control of gene expression that leads to memory storage. Broadly speaking, these epigenetic mechanisms encompass changes in chromatin structure, such as posttranslational histone modifications and DNA methylation. Many studies have shown that histone acetylation is dynamically regulated after experience and that it acts as a permissive switch to allow gene transcription. These studies have established a dichotomy where permissive gene transcription results in memory enhancement and restrictive gene transcription in memory impairment. Other studies have focused on DNA methylation, specifically on the promoter region of genes, where it is associated with gene inactivation. Like histone acetylation, it has been shown that DNA methylation is regulated after experience, and can be dynamically regulated, although it is thought to be a more stable mark than histone acetylation. The relationship between levels of DNA methylation and memory impairment or enhancement is unclear and will require future study. Many other chromatin modifications play a role in experience-induced gene regulation, such as histone methylation and phosphorylation, as well as substitution by histone variants. Ultimately, these modifications in chromatin structure act in concert, in a potential combinatorial code, to regulate gene-specific transcription that results in memory consolidation.

Keywords Combinatorial chromatin code · DNA methylation · Electroconvulsive treatment · Histone acetylation · Histone methylation · Histone phosphorylation · Long-term memory · Long-term potentiation · Memory consolidation · Synaptic plasticity

M.A. Estevez and T. Abel (✉)
Department of Biology, University of Pennsylvania, 433 South University Avenue, Philadelphia, PA 19104, USA
e-mail: mestevez@sas.upenn.edu, abele@sas.upenn.edu

A. Petronis and J. Mill (eds.), *Brain, Behavior and Epigenetics*,   267
Epigenetics and Human Health, DOI 10.1007/978-3-642-17426-1_13,
© Springer-Verlag Berlin Heidelberg 2011

Unlike most science jargon, *memory* is a common term used in everyday life. Nevertheless, *memory* is rather abstract and not uniformly defined. As scientists, we describe it as both a behavioral adaptation and information storage, which come as a result of experience. In terms of information storage, there are different stages for memory that have been described: *acquisition, consolidation*, and *retrieval*. Memory acquisition refers simply to learning, that is, the encoding of information after an experience. Memory retrieval is the remembering of the experience, which is where a behavioral adaptation can be measured. In between these two temporally spaced stages lies memory consolidation. Memory consolidation is the establishment of *long-term* memory, lasting days, weeks, or even years after acquisition. Somehow the coded information is stabilized into a more persistent state. Not all information learned is consolidated, however, as most experiences are not committed to long-term storage. This labile information is referred to as *short-term* memory, which can only be retrieved in a short span of time after acquisition.

The study of the underlying mechanisms of memory consolidation is a daunting task. Firstly, the code for memory is not understood. Secondly, several memory systems have evolved to store different types of information. For instance, reflex conditioning depends on cerebellar circuitry, conditioned emotional responses depend on amygdalar circuitry, and cognitive or relational learning depends on hippocampal circuitry (Rugg 1997). Furthermore, consolidation is not a single process but a family of processes, as there is a distinction between synaptic or cellular consolidation versus system consolidation. At the level of a synapse or cell, consolidation occurs in a matter of minutes or hours, whereas at a system level, consolidation occurs in the time frame of days or weeks. In the latter, it is believed that the circuitries of the brain that encode memory are reorganized and that the information storage is displaced from the circuitry where it was encoded, e.g., the hippocampus, to a more permanent site of retention, e.g., the neocortex (Dudai 2004).

Memory research has mostly focused on studying cellular correlates and molecular components in neurons that underlie memory storage via *synaptic* or *cellular consolidation*. Moreover, the study of memory has focused on declarative memory – the memory of facts and places that is dependent on hippocampus and cortex for consolidation and maintenance. One of the first steps in understanding the molecular composition of memory came in the 1960s and 1970s when several groups showed that protein synthesis inhibitors block formation of long-term, but not short-term, memory consolidation in fish and rodents (e.g., Agranoff et al. 1966; Barondes and Cohen 1967). These initial studies looked at discrimination tasks based on reward, which are dependent on hippocampus. Although the time window for protein synthesis inhibitor to have amnesic effects is variable (Gold 2006), these initial studies establish that protein synthesis is needed immediately after the learning experience.

Not surprisingly, transcription immediately after the learning experience is also required for memory consolidation (Squire and Barondes 1970; Neale et al. 1973) and also 3–6 h after training (Igaz et al. 2002). Seemingly paradoxically, electroconvulsive stimulation, which causes increased transcription of immediate early genes (Saffen et al. 1988; Morgan et al. 1987), is an amnesic treatment. So, whereas long-term changes in synaptic plasticity and memory require transcription and translation of these early gene products, indiscriminate, mass neuronal transcriptional activation impedes memory formation. This suggests that some level of specificity of neuronal activity and consequent gene regulation is required for memory, while mass neuronal activity masks the storage of memory. Many of these early genes that are induced during learning or mass neuronal stimulation are transcription factors, which are then able to initiate another wave of transcription. The products of these transcriptional waves result in long-lasting changes in synaptic strength, which is widely understood as a cellular correlate of memory.

13.1 Long-Term Potentiation as a Correlate of Long-Term Memory

Activity-dependent changes in synaptic strength in the hippocampus are thought to underlie memory storage and the acquisition of learned behaviors. One intensely studied form of synaptic plasticity is long-term potentiation (LTP), a persistent, activity-dependent form of synaptic enhancement that is a model for certain types of long-term memory (Bliss and Collingridge 1993; Martin et al. 2000; Neves et al. 2008). LTP in the CA1 region of the hippocampus has distinct temporal phases (Nguyen and Woo 2003): a transient, early phase (E-LTP) that lasts 1–2 h and a late phase (L-LTP) that lasts for up to 8 h in hippocampal slices (Frey et al. 1993) and for days in the intact animal (Abraham et al. 1993). Both E-LTP and L-LTP in the CA1 region depend on the N-methyl D-aspartate (NMDA) receptor and on the activation of kinases such as calcium/calmodulin-dependent protein kinase II (CaMKII), whereas L-LTP (but not E-LTP) shares with long-term memory a requirement for transcription and translation (Frey et al. 1988, 1993, 1996; Frey and Morris 1997; Huang and Kandel 1994, 1995; Huang et al. 1996; Nguyen et al. 1994; Nguyen and Kandel 1997; Nguyen and Woo 2003).

Studies in *Aplysia* and *Drosophila* have been important in establishing a role for the cyclic adenosine monophosphate (cAMP)–protein kinase A (PKA) pathway in memory consolidation (Carew 1996). This pathway leads to activation by phosphorylation of the cAMP response element-binding protein (CREB), a transcriptional activator for many immediate early genes. It has been shown in these invertebrate models that not only does inactivation of CREB disrupt long-term memory, but CREB activation enhances it. The role for CREB in mammalian memory was later elucidated using a mouse genetic approach, where two CREB isoforms, namely α and δ, were deleted from the genome resulting in memory impairment (Bourtchuladze et al. 1994). Moreover, CREB overexpression also results in *enhanced* memory consolidation in rats (Josselyn et al. 2001). Together with comparable data from invertebrate models, these studies demonstrate that CREB has a key role in modulating memory consolidation.

Considering the limited time window for protein synthesis and transcription inhibitors blocking memory consolidation, and also the short half-life of mRNA and protein, it is puzzling how the gene products made in this time window result in the long-lasting neuronal changes of memory consolidation. Certainly, these gene products must pave the way for mechanisms required to maintain memory. A widely accepted view is that these activity-dependent gene products result in lasting changes in synaptic morphology and strength. However, recent studies suggest that persistent changes in gene expression may also underlie the maintenance of memory.

Recently, much attention has shifted to the regulation of the state of *chromatin* for gene regulation during memory consolidation. Chromatin, the complex of genomic DNA with packaging proteins, exists in different states where genes or gene clusters are either expressed or repressed. Chromatin exists in different states, grossly identified as euchromatin and heterochromatin. The regulation of these states of chromatin has been studied to explain the regulation of gene expression in different cell types and the maintenance of chromosomal regions such as telomeres and centromeres. During cell differentiation, chromatin is silenced or activated to regulate the expression of genes according to a specific cell type. These chromatin states are considered extremely stable in terminally differentiated, postmitotic cells, accounting for the maintenance of the identity of the differentiated cell. However, it has become evident that some chromatin changes are quite dynamic in postmitotic cells, such as neurons and immune cells that undergo gene expression changes in response to experience (e.g., Borrelli et al. (2008) review epigenetic control in neuronal plasticity; Placek et al. (2009) review epigenetic control in CD4+ T cell activation). Chromatin regulation is possible through covalent modifications in nucleosomal proteins known as histones, and also the DNA itself. Some of these modifications are more labile, such as histone acetylation, while others such as DNA methylation are much more stable. Here, we focus on the role of these chromatin modifications during memory consolidation.

13.2 Histone Acetylation

Histones are basic proteins that are modified by acetylation, phosphorylation, methylation, ubiquitination, and sumoylation of their amino-terminal tails (Strahl and Allis 2000; Peterson and Laniel 2004). A groundbreaking finding in the field of memory was to show that inhibition of histone deacetylation *enhances* memory, which is reminiscent of the effect of CREB overexpression (Levenson et al. 2004; Fischer et al. 2007; Alarcón et al. 2004; Vecsey et al. 2007; Stefanko et al. 2009). Because the increase of acetylated histones in response to histone deacetylase inhibitor is global, and not cell- or gene-specific, it suggests that histone acetylation alone, unlike mass neuronal activity, is not sufficient for gene expression. Moreover, it suggests that the specificity of neuronal activity confers memory consolidation, while histone acetylation is a gate for this to occur.

In the seminal study by Levenson et al. (2004), the authors use the contextual fear conditioning paradigm, a hippocampus-dependent association task, to investigate the role of histone acetylation in hippocampus-dependent memory. One of their major findings is that training in this association task leads to a significant increase in acetyl-H3 in area CA1 of the hippocampus, but not acetyl-H4. Also, pre-exposure to the context – which blocks the association of context and shock – does not result in increased acetyl-H3, but does increase acetyl-H4. Moreover, both phorbol ester and forskolin treatments, which activate protein kinase C (PKC) and protein kinase A (PKA), respectively, mimic this acetyl-H3 increase without acetyl-H4 increase, suggesting a role for these pathways in association-dependent histone acetylation. In a later study, they show that DNA methylation is required for the phorbol ester-induced H3 acetylation (Levenson et al. 2006). It should be noted, however, that global changes in acetylation may not correlate to gene-specific changes, as forskolin induces acetylation of histone H4, but not H3, in the *Bdnf* promoter IV in cultured neuroblastoma cells (He et al. 2010).

The MAPK pathway is necessary for the increase in acetyl-H3 (Levenson et al. 2004), and the study proposes that the PKA and PKC pathways converge upstream of the MAPK pathway. Another study by the same group also implicates the MAPK pathway in histone H3 phosphorylation, which is also induced by the contextual fear conditioning paradigm (Chwang et al. 2006). The work by Levenson et al. (2004) also shows that broad-spectrum HDAC inhibitors, namely sodium butyrate (NaB) and trichostatin A (TSA), enhance a form of hippocampal LTP. The LTP protocol that the authors use is two 100-Hz stimuli, spaced by 20 s. This LTP protocol is not particularly robust, and also not PKA-dependent (Abel et al. 1997), although it is sufficient to elicit a long-lasting potentiation of synaptic strength. Lastly, a major finding in the study is that sodium butyrate administered intraperitoneally is able to enhance long-term (24 h) associative memory (contextual fear conditioning) but not short-term (1 h) memory.

A study by Fischer et al. (2007) expands on this previous study by showing residue-specific histone acetylation and changes in synaptic morphology. In their study, they use a neurodegenerative disease mouse model and show that environmental enrichment rescues learning and memory deficits. Unlike the Levenson study, this study looks at histone acetylation and synaptic spine morphology after environmental enrichment and not after associative learning. The authors show a significant increase in acetylation of specific residues in histones H3 and H4, 24 h or 2 weeks after environmental enrichment. In the hippocampus, some increases return to baseline at 2 weeks (Ac-H3K14, Ac-H4K8, and Ac-H4K12), whereas some stay elevated after 2 weeks (Ac-H3K9 and Ac-H4K5) not only in hippocampus, but also in cortex, which is congruent with a role for the cortex in remote memory storage. Also, methyl-H3K4 is elevated at 24 h and at 2 weeks after enrichment in cortex only. Together with the previous studies, these findings suggest that environmental enrichment acts in a manner similar to histone deacetylase inhibitors to increase histone acetylation and enhance contextual memory and modulate synaptic morphology.

13.3 Histone Acetyltransferases and Histone Deacetylases

The study of the transcriptional coactivator, and histone acetyltransferase (HAT), CREB-binding protein (CBP) in memory consolidation came with the recognition of the importance of histone acetylation in memory, together with the established role for cAMP/PKA/CREB signaling in this process. Also, along with CBP, other factors with histone acetyltransferase activity such as p300, a CBP homologue, and p300/CBP-associated factor (PCAF) became targets of memory studies. CBP and p300 are large and widely expressed multidomain transcriptional coactivators with HAT activity. A role for CBP in synaptic plasticity first came from studies in *Aplysia* (Guan et al. 2002). The role of these transcriptional coactivators in cognition had already been recognized, as mutations in the human CBP or p300 genes map with Rubenstein–Taybi syndrome (RTS) (Petrij et al. 1995; Roelfsema et al. 2005). Different loss-of-function and dominant-negative CBP and p300 mouse models have been used to study the role of these factors in memory. One such study uses heterozygous *Cbp*-mutant mice, which express a truncated CBP protein that lacks the C-terminus, thus inhibiting CBP function and resulting in RTS-like phenotypes (Oike et al. 1999). This RTS mouse model has impaired long-term memory in passive avoidance, fear conditioning, and object recognition, demonstrating a role for CBP in memory consolidation (Bourtchuladze et al. 2003; Oike et al. 1999).

In a haploinsufficiency model of RTS carrying a single null allele of *Cbp* (Tanaka et al. 1997, 2000), deficits in long-term memory for object recognition and fear conditioning are observed, and these deficits are ameliorated by histone deacetylase (HDAC) inhibitor treatment (Alarcón et al. 2004). This is the first study to implicate CBP in HDAC inhibitor-mediated synaptic strengthening and memory enhancement. The authors show that this heterozygous null mutant mouse, $Cbp^{+/-}$, which only has one functional allele of *Cbp*, has deficits in long-term contextual associative memory and in hippocampal LTP. These memory and plasticity impairments are rescued by an HDAC inhibitor, suggesting that CBP-mediated histone acetylation is required for memory consolidation and LTP. They also show that the mice have a significant, constitutional 50% decrease of acetylated histone H2B, while there are no changes in the other core nucleosome histones (H2A, H3, and H4). It is interesting that the target of acetylation in these *Cbp* mutants (namely, H2B) is different than the target of acetylation induced by environmental enrichment (H3 and H4), associative learning (H3), or nonassociative context exposure (H4). This suggests that multiple histones are required to form a code for memory formation. This also highlights the difficulty in assessing a role for acetylation of a specific histone, or histone residue, at a whole genome scale as opposed to individual target genes.

These results suggest that CBP and its HAT activity have a role in long-term memory. However, the developmental abnormalities and broad effects of the *Cbp* mutants described above make it difficult to draw conclusions on an adult role for CBP. Moreover, these mutants still have a functional copy of the *Cbp* gene. To address these concerns, two studies using transgenic mouse models with regulated expression of dominant-negative CBP constructs have confirmed a role for CBP in memory storage without confounding developmental abnormalities (Korzus et al. 2004; Wood et al. 2005). One of these constructs, CBPΔ1, lacks the HAT domain of CBP and has deficits in long-term contextual memory but not short-term contextual memory, implicating HAT activity of CBP in memory consolidation (Wood et al. 2005). Moreover, another *Cbp* mutant that lacks the ability to interact with phospho-CREB, $Cbp^{kix/kix}$, also has a contextual memory deficit without a developmental phenotype (Wood et al. 2006).

The study by Vecsey et al. (2007) uses the $Cbp^{kix/kix}$ mutant to implicate the CREB–CBP interaction in HDAC inhibitor-mediated memory enhancement. The authors show that a mutant CREB mouse lacking two isoforms of the transcription factor (α and δ), $Creb\alpha\delta^{-/-}$, (Bourtchuladze et al. 1994) and $Cbp^{kix/kix}$ (Wood et al. 2006), both of which exhibit deficits in HDAC inhibitor-mediated memory and LTP enhancements. This finding suggests that the recruitment of CBP by CREB is necessary for HDAC-mediated memory and LTP enhancement.

The role of p300 in memory was also addressed by using similar approaches as in the case for CBP. Two published studies look at different p300 mutant mouse models in contextual memory. A study by Oliveira et al. (2007) uses a transgenic dominant-negative approach, equivalent to the CBPΔ1 mutant, p300Δ1, which is expressed in forebrain neurons to block p300 function. Mice expressing this dominant negative, which lacks the HAT domain of the protein, have deficits in long-term contextual memory but not in short-term memory. Viosca et al. (2010) use a heterozygous null, p300$^{+/-}$, to assess the role of p300 in RTS etiology. While these mice have some developmental abnormalities, they did not exhibit deficits in contextual or spatial memory consolidation. The mice did, however, show impairment in relearning a spatial memory (water maze transfer task – where the mice have to relearn a new position for the platform in the Morris water maze). This learning deficit reflects a higher order role for p300 in plasticity or reorganization of a previous memory. This deficit could be at either a cellular- or system-level consolidation.

Another study related to HAT activity suggests a role for PCAF in memory acquisition, but not consolidation (Duclot et al. 2010). This study uses PCAF null mice in a spatial working memory task.

While the roles of CBP and p300 had been widely studied in the context of histone acetylation and memory, the target of the HDAC inhibitors implicated in memory enhancement had not been identified. HDACs comprise a large superfamily with mainly three classes. Both class I and class II HDACs are NAD-independent, whereas class III HDACs, also called sirtuins, are NAD-dependent. Both TSA and NaB inhibit largely class I and II HDACs, but within these are many HDACs that are expressed in the brain.

A recent study identifies HDAC2, a class I HDAC, as the main target of HDAC inhibitor-mediated memory enhancement (Guan et al. 2009). The study uses both *Hdac2* knockouts, as well as HDAC1 and HDAC2 overexpressors (OE). While the HDAC2 OE shows impairment in long-term contextual fear memory, the HDAC1 OE does not. Moreover, the impairment in HDAC2 OE memory is rescued with

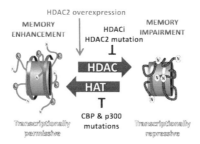

Fig. 13.1 *Role of histone acetylation in memory consolidation.* The balance of histone acetylation is regulated by histone deacetylases (HDACs) and histone acetyl transferases (HATs). Acetylation of histones by HATs allows for a more transcriptionally permissive state of chromatin. Conversely, deacetylated or hypoacetylated histones lead to a tight bond with DNA that is transcriptionally repressive. Manipulations such as HDAC inhibitor (HDACi) treatment or HDAC2 loss-of-function mutation favor the more transcriptionally permissive hyperacetylated state and result in memory enhancement. Likewise, CBP and p300 loss-of-function mutations and dominant-negative transgene expression lead to a more transcriptionally repressive hypoacetylated state that results in memory impairment

HDAC inhibitor treatment. Histone H4K12 acetylation was significantly reduced in the HDAC2 OE but not HDAC1 OE. This residue is also acetylated in response to environmental enrichment (Fischer et al. 2007). In the *Hdac2* knockout, the authors see an enhancement in long-term contextual memory, reminiscent of HDAC inhibitor-mediated enhancement. This knockout has increased acetylation of Histone H4K5 and H4K12, as well as H2B, this last one in congruence with the HDAC inhibitor increase of acetyl H2B (Alarcón et al. 2004). In addition, chromatin immunoprecipitation with HDAC2 antibody shows association of this deacetylase with many plasticity-related genes, such as *Bdnf*, *Egr1*, and *Fos*. The study also shows that in the HDAC2 OE mice there is decreased dendritic spine density and synapse number, while the HDAC knockout mice have an increased synapse number. Overall, this study shows that HDAC2 is a target for HDAC inhibitor-mediated memory enhancement.

As we discuss later, histone acetylation is merely a component of a larger combinatorial epigenetic code, but it has proved to be quite an important component. What is more impressive about the studies on histone acetylation is that they all seem to agree that there is a balance between hyperacetylated and hypoacetylated states of histones, where the hyperacetylated state facilitates memory and synaptic plasticity, and the hypoacetylated state impairs it (Fig. 13.1).

13.4 Other Histone Posttranslational Modifications

Aside from acetylation, another histone modification that has been linked to memory consolidation is histone methylation. A recent study demonstrates that trimethyl-H3K4 is upregulated in hippocampus 1 h after associative learning and returns to baseline levels at 24 h (Gupta et al. 2010). Mice deficient in Mll (H3K4 methyltransferase) have an associative memory deficit. Interestingly, an HDAC inhibitor (NaB) increased trimethyl-H3K4 and decreased dimethyl-H3K9. While H3K4 trimethylation is dependent on association of context and shock, H3K9 dimethylation occurs with context exposure alone. Mll complexed with Eed regulates neuronal plasticity, histone methylation, and HDAC recruitment (Kim et al. 2007). *Egr1* and *Bdnf* promoters show increased trimethyl-H3K4, altered DNA methylation, and methyl-cytosine-binding protein 2 (MeCP2) binding after contextual learning (Gupta et al. 2010). This work suggests that histone methylation results in increased DNA methylation that recruits MeCP2, paradoxically, to increase gene transcription. Interestingly, H3K9 dimethylation was also identified as the target of histone methyltransferase G9a, which has a role in cocaine-induced plasticity (Maze et al. 2010). Moreover, conditional deletion of G9a in forebrain neurons leads to reduced exploratory behavior and other behavioral abnormalities, suggesting a role for this histone methyltransferase in transcriptional homeostasis (Schaefer et al. 2009).

As alluded to previously, histone phosphorylation, another type of histone post-translational modification, may also have a role in memory consolidation. Although it is still unclear as to whether an increase in phosphorylation is required for memory consolidation, it has been shown that histone phosphorylation increases with novel context, more so in an associative fear paradigm (Chwang et al. 2006). This increase, like the increase in histone acetylation, is dependent on the MAPK pathway. Because the same pathways regulate both acetylation and phosphorylation, and because phosphorylation increases with experience, it suggests that phosphorylation of histones, along with acetylation, regulates gene expression and therefore memory consolidation. This is addressed by a study showing that protein phosphatase 1 (PP1) is able to directly recruit epigenetic machinery, namely HDAC1 and histone demethylase JMJD2A to target genes (Koshibu et al. 2010). Inhibition of PP1 results in increased histone phosphorylation, methylation, and acetylation. Moreover, inhibition of PP1 results in enhanced long-term object recognition memory, as well as long-term spatial memory. This study suggests that histone deacetylases, demethylases, and phosphatases exist in a complex that works in concert to silence gene expression. Conversely, relief of this inhibition results in addition of these posttranslational marks to histones: acetylation, phosphorylation, and methylation.

13.5 Histone Variants

Gross changes in histone variant composition of the nucleosome in neurons occur mainly throughout development from Day 3 (E19) to Day 30 (P30). Nevertheless, compositions of H2A.1 and H2A.2, as well as H3.2 and H3.3, change with aging, where H2A.1 and H3.2 decrease with age, and H2A.2 and H3.3 increase with age (Pina and Suau 1987).

Local changes in histone variants are thought to be associated with active promoter and other regulatory regions (Jin et al. 2009). Specifically nucleosomes containing variants H3.3 and H2A.Z are enriched in so-called nucleosome-free regions of active promoters, enhancers, and insulator regions. This report hypothesizes that the H3.3- and H2A.Z-containing nucleosomes are less stable than those containing the standard variants and therefore allow for dissociation from DNA, making the DNA sequence accessible to transcription factors. Although purely speculative, since there are no reported studies to confirm, it can be postulated that upon experience there is an exchange of histone variant composition. This would allow an enrichment of H3.3 and H2A.Z in active regions, leading to increased transcription and changes in gene expression that would ultimately affect behavior.

13.6 DNA Methylation

Many of the histone modifications described that result from learning are transient and do not explain persistent changes in gene expression, as they typically return to baseline levels before memory retrieval. Another epigenetic mark, DNA methylation, which occurs in cytosine residues, is considered more stable. DNA methylation has a demonstrated role in development and is thought to be static in nondividing, postmitotic, terminally differentiated cells. DNA methylation occurs only in cytosines that are followed by a guanine; this dinucleotide is abbreviated as CpG, where the p represents the phosphate group that covalently links the two nucleotides on the same strand. This nomenclature differentiates it from the CG base pair where each nucleotide is on opposite strands and bound primarily by noncovalent hydrogen bonds. The opposite strand of the CpG dinucleotide does, however, has a complementary CpG, which can also be methylated. CpG dinucleotides are disproportionately rare but cluster in regions in and around genes called CpG islands.

Because it was thought that DNA methyltransferases (DNMTs) do not have a role in postmitotic cells, they were not thought to be expressed in these cell populations. However, reports have shown that DNMTs are indeed highly expressed in neurons (Goto et al. 1994). Even after this report, it was unclear what the role of DNMTs was in neurons. It was speculated that these enzymes might have a role in DNA repair or neurodegeneration (Brooks et al. 1996; Endres et al. 2000). It should be noted that DNMTs are classified into two types: maintenance DNMTs, such as DNMT1, which methylate hemimethylated DNA – typically during DNA replication, and de novo DNMTs, such as DNMT3A and DNMT3B, which methylate DNA where neither strand is methylated.

A seminal study by Levenson et al. (2006) shows a role for DNMTs in plasticity-related gene regulation. This study relies on pharmacological DNMT inhibition, which decreases DNA methylation of plasticity-related gene *Reelin*, suggesting that this gene is actively methylated. Importantly, the DNMT inhibition has region-specific effects, as it increases unmethylated DNA in one CpG island of the *Bdnf* promoter I, but has no change in another CpG island of the same promoter. The study goes on to show that activation of the protein kinase C (PKC) pathway also decreases DNA methylation of the *Reelin* promoter and increases mRNA expression of the *Dnmt3a* gene, but not *Dnmt1*. These data, together with the standing notion that DNA methylation is inhibitory, suggest that activity that leads to PKC activation leads to *Reelin* expression through decreased DNA methylation, and at the same time *Dnmt3a* expression is increased creating a negative feedback loop. However, DNMT inhibition blocks PKC-induced histone H3 acetylation, suggesting that DNA methylation recruits histone acetyltransferases, and therefore leads to transcriptional activation, whereas DNA methylation is canonically linked to transcriptional repression. This study also shows that blocking DNA methylation blocks L-LTP, which is also paradoxical, because L-LTP is associated with increased gene expression.

A follow-up study by the same research group (Miller and Sweatt 2007) looked at the role of methylation in memory formation. The mRNA expression of both *Dnmt3a* and *Dnmt3b* is increased after a contextual fear conditioning paradigm, even after subtracting context alone exposure. An interesting finding is that they are able to substantially and significantly impair long-term associative memory using DNMT inhibitors immediately after training, and that this impairment is transient. Animals are retrained without DNMT inhibitors after testing, and on the second day of testing they perform as well as controls perform on the first day of testing. This is a remarkable finding that shows the plasticity of DNA methylation, while it is widely considered to be a static mark. As stated earlier, *Reelin* gene methylation decreases with PKC activity (Levenson et al. 2006). Other genes whose methylation has been shown to be regulated are *PP1* (Miller and Sweatt 2007), *Bdnf* (Lubin et al. 2008), and *Arc* (Penner et al. 2010). *Bdnf* methylation, like *Reelin*, decreases with experience – contextual fear training, in this case – which results in higher *Bdnf* mRNA (Lubin et al. 2008). *PP1* methylation increases with experience, which results in lower *PP1* mRNA (Miller and Sweatt 2007). *Arc* is differentially methylated in promoter and intragenic regions, and this pattern is reversed from the CA1 neurons to the DG neurons of the hippocampus. Upon novel context exploration, *Arc* promoter methylation is decreased in the CA1 region, but increased in the DG region. However, in both hippocampal regions *Arc* mRNA increases with exploration (Penner et al. 2010).

As with the case of the *Hdac2* knockout recapitulating the phenotypes of HDAC pharmacological inhibition, Feng et al. (2010) show that a conditional forebrain deletion of both *Dnmt1* and *Dnmt3a* genes recapitulates the effects of pharmacological inhibitors of these enzymes in LTP, and memory. The conditional double knockout shows grossly normal synaptic properties, although it has a reduced hippocampal volume. These mutant mice show an impairment in LTP $(2 \times 100$ Hz, 20 s interval) and an enhancement in long-term depression (LTD). The mice also show deficits in spatial learning, long-term spatial memory, and in long-term contextual fear memory. Not surprisingly, overall DNA methylation levels are reduced in the conditional double knockout. Also, DNA methylation at a gene-specific level was also found to be decreased, with a concomitant increase in gene expression, as is the case for *Stat1*. Together with the previous studies looking at pharmacological inhibition of DNMTs, this study demonstrates the importance of regulated gene methylation in activity-dependent gene expression that leads to synaptic plasticity and memory. However, the findings are contradictory to the notion that inhibition of DNA methylation, by virtue of an overall increase in transcription, would result in memory and plasticity enhancements, when in fact they are impairments.

Until recently, the identity of an active neuronal DNA demethylase was not known. *Gadd45b* is a gene that is induced in the brain in response to electroconvulsive treatment (Ploski et al. 2006), and it has had a known role in DNA damage growth arrest. Ma et al. (2009) show that neural activity induces *Gadd45b* expression in the mature hippocampus. Gadd45b was shown to be required for electroconvulsive therapy-induced demethylation of *Bdnf* promoter IX and *Fgf-1*. Furthermore, Gadd45b was found to associate with these gene regions, suggesting that it may itself act as a demethylase. Additionally, Gadd45b is required for activity-dependent adult neurogenesis, possibly through demethylation. Because no global demethylation is detected, it is postulated that Gadd45b is recruited to specific loci. Further studies on the role of Gadd45b are needed to elucidate its role in activity-dependent plasticity and memory.

Most of the studies on DNA methylation have focused on the hippocampus, and relatively transient changes in methylation status. Memory consolidation, however, may necessitate more permanent modes of memory storage. One mechanism of long-term memory storage that we discussed earlier is system consolidation, which involves the reorganization of information in brain circuitries. The most prominent example being the storage of declarative memory consolidated in the hippocampus, reorganized into the cortex. Empirical evidence of hippocampal lesions that result in anterograde amnesia (inability to form new memories) but have no effect on retrograde amnesia, supports this idea. The term for this type of memory that goes beyond days and into weeks and years is remote memory, and it is tightly associated with the cortex. Methylation, as a relatively stable epigenetic mark, is a good candidate to effect long-lasting changes in gene expression in cortical neurons. Miller et al. (2010) show that indeed gene-specific hypermethylation is induced in cortical neurons of rats, following a single, hippocampus-dependent associative learning experience. They go on to show that remote memory can be disrupted by intracortical DNMT inhibition 1 month after the learning experience.

Unlike histone acetylation, but similar to electroconvulsive treatment (ECT), DNA methylation remains somewhat of a paradox. Blocking DNMTs results in less methylation, which leads to broad gene activation and therefore would logically be associated with facilitating plasticity and memory. However, we see that DNMT inhibition, like ECT, leads to memory impairment (Fig. 13.2). With DNMT inhibition, some genes are indeed activated: *Reelin*, *Bdnf*, and *Arc*, and some are not: *PP1*. Of course the genes that are activated are positively associated with plasticity, whereas PP1 has been shown to lead to gene repression, leaving the paradox in place. One explanation for this paradox is that DNA hypomethylation is sufficient for broad transcriptional activation, in the same manner as ECT, whereas histone hyperacetylation is permissive of transcription, but not sufficient, and the refinement necessary for transcription specificity, and therefore plasticity, is determined

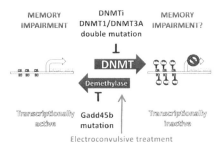

Fig. 13.2 *Role of DNA methylation in memory consolidation.* The balance of DNA methylation is regulated by DNA methyltransferases (DNMTs) and DNA demethylases. Unmethylated or hypomethylated DNA leads to active transcription, and hypermethylated DNA leads to transcriptional inactivation. DNMT inhibitors (DNMTi) and a conditional double knockout for DNMT1 and DNMT3A result in a hypomethylated state with increased transcription, which results in memory impairment. Gadd45b mediates DNA demethylation, and a Gadd45b conditional knockout presents increased methylation and decreased gene transcription. Electroconvulsive treatment demethylates DNA through Gadd45b

by other factors. ECT has indeed been shown to actively demethylate DNA through Gadd45b, as discussed earlier (Ma et al. 2009). It is possible that some gene targets not yet studied in the context of DNA methylation may also explain this discrepancy. Also, future studies of the role of Gadd45b in demethylation may also clarify some uncertainties.

13.7   Combinatorial Chromatin Code

The idea of a histone code for gene expression is not a new concept, as it precedes this explosion of epigenetics in neuroscience research. What neuroscientists are considering now is how the histone code, together with DNA methylation, and histone variants form a combinatorial chromatin code that is relevant to synaptic plasticity and memory consolidation (Table 13.1).

Many studies show an interdependence of these epigenetic marks: PP1, a phosphatase that recruits a histone deacetylase and a histone demethylase (Koshibu et al. 2010), histone methylation leading to changes in DNA methylation (Gupta et al. 2010), and DNA methylation leading to histone acetylation (Levenson et al. 2006; Miller et al. 2008). What remains a question is how the transient changes in histone posttranslational modifications and DNA methylation that are observed in response to activity lead to a lasting retention of information. Nevertheless, this interplay of epigenetic marks highlights the complexity of elucidating a code. What we can recognize is that there are key players in this code – dubbed *writers* and *erasers* by Borrelli et al. (2008). The writers are those enzymes that add epigenetic marks: HATs, DNMTs, histone methyltransferases, and kinases; and the erasers take away those marks: HDACs, demethylases, and phosphatases. Moreover, these marks must be able to be *read* or decoded – task that is

Table 13.1 Effect of pharmacological or genetic manipulations on memory consolidation

Manipulation or mouse model	Epigenetic mechanism	Study	Effect on long-term memory
HDAC inhibition	↑ Histone acetylation	Levenson et al. (2004)	Enhancement
$Creb\alpha\delta^{-/-}$	↓ Histone acetylation (through disruption of CBP interaction)	Bourtchuladze et al. (1994), Vecsey et al. (2007)	Impairment
Cbp KO	↓ Histone acetylation	Oike et al. (1999), Bourtchuladze et al. (2003)	Impairment
$Cbp^{+/-}$	↓ Histone acetylation	Alarcón et al. (2004)	Impairment
Cbp{HAT-}	↓ Histone acetylation	Korzus et al. (2004)	Impairment
CbpΔ1	↓ Histone acetylation	Wood et al. (2005)	Impairment
$Cbp^{kix/kix}$	↓ Histone acetylation	Wood et al. (2006)	Impairment
p300 Δ1	↓ Histone acetylation	Oliveira et al. (2007)	Impairment
$p300^{+/-}$	↓ Histone acetylation	Viosca et al. (2010)	No change (Impairment in relearning)
Pcaf KO	↓ Histone acetylation	Duclot et al. (2010)	Impairment (acquisition)
Hdac2 KO	↑ Histone acetylation	Guan et al. (2009)	Enhancement
Hdac1 OE	↓ Histone acetylation	Guan et al. (2009)	No change
Hdac2 OE	↓ Histone acetylation	Guan et al. (2009)	Impairment
Mll KO	↓ Histone methylation	Gupta et al. (2010)	Impairment
NIPP1	↑ Histone phosphorylation	Koshibu et al. (2010)	Enhancement
DNMT inhibition	↓ DNA methylation	Levenson et al. (2006), Miller and Sweatt (2007)	Impairment
Dnmt1/Dnmt3a KO	↓ DNA methylation	Feng et al. (2010)	Impairment
ECT	↓ DNA methylation (through Gadd45b)	Duncan (1949), Ma et al. (2009)	Impairment

Several mouse models and other manipulations in rodents have consistently demonstrated that epigenetic mechanisms are able to modulate memory consolidation. The table summarizes each manipulation, with its effect on epigenetic state, and its ultimate memory phenotype

performed through protein domains such as bromo and chromo domains that recognize these marks. The interplay of these marks comes in that many of the domains that *read* them are in writers and erasers themselves. HATs have bromo domains that recognize histone acetylation and therefore propagate this mark. HDACs are recruited by MeCP2, which recognizes methylated DNA. Ultimately, much of this code will be deciphered through high throughput proteomics and methyl-cytosine sequencing.

13.8 Higher Order Chromatin Structure

Recent evidence shows that CBP recruitment is not only in gene promoter regions, but also in enhancer regions, which play a more central role in multiple gene regulation (Kim et al. 2010). The presence of CBP in these regions, outside of promoters, prompts the question of the role of these enhancers in memory consolidation. When we think of gene regulation, our vision is somewhat limited by the depictions that we use. The nucleus is a very crowded space, and subnuclear chromosomal arrangements are important for the regulation of gene expression. Enhancer and insulator regions have special importance as they can modulate expression in this crowded space, with enhancers aiding in gene activation by bringing elements together, and insulators aid in separating elements and avoiding spurious gene activation. Chromosomal organizers, such as SATB1 (Cai et al. 2006), may well be the target of regulation in response to neuronal activity. DNA is held in large loops thanks to these organizers, and these loops have torsional strains if they are actively transcribed. So another level of regulation to consider is the role of topoisomerases, and alternative DNA structures, in gene regulation. Future studies will elucidate the role of these higher order structures in activity-dependent regulation of transcription.

13.9 Concluding Remarks

As stated in a review by Roth and Sweatt (2009), the field of epigenetics in neuroscience has created a paradigm shift in the locus of plasticity. Much attention had been given to the synapse and to synapse-specific regulation. Now we have compelling evidence for a role of the nucleus in modulating plasticity. These recent findings on regulation of plasticity at the level of the nucleus do not allow us to discard the concept of synapse-specific regulation. There are certainly different tiers of regulation where one nucleus with one genome is able to somehow orchestrate synapse-specific plastic changes. Epigenetic marks are able to explain persistent changes in gene expression, but they do not explain how those changes translate to the synapse. However, examples like BDNF expression give us an idea of how this can occur. *Bdnf* transcription is regulated by DNA methylation, histone methylation, and histone acetylation (Lubin et al. 2008; Gupta et al. 2010; He et al. 2010), and its mRNA once transcribed has another level of regulation: dendritic trafficking (reviewed in Lu 2003; Tongiorgi 2008). This is regulated by mRNA-binding proteins that can target the message to specific synapses and also by regulating local translation at those synapses. Lastly, there is a vast virtually uncharacterized collection of noncoding RNAs whose gene regulation would certainly also depend on the state of chromatin. These RNAs can modulate mRNA permanence and therefore provide another means for regulation that has not been fully incorporated into the big picture (Mercer et al. 2008). Overall, the regulation of the state of chromatin as part of neuronal plasticity is a burgeoning field, and specifically for memory, it has had a profound impact in our understanding of long-term information storage.

References

Abel T, Nguyen PV, Barad M, Deuel TAS, Kandel ER, Bourtchouladze R (1997) Genetic demonstration of a role for PKA in the late phase of LTP and in hippocampus-based long-term memory. Cell 88(5):615–626

Abraham WC, Mason SE, Demmer J, Williams JM, Richardson CL, Tate WP, Lawlor PA, Dragunow M (1993) Correlations between immediate early gene induction and the persistence of long-term potentiation. Neuroscience 56(3):717–727

Agranoff BW, Davis RE, Brink JJ (1966) Chemical studies on memory fixation in goldfish. Brain Res 1(3):303–309

Alarcón JM, Malleret G, Touzani K, Vronskaya S, Ishii S, Kandel ER, Barco A (2004) Chromatin acetylation, memory, and LTP are impaired in CBP+/− mice: a model for the cognitive deficit in rubinstein-taybi syndrome and its amelioration. Neuron 42(6):947–959

Barondes SH, Cohen HD (1967) Comparative effects of cycloheximide and puromycin on cerebral protein synthesis and consolidation of memory in mice. Brain Res 4(1):44–51

Bliss TV, Collingridge GL (1993) A synaptic model of memory: long-term potentiation in the hippocampus. Nature 361(6407):31–39

Borrelli E, Nestler EJ, Allis CD, Sassone-Corsi P (2008) Decoding the epigenetic language of neuronal plasticity. Neuron 60(6):961–974

Bourtchuladze R, Frenguelli B, Blendy J, Cioffi D, Schutz G, Silva AJ (1994) Deficient long-term memory in mice with a targeted mutation of the cAMP-responsive element-binding protein. Cell 79(1):59–68

Bourtchuladze R, Lidge R, Catapano R, Stanley J, Gossweiler S, Romashko D, Scott R, Tully T (2003) A mouse model of rubinstein-taybi syndrome: defective long-term memory is ameliorated by inhibitors of phosphodiesterase 4. Proc Natl Acad Sci USA 100(18):10518–10522

Brooks P, Marietta C, Goldman D (1996) DNA mismatch repair and DNA methylation in adult brain neurons. J Neurosci 16(3):939–945

Cai S, Lee CC, Kohwi-Shigematsu T (2006) SATB1 packages densely looped, transcriptionally active chromatin for coordinated expression of cytokine genes. Nat Genet 38(11):1278–1288

Carew TJ (1996) Molecular enhancement of memory formation. Neuron 16(1):5–8

Chwang WB, O'Riordan KJ, Levenson JM, Sweatt JD (2006) ERK/MAPK regulates hippocampal histone phosphorylation following contextual fear conditioning. Learn Mem 13(3):322–328

Duclot F, Jacquet C, Gongora C, Maurice T (2010) Alteration of working memory but not in anxiety or stress response in p300/CBP associated factor (PCAF) histone acetylase knockout mice bred on a C57BL/6 background. Neurosci Lett 475(3):179–183

Dudai Y (2004) The neurobiology of consolidations, or, how stable is the engram? Annu Rev Psychol 55:51–86

Duncan CP (1949) The retroactive effect of electroshock on learning. J Comp Physiol Psychol 42(1):32–44

Endres M, Meisel A, Biniszkiewicz D, Namura S, Prass K, Ruscher K, Lipski A, Jaenisch R, Moskowitz MA, Dirnagl U (2000) DNA methyltransferase contributes to delayed ischemic brain injury. J Neurosci 20(9):3175–3181

Feng J, Zhou Y, Campbell SL, Le T, Li E, Sweatt JD, Silva AJ, Fan G (2010) Dnmt1 and Dnmt3a maintain DNA methylation and regulate synaptic function in adult forebrain neurons. Nat Neurosci 13(4):423–430

Fischer A, Sananbenesi F, Wang X, Dobbin M, Tsai LH (2007) Recovery of learning and memory is associated with chromatin remodelling. Nature 447(7141):178–182

Frey U, Morris RG (1997) Synaptic tagging and long-term potentiation. Nature 385(6616):533–536

Frey U, Krug M, Reymann KG, Matthies H (1988) Anisomycin, an inhibitor of protein synthesis, blocks late phases of LTP phenomena in the hippocampal CA1 region in vitro. Brain Res 452(1–2):57–65

Frey U, Huang YY, Kandel ER (1993) Effects of cAMP simulate a late stage of LTP in hippocampal CA1 neurons. Science 260(5114):1661–1664

Frey U, Muller M, Kuhl D (1996) A different form of long-lasting potentiation revealed in tissue plasminogen activator mutant mice. J Neurosci 16(6):2057–2063

Gold PE (2006) The many faces of amnesia. Learn Mem 13(5):506–514

Goto K, Numata M, Komura JI, Ono T, Bestor TH, Kondo H (1994) Expression of DNA methyltransferase gene in mature and immature neurons as well as proliferating cells in mice. Differentiation 56(1–2):39–44

Guan Z, Giustetto M, Lomvardas S, Kim JH, Miniaci MC, Schwartz JH, Thanos D, Kandel ER (2002) Integration of long-term-memory-related synaptic plasticity involves bidirectional regulation of gene expression and chromatin structure. Cell 111(4):483–493

Guan JS, Haggarty SJ, Giacometti E, Dannenberg JH, Joseph N, Gao J, Nieland TJ, Zhou Y, Wang X, Mazitschek R et al (2009) HDAC2 negatively regulates memory formation and synaptic plasticity. Nature 459(7243):55–60

Gupta S, Kim SY, Artis S, Molfese DL, Schumacher A, Sweatt JD, Paylor RE, Lubin FD (2010) Histone methylation regulates memory formation. J Neurosci 30(10):3589–3599

He DY, Neasta J, Ron D (2010) Epigenetic regulation of BDNF expression via the scaffolding protein RACK1. J Biol Chem 285(25):19043–19050

Huang YY, Kandel ER (1994) Recruitment of long-lasting and protein kinase A-dependent long-term potentiation in the CA1 region of hippocampus requires repeated tetanization. Learn Mem 1(1):74–82

Huang YY, Kandel ER (1995) D1/D5 receptor agonists induce a protein synthesis-dependent late potentiation in the CA1 region of the hippocampus. Proc Natl Acad Sci USA 92(7):2446–2450

Huang YY, Nguyen PV, Abel T, Kandel ER (1996) Long-lasting forms of synaptic potentiation in the mammalian hippocampus. Learn Mem 3(2–3):74–85

Igaz LM, Vianna MR, Medina JH, Izquierdo I (2002) Two time periods of hippocampal mRNA synthesis are required for memory consolidation of fear-motivated learning. J Neurosci 22(15): 6781–6789

Jin C, Zang C, Wei G, Cui K, Peng W, Zhao K, Felsenfeld G (2009) H3.3/H2A.Z double variant-containing nucleosomes mark 'nucleosome-free regions' of active promoters and other regulatory regions. Nat Genet 41(8):941–945

Josselyn SA, Shi C, Carlezon WA Jr, Neve RL, Nestler EJ, Davis M (2001) Long-term memory is facilitated by cAMP response element-binding protein overexpression in the amygdala. J Neurosci 21(7):2404–2412

Kim SY, Levenson JM, Korsmeyer S, Sweatt JD, Schumacher A (2007) Developmental regulation of eed complex composition governs a switch in global histone modification in brain. J Biol Chem 282(13):9962–9972

Kim TK, Hemberg M, Gray JM, Costa AM, Bear DM, Wu J, Harmin DA, Laptewicz M, Barbara-Haley K, Kuersten S et al (2010) Widespread transcription at neuronal activity-regulated enhancers. Nature 465(7295):182–187

Korzus E, Rosenfeld MG, Mayford M (2004) CBP histone acetyltransferase activity is a critical component of memory consolidation. Neuron 42(6):961–972

Koshibu K, Graff J, Jouvenceau A, Dutar P, Mansuy IM (2010) Protein phosphatase 1-dependent transcriptional programs for long-term memory and plasticity. Learn Mem 17(7):355–363

Levenson JM, O'Riordan KJ, Brown KD, Trinh MA, Molfese DL, Sweatt JD (2004) Regulation of histone acetylation during memory formation in the hippocampus. J Biol Chem 279(39): 40545–40559

Levenson JM, Roth TL, Lubin FD, Miller CA, Huang IC, Desai P, Malone LM, Sweatt JD (2006) Evidence that DNA (cytosine-5) methyltransferase regulates synaptic plasticity in the hippocampus. J Biol Chem 281(23):15763–15773

Lu B (2003) BDNF and activity-dependent synaptic modulation. Learn Mem 10(2):86–98

Lubin FD, Roth TL, Sweatt JD (2008) Epigenetic regulation of BDNF gene transcription in the consolidation of fear memory. J Neurosci 28(42):10576–10586

Ma DK, Jang MH, Guo JU, Kitabatake Y, Chang ML, Pow-Anpongkul N, Flavell RA, Lu B, Ming GL, Song H (2009) Neuronal activity-induced Gadd45b promotes epigenetic DNA demethylation and adult neurogenesis. Science 323(5917):1074–1077

Martin SJ, Grimwood PD, Morris RG (2000) Synaptic plasticity and memory: an evaluation of the hypothesis. Annu Rev Neurosci 23:649–711

Maze I, Covington HE 3rd, Dietz DM, LaPlant Q, Renthal W, Russo SJ, Mechanic M, Mouzon E, Neve RL, Haggarty SJ et al (2010) Essential role of the histone methyltransferase G9a in cocaine-induced plasticity. Science 327(5962):213–216

Mercer TR, Dinger ME, Mariani J, Kosik KS, Mehler MF, Mattick JS (2008) Noncoding RNAs in long-term memory formation. Neuroscientist 14(5):434–445

Miller CA, Sweatt JD (2007) Covalent modification of DNA regulates memory formation. Neuron 53(6):857–869

Miller CA, Campbell SL, Sweatt JD (2008) DNA methylation and histone acetylation work in concert to regulate memory formation and synaptic plasticity. Neurobiol Learn Mem 89(4):599–603

Miller CA, Gavin CF, White JA, Parrish RR, Honasoge A, Yancey CR, Rivera IM, Rubio MD, Rumbaugh G, Sweatt JD (2010) Cortical DNA methylation maintains remote memory. Nat Neurosci 13(6):664–666

Morgan JI, Cohen DR, Hempstead JL, Curran T (1987) Mapping patterns of c-fos expression in the central nervous system after seizure. Science 237(4811):192–197

Neale JH, Klinger PD, Agranoff BW (1973) Camptothecin blocks memory of conditioned avoidance in the goldfish. Science 179(79):1243–1246

Neves G, Cooke SF, Bliss TV (2008) Synaptic plasticity, memory and the hippocampus: a neural network approach to causality. Nat Rev Neurosci 9(1):65–75

Nguyen PV, Kandel ER (1997) Brief theta-burst stimulation induces a transcription-dependent late phase of LTP requiring cAMP in area CA1 of the mouse hippocampus. Learn Mem 4(2):230–243

Nguyen PV, Woo NH (2003) Regulation of hippocampal synaptic plasticity by cyclic AMP-dependent protein kinases. Prog Neurobiol 71(6):401–437

Nguyen PV, Abel T, Kandel ER (1994) Requirement of a critical period of transcription for induction of a late phase of LTP. Science 265(5175):1104–1107

Oike Y, Hata A, Mamiya T, Kaname T, Noda Y, Suzuki M, Yasue H, Nabeshima T, Araki K, Yamamura K (1999) Truncated CBP protein leads to classical rubinstein-taybi syndrome phenotypes in mice: Implications for a dominant-negative mechanism. Hum Mol Genet 8(3):387–396

Oliveira AM, Wood MA, McDonough CB, Abel T (2007) Transgenic mice expressing an inhibitory truncated form of p300 exhibit long-term memory deficits. Learn Mem 14(9):564–572

Penner MR, Roth TL, Chawla MK, Hoang LT, Roth ED, Lubin FD, Sweatt JD, Worley PF, Barnes CA (2010) Age-related changes in arc transcription and DNA methylation within the hippocampus. Neurobiol Aging (in press)

Peterson CL, Laniel MA (2004) Histones and histone modifications. Curr Biol 14(14):R546–R551

Petrij F, Giles RH, Dauwerse HG, Saris JJ, Hennekam RC, Masuno M, Tommerup N, van Ommen GJ, Goodman RH, Peters DJ (1995) Rubinstein-taybi syndrome caused by mutations in the transcriptional co-activator CBP. Nature 376(6538):348–351

Pina B, Suau P (1987) Changes in histones H2A and H3 variant composition in differentiating and mature rat brain cortical neurons. Dev Biol 123(1):51–58

Placek K, Coffre M, Maiella S, Bianchi E, Rogge L (2009) Genetic and epigenetic networks controlling T helper 1 cell differentiation. Immunology 127(2):155–162

Ploski JE, Newton SS, Duman RS (2006) Electroconvulsive seizure-induced gene expression profile of the hippocampus dentate gyrus granule cell layer. J Neurochem 99(4):1122–1132

Roelfsema JH, White SJ, Ariyurek Y, Bartholdi D, Niedrist D, Papadia F, Bacino CA, den Dunnen JT, van Ommen GJ, Breuning MH et al (2005) Genetic heterogeneity in rubinstein-taybi syndrome: mutations in both the CBP and EP300 genes cause disease. Am J Hum Genet 76(4):572–580

Roth TL, Sweatt JD (2009) Regulation of chromatin structure in memory formation. Curr Opin Neurobiol 19(3):336–342

Rugg MD (1997) Cognitive neuroscience, vol 1. MIT, Cambridge, MA

Saffen DW, Cole AJ, Worley PF, Christy BA, Ryder K, Baraban JM (1988) Convulsant-induced increase in transcription factor messenger RNAs in rat brain. Proc Natl Acad Sci USA 85(20):7795–7799

Schaefer A, Sampath SC, Intrator A, Min A, Gertler TS, Surmeier DJ, Tarakhovsky A, Greengard P (2009) Control of cognition and adaptive behavior by the GLP/G9a epigenetic suppressor complex. Neuron 64(5):678–691

Squire LR, Barondes SH (1970) Actinomycin-D: effects on memory at different times after training. Nature 225(5233):649–650

Stefanko DP, Barrett RM, Ly AR, Reolon GK, Wood MA (2009) Modulation of long-term memory for object recognition via HDAC inhibition. Proc Natl Acad Sci USA 106(23): 9447–9452

Strahl BD, Allis CD (2000) The language of covalent histone modifications. Nature 403(6765): 41–45

Tanaka Y, Naruse I, Maekawa T, Masuya H, Shiroishi T, Ishii S (1997) Abnormal skeletal patterning in embryos lacking a single cbp allele: a partial similarity with rubinstein-taybi syndrome. Proc Natl Acad Sci USA 94(19):10215–10220

Tanaka Y, Naruse I, Hongo T, Xu M, Nakahata T, Maekawa T, Ishii S (2000) Extensive brain hemorrhage and embryonic lethality in a mouse null mutant of CREB-binding protein. Mech Dev 95(1–2):133–145

Tongiorgi E (2008) Activity-dependent expression of brain-derived neurotrophic factor in dendrites: facts and open questions. Neurosci Res 61(4):335–346

Vecsey CG, Hawk JD, Lattal KM, Stein JM, Fabian SA, Attner MA, Cabrera SM, McDonough CB, Brindle PK, Abel T et al (2007) Histone deacetylase inhibitors enhance memory and synaptic plasticity via CREB:CBP-dependent transcriptional activation. J Neurosci 27(23): 6128–6140

Viosca J, Lopez-Atalaya JP, Olivares R, Eckner R, Barco A (2010) Syndromic features and mild cognitive impairment in mice with genetic reduction on p300 activity: Differential contribution of p300 and CBP to rubinstein-taybi syndrome etiology. Neurobiol Dis 37(1):186–194

Wood MA, Kaplan MP, Park A, Blanchard EJ, Oliveira AM, Lombardi TL, Abel T (2005) Transgenic mice expressing a truncated form of CREB-binding protein (CBP) exhibit deficits in hippocampal synaptic plasticity and memory storage. Learn Mem 12(2):111–119

Wood MA, Attner MA, Oliveira AM, Brindle PK, Abel T (2006) A transcription factor-binding domain of the coactivator CBP is essential for long-term memory and the expression of specific target genes. Learn Mem 13(5):609–617

Chapter 14
Epigenetic Mechanisms in Memory Formation

Johannes M.H.M. Reul, Andrew Collins, and María Gutièrrez-Mecinas

Abstract Formation of memories of events in our lives is one of the principal functions of the brain. We make particularly strong memories of events with an emotional impact. Glucocorticoid hormones, secreted in response to the stressful event, have been identified as playing an important role in the acquisition and consolidation of such memories. In recent years, significant advances have been made in the identification of the signaling and epigenomic mechanisms in the hippocampus underlying memory formation. Evidence has been accumulating for a principal role of the NMDA–ERK MAPK signaling pathway and its downstream effector molecules MSK1 and Elk-1. Activation of this signaling cascade results in the phosphorylation, acetylation, and possibly methylation of histone molecules within the chromatin structure and in the induction of immediate-early (e.g., c-Fos) and many other genes required for the molecular and cellular adaptation of the affected neurons. Glucocorticoid hormones via the glucocorticoid receptor (GR) enhance memory formation through facilitation of ERK MAPK signaling to the chromatin leading to the enhancement of epigenomic mechanisms and cognitive performance. Thus, formation of strong memories of emotional events involves an interaction between the GR and the NMDA/ERK/MSK1 and Elk-1 signaling pathways resulting in optimization of epigenomic changes in hippocampal neurons to allow the induction of required neuroplasticity changes.

Keywords Acetylation · Behavior · c-fos · Chromatin · Cognition · Elk-1 · ERK · Glucocorticoid · Histone · Learning and memory · MAPK · MSK · NMDA · Phosphorylation · Resilience · Stress

J.M.H.M. Reul (✉), A. Collins, and M. Gutièrrez-Mecinas
Henry Wellcome Laboratories for Integrative Neuroscience and Endocrinology, University of Bristol, Dorothy Hodgkin Building, Whitson Street, Bristol BS1 3NY, UK
e-mail: Hans.Reul@bristol.ac.uk

A. Petronis and J. Mill (eds.), *Brain, Behavior and Epigenetics*,
Epigenetics and Human Health, DOI 10.1007/978-3-642-17426-1_14,
© Springer-Verlag Berlin Heidelberg 2011

One of the principal functions of the brain is the formation of memories of experienced events. Particularly, memories of emotional events are strong and sometimes lasting for life. Possibly, importance is given to such memories because they help the organism to adapt and respond better if similar events would reoccur in the future. Therefore, mostly memories are beneficial for survival, health, and well-being. However, disruptions in this cognitive process may play a role in stress-related psychiatric disorders such as major depression and posttraumatic stress disorder (PTSD).

The neurobiological mechanisms underlying learning and memory have been mostly studied in rodents such as rats and mice. Well-known learning and memory paradigms include the Morris water maze, the radial maze and the forced swim test. In these tests the animal learns to choose the most appropriate behavioral response to enhance the chance of survival [finding the platform in the Morris water maze (Morris 1984); conservation of energy by floating in the forced swim test (Bilang-Bleuel et al. 2005; De Pablo et al. 1989; Korte 2001; West 1990)] and reward (food in the radial maze)]. Clearly, many of these behavioral tests involve aversive and anxiogenic conditions (e.g., novelty, fear, and sleep deprivation), and stress hormones such as glucocorticoid hormones (corticosterone in rats and mice) are secreted during the learning sessions (Bilang-Bleuel et al. 2005; Droste et al. 2008; Peñalva et al. 2003). Thus, secretion of glucocorticoids and other stress hormones (e.g., adrenalin and noradrenalin) is inherent to most behavioral tests in rodents.

Notably, the stress response and the learning and memory processes have in the past been separately described, but it may be argued that they actually constitute highly integrated biological mechanisms. It has been shown that the released glucocorticoid hormones strongly facilitate the formation of memories of the experienced event. The memory-enhancing effects of glucocorticoid hormones have been described in many behavioral tests such as Morris water maze behavior (Oitzl and De Kloet 1992), fear conditioning (Roozendaal et al. 2006), the forced swim test (Bilang-Bleuel et al. 2005; De Kloet et al. 1988; Korte 2001; Korte et al. 1996) and others (Beylin and Shors 2003; Smeets et al. 2009). Although these facilitatory actions of glucocorticoids have been known for many years, the question of how glucocorticoids act on learning and memory processes has remained unanswered. However, recent findings based on signaling and epigenomic studies have substantially increased our insight into the underlying mechanisms of glucocorticoid action on learning and memory.

14.1   Gene Transcription-Related Epigenetic Mechanisms

It is now well established that gene transcription is largely controlled by epigenetic mechanisms at the chromatin level. Epigenetic mechanisms affecting the chromatin structure and function include the covalent modifications of histone molecules and the methylation of DNA. Here we will focus on the role of histone modifications. Histone proteins such as histone H3 have evolutionary highly conserved N-terminal tails which stand out from the nucleosome and can be subjected to posttranslational modifications such as acetylation, phosphorylation, methylation and others (Strahl and Allis 2000).

These histone modifications, and more importantly the combination of various histone modifications, determine the functional state of the chromatin. The acetylation of Lysine amino acids in histone H3 and H4 is seen in open, transcriptionally active chromatin (Strahl and Allis 2000). Some immediate-early genes such as *c-fos* and *c-jun* (Clayton et al. 2000), and other genes [e.g., matrix metalloprotease-1 (MMP-1) (Martens et al. 2003)] require the phosphorylation of Serine-10 (S10p) combined with the acetylation of Lysine-14 (K14ac) for induction of gene expression. The specific combination of histone H3 modification may be required for the recruitment of specific nuclear factors to the chromatin to allow induction of transcription. The methylation of histone H3 tails is associated with transcriptional activation as well as gene silencing. Methylation of the H3K4 mark results in gene activation whereas H3K9 and H3K27 methylation leads to gene silencing (Akbarian and Huang 2008). The combination of the H3K9 methylation and H3S10 phosphorylation marks is associated with gene silencing (Sabbattini et al. 2007). As the combinatorial H3S10p-K14ac marks are thought to play a role in the local opening of condensed, inactive chromatin these histone modifications may be crucial for the transcriptional activation of dormant genes (Cheung et al. 2000; Clayton et al. 2000). However, whether the H3S10p-K14ac marks are required for any gene located in condensed, heterochromatin seems questionable. Even the necessity of these histone marks for the induction of *c-fos* may depend on the cell type or tissue under investigation (see below).

14.2 Psychologically Salient Events Evoke Gene Transcription-Related Histone Modifications in the Brain

It was a serendipitous finding around the turn of the millennium when we found the H3S10p mark in neurons of the rat and mouse brain (Bilang-Bleuel et al. 2000). Using an antibody against H3S10p (also recognizing H3S10p acetylated at Lys14, i. e. H3S10p-K14ac [(Chandramohan et al. 2007), Chandramohan and Reul, unpublished observations] neurons were found showing a speckled nuclear immunostaining pattern. These neurons were mainly found in the dentate gyrus of the hippocampus and there were only few neurons scattered in the amygdala, neocortex and striatum (Bilang-Bleuel et al. 2005; Chandramohan et al. 2007). Our studies indicated that histone H3 if phosphorylated at Ser10 will be acetylated at Lys14, thus forming H3S10p-K14ac (Chandramohan et al. 2007). As we were interested in how animals adapt to and learn from psychologically stressful events we studied whether such challenges would affect the number of neurons expressing H3S10p-K14ac. Challenging rats or mice with forced swimming, a predator or a novel environment, led to a substantial rise in the number of H3S10p-K14ac-positive neurons specifically in the dentate gyrus (Bilang-Bleuel et al. 2005; Chandramohan et al. 2007, 2008). The increase peaked at 1–2 h after the challenge and returned to baseline levels after approximately 4 h (Chandramohan et al. 2007, 2008). Thus, the response was relatively fast and transient showing that epigenetic changes underlying gene expression can be highly dynamic. Morris water maze learning [Chandramohan and Reul, unpublished observations; (Chwang et al. 2007)] and fear conditioning [Chandramohan Y, Sacchetti B, Strata P, and Reul JMHM, unpublished observations; (Chwang et al. 2007)] also resulted in increases in the number of H3S10p-K14ac-expressing neurons in the dentate gyrus. The question arose why the combinatorial H3S10p-K14ac mark in dentate neurons responded similarly to such different stimuli? The response pattern of H3S10p-K14ac-positive neurons in the dentate gyrus indeed does not give clues about the challenge the animal has undergone; see for instance references (Bilang-Bleuel et al. 2005; Chandramohan et al. 2007, 2008). These findings nonetheless correspond with the role of the dentate gyrus in learning and memory processes.

14.3   Sparse Epigenetic Responses in the Dentate Gyrus

The dentate gyrus represents a part of the hippocampus which is one of the principal structures of the limbic system. It plays a major role in learning and memory processes. As the main neuroanatomical gate of the hippocampus, the dentate gyrus receives inputs from the entorhinal cortex, the principal neocortical region that feeds integrated sensory and other information into the limbic system (Witter 2007). After processing, the dentate neurons pass this information on to pyramidal neurons in the other hippocampal cell fields (mainly CA3) where the information is integrated with other, stimulus-specific information for further processing to yield appropriate physiological and behavioral responses and, ultimately, memory formation of the event (Rolls and Kesner 2006; Treves and Rolls 1994). Thus, when animals are challenged, as a result of the sensory information flow, granule neurons in the dentate gyrus are activated. GABAergic interneurons exert a high tonic inhibitory control on dentate granule neurons and therefore only relatively few granule cells ($<5\%$) become activated. Such sparse activation occurs irrespective of the stimulus (e.g., novelty, forced swimming, Morris water maze learning; in contrast, strong depolarizing agents, such as kainate, or electroconvulsive shocks evoke an all-out activation) (Bilang-Bleuel et al. 2005; Chandramohan et al. 2007, 2008; Chawla et al. 2005; Rolls and Kesner 2006). Indeed, recently we showed that GABA is an important modulator of baseline and novelty-evoked H3S10p-K14ac and c-Fos in dentate neurons (Papadopoulos et al. 2008) (see below). Thus, the neuronal activation pattern in the dentate gyrus seems to be a reflection of the degree to which prominence is given to afferent sensory stimuli. It appears that the enhanced H3S10p-K14ac expression in dentate granule neurons after such stimuli is part of the sparse activation response of this hippocampal region.

Despite the abundance of evidence favoring a role of the H3S10p-K14ac marks in gene activation, until now surprisingly few genes have been identified whose expression depends on these epigenetic marks. Mahadevan et al. demonstrated in in vitro cell culture experiments that phosphoacetylated histone H3 is associated with the induction of the immediate-early genes *c-fos* and *c-jun* (Clayton et al. 2000). Later studies of

Martens and colleagues showed that H3S10p is involved in MMP-1 induction (Martens et al. 2003). We showed for the first time in vivo that the H3S10p-K14ac marks in rat and mouse dentate granule neurons are associated with c-Fos induction (Chandramohan et al. 2007, 2008; Gutierrez-Mecinas et al. 2009). A first indication was founded on the strictly parallel changes in H3S10p-K14ac-positive and c-Fos-positive neurons after various experimental manipulations and the colocalization of the epigenetic mark and gene product in the same dentate neurons based on immunofluorescence analyses (Chandramohan et al. 2007, 2008). Recently, using chromatin immunoprecipitation (ChIP) and qPCR we showed that forced swimming indeed evoked the combinatorial histone marks in the *c-fos* promoter region in dentate neurons (Gutierrez-Mecinas et al. 2009). Moreover, forced swimming also resulted in histone H4 hyperacetylation, but not H3 hyperacetylation, in this promoter (Gutierrez-Mecinas et al. 2009). A similar pattern of histone modification marks has been reported for the hippocampal *c-fos* promoter after electroconvulsive shock treatment which is known to elicit a full-blown c-Fos induction in the hippocampus including the dentate gyrus (Tsankova et al. 2004). In contrast, the neocortex known as well to induce c-Fos after forced swimming (Bilang-Bleuel et al. 2002) presented a different pattern of epigenetic marks at the c-fos promoter. ChIP revealed hyperacetylation of H4 in the c-fos promoter after forced swimming but no changes in H3S10p-K14ac and acetylated H3 (Gutierrez-Mecinas et al. 2009). These observations confirm earlier findings that the rise in H3S10p-K14ac observed after psychological challenges such as forced swimming and novelty is exclusively occurring in the dentate gyrus and is not seen elsewhere in the brain (Bilang-Bleuel et al. 2005; Chandramohan et al. 2007, 2008). Thus, in different neuronal populations in the brain, expression of the same gene may be driven by epigenetically diverse mechanisms. Furthermore, in different neurons, epigenetic mechanisms controlling expression of the gene may be steered by distinct signaling pathways.

14.4 Signaling to the Chromatin Involves Integration of Extracellular and Intracellular Pathways

14.4.1 Involvement of the NMDA Receptor and Glucocorticoid Receptor

For survival, an organism needs to adapt to and learn from challenges imposed by its environment. In recent years a picture is emerging that cognitive processing of environmental challenges involves changes in epigenetic mechanisms and gene expression profiles in multiple populations of neurons. The environment impacts on these intranuclear events through a coordinated activation of extracellular (e.g., hormones and neurotransmitters) and intracellular signaling pathways. It is however still early days with regard to our understanding how epigenetic mechanisms are steered by signaling molecules. Recently we reported that the neurotransmitter glutamate and the glucocorticoid hormone corticosterone (acting through the

N-methyl-D-aspartate (NMDA) receptor and the glucocorticoid receptor (GR), respectively) are both required for the forced swimming- and novelty-induced histone H3 phosphoacetylation and c-Fos induction in dentate neurons (Bilang-Bleuel et al. 2005; Chandramohan et al. 2007, 2008). The requirement for activation of both pathways was additionally substantiated by the finding that the sole injection of rats with a GR-occupying dose of corticosterone was ineffective (Chandramohan et al. 2007). Glucocorticoid hormone action via the mineralocorticoid receptor and the gaseous messenger nitric oxide is not involved (Chandramohan et al. 2007, 2008), suggesting specificity in participating mediators.

14.5 GABAergic Control of Dentate Gyrus Epigenomic Responses

On the basis of electrophysiological and computational studies, it is thought that the encoding of sensory information within the dentate gyrus is conducted orthogonally by sparsely distributed granule neurons (Rolls and Kesner 2006). The sparse neuronal activation pattern is required for appropriate information processing (Leutgeb et al. 2007; Rolls and Kesner 2006) and involves an important role of the strong tonic inhibitory control exerted by local GABAergic interneurons (Rolls and Kesner 2006; Treves and Rolls 1994). Thus, granule neurons are only excited if the stimulus is strong enough to overcome the GABAergic inhibitory tone. The excitation is brought about by glutamate acting via NMDA receptors (Collingridge and Singer 1990; McHugh et al. 2007; Richter-Levin et al. 1995; Treves and Rolls 1994).

Aspsychological challenges evoke a sparse pattern of H3S10p-K14ac and c-Fos in dentate granule neurons, we hypothesized that GABA may be an important modulator of such epigenomic responses. We found that pretreatment of rats with the benzo Lorazepam, an indirect GABA-A receptor agonist, dose-dependently blocked the effect of a novel cage challenge on histone H3 phosphoacetylation and c-Fos induction in dentate neurons (Papadopoulos et al. 2008). This inhibition was accomplished at a dose of the benzo that was found to be anxiolytic but not sedative. Conversely, the partial inverse GABA-A agonist FG-7142, a drug that is known to attenuate the GABAergic inhibition of dentate granule neurons, profoundly enhanced baseline levels as well as novelty-induced increases in the number of H3S10p-K14ac- and c-Fos-positive dentate neurons (Papadopoulos et al. 2008). Corresponding with previous reports, after FG-7142 the rats showed anxiety-like behavior and hypervigilance in the novel cage. Furthermore, the FG-7142-evoked enhancements in epigenomic changes were found to be completely blocked by the NMDA receptor antagonist MK-801, which underscores the critical importance of this glutamate receptor in dentate granule neuron activation (Papadopoulos et al. 2008).

These observations confirm that GABA functions as a major controller in the dentate gyrus. This function precipitates at least in part through its modulation of epigenomic responses in the granule neurons. Thus, regulators of GABA activity in the dentate gyrus may modulate the extent to which salience is given to incoming sensory information.

14.6 ERK–MSK Signaling Drives the Histone H3S10 Phosphorylation Mark

In general, relatively little is known about the signaling mechanisms involved in the activation or inhibition of histone modifying enzymes. The signaling cascade mediating the phosphorylation and acetylation of histone H3 has, however, been rather well established. Pharmacological and mutant mouse studies have indicated the involvement of the extracellular signal-regulated kinases ERK1/2 and the mitogen- and stress-activated kinases MSK1/2 (Chandramohan et al. 2008). ERK1/2 has been shown to be activated by phosphorylation via the mitogen-activated protein kinase (MAPK) pathway after NMDA receptor stimulation (Sweatt 2004). pERK1/2 (as well as p38MAPK) can phosphorylate MSK1 at Ser-360, Thr-581, and Thr-700 after which MSK1 will autophosphorylate itself at multiple sites resulting in full catalytic – H3S10 kinase – activity (Arthur 2008; Hauge and Frodin 2006). Dentate gyrus neurons are known to express NMDA receptors, ERK1/2 and MSK1, but it was unclear whether pERK1/2, pMSK1, H3S10p-K14ac, and c-Fos would actually come to expression in the same neurons after a psychological challenge. The often practiced Western blot analysis would, of course, not provide any clues in this regard. Recently, in a series of immunofluorescence studies we could demonstrate the colocalization of pERK and pMSK1 in dentate granule neurons (Gutierrez-Mecinas et al. 2009). Moreover, we could show that pERK1/2, pMSK1, and H3S10p-K14ac are expressed in the same dentate neurons after a forced swim challenge providing clear evidence that H3S10 phosphorylation is the result of NMDA/ERK1/2/MSK1 signaling in these neurons (Gutierrez-Mecinas et al. 2009) (Fig. 14.1). In addition, neither expression of another MSK kinase, i.e., phospho-p38MAPK, nor expression of the MSK-related kinase, pRSK1/2, was found in dentate granule neurons (Gutierrez-Mecinas et al. 2009). Thus, there is specificity in the signaling mechanisms recruited to convey environmental challenges to the neuronal chromatin.

14.7 Establishment of the Combinatorial H3S10p-K14ac Marks: K14 Acetylation of H3S10p

Some time ago, we proposed on the basis of the following observations that pCREB-CBP may be responsible for the K14 acetylation in H3S10p (Chandramohan et al. 2008; Reul and Chandramohan 2007; Reul et al. 2009) (1) psychological challenges such as forced swimming result in a strongly increased phosphorylation of the transcription factor CREB in dentate gyrus neurons (Bilang-Bleuel et al. 2002); (2) MSK is, in addition to a H3S10 kinase, also a CREB kinase (Arthur and Cohen 2000); (3) the

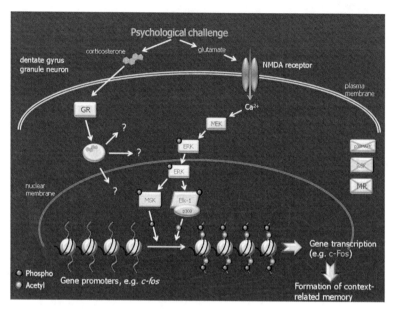

Fig. 14.1 A psychological challenge impacts on epigenomic mechanisms and memory formation through convergent activation of the GR- and NMDA–ERK-driven MSK1 and Elk-1 signaling pathways. Activation of these pathways leads to S10-phosphorylation and K14-acetylation of histone H3, hyperacetylation of histone H4, transcriptional induction of c-Fos (and other genes) in a distinct population of mature dentate granule neurons (Bilang-Bleuel et al. 2005; Chandramohan et al. 2007, 2008; Gutierrez-Mecinas et al. 2009), and the encoding of contextual memory of the endured event. Our research has shown that factors such as the MSK kinase p38MAPK, the MSK-related kinase RSK, and the glucocorticoid-binding mineralocorticoid receptor (MR) are not involved in the observed epigenetic, gene expression, and cognitive phenomena

c-fos gene promoter contains a CRE site; and (4) pCREB is able to recruit CREB-binding protein (CBP/p300, proteins with histone acetyl transferase (HAT) activity) to the promoter (Schiltz et al. 1999). However, after forced swimming phosphorylation of CREB takes place in virtually all dentate gyrus neurons (Bilang-Bleuel et al. 2002), which is in stark contrast to the sparse H3S10p-K14ac and c-Fos induction. Therefore, although a role of pCREB/CBP cannot be entirely excluded, pCREB may be playing a more general, neuroprotective role (Papadia et al. 2005) in the dentate gyrus after a psychological challenge. Recently, we discovered that challenges such as forced swimming and novelty result in the phosphorylation of the E twenty-six (ETS)-domain protein Elk-1 [Ets-like protein-1 (Sharrocks 2001; Shaw and Saxton 2003; Yordy and Muise-Helmericks 2000)] specifically in pERK1/2/pMSK1/H3S10p-K14ac/c-Fos-positive neurons of the dentate gyrus (Gutierrez-Mecinas et al. 2009). According to in vitro studies Elk-1 can be activated through ERK MAPK signaling (Yang et al. 2003a, b). Moreover, pElk-1 bound to the Elk-1-binding site within the serum response element (SRE) of the *c-fos* promoter recruits HATs like p300 to the promoter that subsequently acetylate histone molecules in adjacent nucleosomes (Li et al. 2003a; O'Donnell et al. 2008). Thus, ERK1/2-driven Elk-1 phosphorylation in dentate neurons may drive the acetylation of H3S10p (and H4) in the *c-fos* promoter (Fig. 14.1). This notion is supported by our recent immunofluorescence data showing the colocalization of pElk-1 with pERK1/2, pMSK1, H3S10p-K14ac, and c-Fos.

14.8 Glucocorticoid Receptor Involvement in Histone H3 Phosphoacetylation and c-fos Gene Expression in Dentate Gyrus Neurons

In a series of studies, we demonstrated that the establishment of the combinatorial H3S10p-K14ac marks and consequent c-Fos induction in dentate gyrus neurons requires in addition to signaling through the NMDA/ERK1/2/MSK1 and Elk-1 pathway also a GR-mediated action (Bilang-Bleuel et al. 2005; Chandramohan et al. 2007, 2008). Presently, however, it is unclear at which level(s) the distinct signaling pathways are interacting (Fig. 14.1). Classically, GRs act as ligand-dependent transcription factors altering gene expression through interaction with glucocorticoid responsive elements (GREs) in promoter regions of glucocorticoid responsive genes. As challenge-induced H3 phosphoacetylation is rather quick (significant increases within 15 min), a role of a glucocorticoid-induced gene product is unlikely. However, GRs may also be acting through nongenomic mechanisms. GRs can interact with different signaling pathways among which the MAPK ERK signaling pathway (Revest et al. 2005). Similar to the demonstrated interaction of the progesterone receptor (PR) with ERK1/2 to produce MSK activation (Vicent et al. 2006), we propose, based on the strong similarity between the GR and the PR, that the GR may be required for the full activation of MSK1. Alternatively, GRs have been shown to recruit chromatin-remodeling proteins such as ATP-dependent chromatin-remodeling complexes and histone modifying enzymes such as HATs (e.g., pCAF), thereby promoting chromatin decondensation, histone acetylation, and transcriptional activation (Hebbar and Archer 2003; Kinyamu and Archer 2004; Li et al. 2003b). Thus, GRs interact with signaling pathways and the chromatin in a highly complex manner and clearly more research is required. Yet, it appears that activated GRs are of crucial importance in the facilitation of NMDA/ERK/MSK and Elk-1 signaling to the chromatin.

14.9 Importance of H3S10p-K14ac-Associated Gene Expression in Dentate Gyrus Granule Neurons in Hippocampus-Related Memory Formation

Using well-characterized primary antibodies and immunofluorescence analysis it is now possible to demonstrate epigenetic mechanisms linked to specific gene expression events (e.g., c-Fos induction) within single cells in the brain. Moreover, intracellular molecules (e.g., pERK1/2, pMSK1, and pElk-1) can be traced signaling to the chromatin, thereby affecting gene expression. Over the last decade an impressive collection of data have been accumulating that strongly support a role of the combinatorial H3S10p-K14ac epigenetic marks and associated gene expression in hippocampus-associated learning and memory processes. Behavioral tests for hippocampus-associated memory formation include the forced swim test, Morris water maze learning, and contextual fear conditioning. In view of its role in sensory information processing and encoding, the dentate gyrus is critically involved in memory formation in these tests (Rolls and Kesner 2006; Treves and Rolls 1994). With regard to the formation of memories of a forced swim experience [for details on the forced swim test, see (Chandramohan et al. 2008)], a strict requirement was the generation of H3S10p-K14ac and c-Fos in dentate granule neurons after the initial test, thus during the acquisition and consolidation phase of memory formation. If the generation of H3S10p-K14ac and c-Fos in these neurons was disrupted due to NMDA receptor or GR blockade, MEK (MAPK kinase) inhibition (thereby preventing of ERK activation), or MSK1/2 gene knockout, formation of memory of the event was greatly impaired (Chandramohan et al. 2007, 2008; Reul and Chandramohan 2007; Reul et al. 2009). Correspondingly, antagonism of the mineralocorticoid receptor [MR; another glucocorticoid-binding receptor in the brain (Reul and De Kloet 1985)] neither affected memory formation of forced swim experience [as shown before (Veldhuis et al. 1985)] nor H3S10p-K14ac and c-Fos in the dentate gyrus (Chandramohan et al. 2008).

Recently, first epigenetic data have been collected in exercising animals. Long-term voluntary exercise has been shown to result in enhanced cognition, reduced anxiety and impulsiveness, and distinct changes in glucocorticoid hormone responses (Binder et al. 2004; Droste et al. 2007, 2009; van Praag et al. 1999). Indeed, exercising rats show enhanced H3S10p-K14ac and c-Fos responses in their dentate gyrus to forced swimming (and novelty) and make stronger memories of the experienced event (i.e., forced swimming) than the sedentary controls (Collins et al. 2009). Exercised rats show increased hippocampal GR expression (Droste et al. 2007, 2009), which may have led to an enhanced facilitation of ERK1/2/MSK1 and Elk-1 signaling and thus to an enhanced epigenomic impact. This hypothesis is currently under investigation.

There is preliminary evidence that Morris water maze learning involves H3S10p-K14ac and c-Fos induction in dentate neurons (Chandramohan and Reul, unpublished observations). Indeed, using whole hippocampus extracts and Western analysis, Chwang et al. (2007) observed a role of H3S10p in memory formation in the Morris water maze and contextual fear conditioning requiring signaling through ERK1/2 and MSK1. Presently, a role of histone H3 and H4 methylation is emerging. The role of histone methylation is complex as lysine residues can carry up to three methyl groups and the degree of methylation can have implications for chromatin structure and transcriptional activity. Mono-, di-, and trimethyl H3K4 are all associated with transcriptional activation (Akbarian and Huang 2008). However, the monomethylation marks of K9 and K27 of H3 and K20 of H4 are linked with gene activation, whereas the di- and trimethylation marks of these residues are associated with gene repression (Akbarian and Huang 2008). It should be emphasized that these findings are based on in vitro studies and until now only few reports exist on histone methylation-associated changes in neuronal gene expression in vivo [e.g., (Huang et al. 2007; Schaefer et al. 2009)]. We found preliminary evidence for an increased H3K4 methylation of the *c-fos* promoter in the hippocampus after forced swimming (Hesketh and Reul, unpublished observations). McEwen and colleagues recently reported changes in overall levels of H3K4, H3K9, and H3K27 methylation in the brain of acutely and chronically (restraint) stressed rats (Hunter et al. 2009). Conditional mutagenesis of H3K9 methyltransferase complex GLP/G9a in mice resulted in altered exploratory, locomotor, and cognitive behaviors (Schaefer et al. 2009). Gupta et al. demonstrated that H3K4 methylation is involved in the establishment of contextual fear memories (Gupta et al. 2010). Thus, we are only beginning to understand how major life events impact on epigenomic mechanisms in neurons participating in the formation of memories of such events.

14.10 Concluding Remarks

There are now clear indications that epigenetic mechanisms controlling gene transcription play a key role in learning and memory processes. Valuable information has also been gathered about how these epigenetic mechanisms are controlled by intracellular and extracellular signaling pathways. In this chapter, we described the role of NMDA/ERK1/2/MSK1 and Elk-1 signaling, GR activation, and GABA-A-mediated control on histone H3 S10-phosphorylation and K14-acetylation, hyperacetylation of H4, and subsequently induction of c-Fos in dentate granule neurons in response to an emotional or otherwise psychologically stressful event. These epigenomic mechanisms appear to be of critical importance for storing memories of such events. Histone methylation and demethylation events may be playing an important role as well. How glucocorticoid hormones strengthen memory formation is still elusive, but recent evidence suggests that glucocorticoids, in part, may act through facilitation of ERK MAPK signaling in dentate neurons leading to enhanced epigenomic responses in these neurons. Elucidation of these epigenomic processes may be key to resolve psychiatric illnesses such as major depression and anxiety-related disorders [e.g., PTSD (Reul and Nutt 2008)] in a not too distant future.

Acknowledgment Our work described in this paper is supported by the Biotechnology and Biological Sciences Research Council (BBSRC; Grant Reference Number BB/F000510/1) of the United Kingdom.

References

Akbarian S, Huang HS (2008) Epigenetic regulation in human brain-focus on histone lysine methylation. Biol Psychiatry 65:198–203

Arthur JS (2008) MSK activation and physiological roles. Front Biosci 13:5866–5879

Arthur JS, Cohen P (2000) MSK1 is required for CREB phosphorylation in response to mitogens in mouse embryonic stem cells. FEBS Lett 482:44–48

Beylin AV, Shors TJ (2003) Glucocorticoids are necessary for enhancing the acquisition of associative memories after acute stressful experience. Horm Behav 43:124–131

Bilang-Bleuel A, Droste S, Gesing A, Rech J, Linthorst ACE, Reul JMHM (2000) Impact of stress and voluntary exercise on neurogenesis in the adult hippocampus: quantitative analysis by detection of Ki-67. Soc Neurosci Abst 26:1534

Bilang-Bleuel A, Rech J, Holsboer F, Reul JMHM (2002) Forced swimming evokes a biphasic response in CREB phosphorylation in extrahypothalamic limbic and neocortical brain structures. Eur J Neurosci 15:1048–1060

Bilang-Bleuel A, Ulbricht S, Chandramohan Y, De Carli S, Droste SK, Reul JMHM (2005) Psychological stress increases histone H3 phosphorylation in adult dentate gyrus granule neurons: involvement in a glucocorticoid receptor-dependent behavioural response. Eur J Neurosci 22:1691–1700

Binder E, Droste SK, Ohl F, Reul JMHM (2004) Regular voluntary exercise reduces anxiety-related behaviour and impulsiveness in mice. Behav Brain Res 155:197–206

Chandramohan Y, Droste SK, Reul JMHM (2007) Novelty stress induces phospho-acetylation of histone H3 in rat dentate gyrus granule neurons through coincident signalling via the N-methyl-D-aspartate receptor and the glucocorticoid receptor: relevance for c-fos induction. J Neurochem 101:815–828

Chandramohan Y, Droste SK, Arthur JS, Reul JMHM (2008) The forced swimming-induced behavioural immobility response involves histone H3 phospho-acetylation and c-Fos induction in dentate gyrus granule neurons via activation of the N-methyl-D-aspartate/extracellular signal-regulated kinase/mitogen- and stress-activated kinase signalling pathway. Eur J Neurosci 27:2701–2713

Chawla MK, Guzowski JF, Ramirez-Amaya V, Lipa P, Hoffman KL, Marriott LK, Worley PF, McNaughton BL, Barnes CA (2005) Sparse, environmentally selective expression of Arc RNA in the upper blade of the rodent fascia dentata by brief spatial experience. Hippocampus 15:579–586

Cheung P, Tanner KG, Cheung WL, Sassone-Corsi P, Denu JM, Allis CD (2000) Synergistic coupling of histone H3 phosphorylation and acetylation in response to epidermal growth factor stimulation. Mol Cell 5:905–915

Chwang WB, Arthur JS, Schumacher A, Sweatt JD (2007) The nuclear kinase mitogen- and stress-activated protein kinase 1 regulates hippocampal chromatin remodeling in memory formation. J Neurosci 27:12732–12742

Clayton AL, Rose S, Barratt MJ, Mahadevan LC (2000) Phosphoacetylation of histone H3 on c-fos-and c-jun-associated nucleosomes upon gene activation. EMBO J 19:3714–3726

Collingridge GL, Singer W (1990) Excitatory amino acid receptors and synaptic plasticity. Trends Pharmacol Sci 11:290–296

Collins A, Hill LE, Chandramohan Y, Whitcomb D, Droste SK, Reul JMHM (2009) Exercise improves cognitive responses to psychological stress through enhancement of epigenetic mechanisms and gene expression in the dentate gyrus. PLoS ONE 4:e4330

De Kloet ER, De Kock S, Schild V, Veldhuis HD (1988) Antiglucocorticoid RU 38486 attenuates retention of a behaviour and disinhibits the hypothalamic-pituitary adrenal axis at different brain sites. Neuroendocrinol 47:109–115

De Pablo JM, Parra A, Segovia S, Guillamón A (1989) Learned immobility explains the behavior of rats in the forced swim test. Physiol Behav 46:229–237

Droste SK, Chandramohan Y, Reul JMHM (2007) Voluntary exercise impacts on the rat hypothalamic-pituitary-adrenal axis mainly at the adrenal level. Neuroendocrinol 86:26–37

Droste SK, de GL A, HC LSL, Reul JMHM, Linthorst ACE (2008) Corticosterone levels in the brain show a distinct ultradian rhythm but a delayed response to forced swim stress. Endocrinology 149:3244–3253

Droste SK, Collins A, Lightman SL, Linthorst ACE, Reul JMHM (2009) Distinct, time-dependent effects of voluntary exercise on circadian and ultradian rhythms and stress responses of free corticosterone in the rat hippocampus. Endocrinology 150:4170–4179

Gupta S, Kim SY, Artis S, Molfese DL, Schumacher A, Sweatt JD, Paylor RE, Lubin FD (2010) Histone methylation regulates memory formation. J Neurosci 30:3589–3599

Gutierrez-Mecinas M, Collins A, Qian X, Hesketh SA, Reul JMHM (2009) Forced swimming-evoked histone H3 phospho-acetylation and c-Fos induction in dentate gyrus granule neurons involves ERK1/2-mediated MSK1 and Elk-1 phosphorylation. Program No. 777.17. 2009 Neuroscience Meeting Planner. Chicago, IL: Society for Neuroscience, 2009. Online. [This is the reference format recommended by SFN for referencing their abstracts]

Hauge C, Frodin M (2006) RSK and MSK in MAP kinase signalling. J Cell Sci 119:3021–3023

Hebbar PB, Archer TK (2003) Chromatin remodeling by nuclear receptors. Chromosoma 111: 495–504

Huang HS, Matevossian A, Whittle C, Kim SY, Schumacher A, Baker SP, Akbarian S (2007) Prefrontal dysfunction in schizophrenia involves mixed-lineage leukemia 1-regulated histone methylation at GABAergic gene promoters. J Neurosci 27:11254–11262

Hunter RG, McCarthy KJ, Milne TA, Pfaff DW, McEwen BS (2009) Regulation of hippocampal H3 histone methylation by acute and chronic stress. Proc Natl Acad Sci USA 106: 20912–20917

Kinyamu HK, Archer TK (2004) Modifying chromatin to permit steroid hormone receptor-dependent transcription. Biochim Biophys Acta 1677:30–45

Korte SM (2001) Corticosteroids in relation to fear, anxiety and psychopathology. Neurosci Biobehav Rev 25:117–142

Korte SM, De Kloet ER, Buwalda B, Bouman SD, Bohus B (1996) Antisense to the glucocorticoid receptor in hippocampal dentate gyrus reduces immobility in forced swim test. Eur J Pharmacol 301:19–25

Leutgeb JK, Leutgeb S, Moser MB, Moser EI (2007) Pattern separation in the dentate gyrus and CA3 of the hippocampus. Science 315:961–966

Li QJ, Yang SH, Maeda Y, Sladek FM, Sharrocks AD, Martins-Green M (2003a) MAP kinase phosphorylation-dependent activation of Elk-1 leads to activation of the co-activator p300. EMBO J 22:281–291

Li X, Wong J, Tsai SY, Tsai MJ, O'Malley BW (2003b) Progesterone and glucocorticoid receptors recruit distinct coactivator complexes and promote distinct patterns of local chromatin modification. Mol Cell Biol 23:3763–3773

Martens JH, Verlaan M, Kalkhoven E, Zantema A (2003) Cascade of distinct histone modifications during collagenase gene activation. Mol Cell Biol 23:1808–1816

McHugh TJ, Jones MW, Quinn JJ, Balthasar N, Coppari R, Elmquist JK, Lowell BB, Fanselow MS, Wilson MA, Tonegawa S (2007) Dentate gyrus NMDA receptors mediate rapid pattern separation in the hippocampal network. Science 317:94–99

Morris R (1984) Development of a water-maze procedure for studying spatial learning in the rat. J Neurosci Meth 11:47–60

O'Donnell A, Yang SH, Sharrocks AD (2008) MAP kinase-mediated c-fos regulation relies on a histone acetylation relay switch. Mol Cell 29:780–785

Oitzl MS, De Kloet ER (1992) Selective corticosteroid antagonists modulate specific aspects of spatial orientation learning. Behav Neurosci 106:62–71

Papadia S, Stevenson P, Hardingham NR, Bading H, Hardingham GE (2005) Nuclear Ca^{2+} and the cAMP response element-binding protein family mediate a late phase of activity-dependent neuroprotection. J Neurosci 25:4279–4287

Papadopoulos A, Chandramohan Y, Collins A, Droste SK, Nutt DJ, Reul JMHM (2008) GABAergic control of stress-responsive epigenetic and gene expression mechanisms in the dentate gyrus. Eur Neuropsychopharmacol 18:S211–S212

Peñalva RG, Lancel M, Flachskamm C, Reul JMHM, Holsboer F, Linthorst ACE (2003) Effect of sleep and sleep depriviation on serotonergic neurotransmission in the hippocampus: a combined in vivo microdialysis/EEG study in rats. Eur J Neurosci 17:1896–1906

Reul JMHM, Chandramohan Y (2007) Epigenetic mechanisms in stress-related memory formation. Psychoneuroendocrinol 32(Suppl 1):S21–S25

Reul JMHM, De Kloet ER (1985) Two receptor systems for corticosterone in rat brain: microdistribution and differential occupation. Endocrinology 117:2505–2512

Reul JMHM, Nutt DJ (2008) Glutamate and cortisol – a critical confluence in PTSD? J Psychopharmacol 22:469–472

Reul JMHM, Hesketh SA, Collins A, Gutierrez-Mecinas M (2009) Epigenetic mechanisms in the dentate gyrus act as a molecular switch in hippocampus-associated memory function. Epigenetics 4:434–439

Revest JM, Di BF, Kitchener P, Rouge-Pont F, Desmedt A, Turiault M, Tronche F, Piazza PV (2005) The MAPK pathway and Egr-1 mediate stress-related behavioral effects of glucocorticoids. Nat Neurosci 8:664–672

Richter-Levin G, Canevari L, Bliss TV (1995) Long-term potentiation and glutamate release in the dentate gyrus: links to spatial learning. Behav Brain Res 66:37–40

Rolls ET, Kesner RP (2006) A computational theory of hippocampal function, and empirical tests of the theory. Prog Neurobiol 79:1–48

Roozendaal B, Hui GK, Hui IR, Berlau DJ, Mcgaugh JL, Weinberger NM (2006) Basolateral amygdala noradrenergic activity mediates corticosterone-induced enhancement of auditory fear conditioning. Neurobiol Learn Mem 86:249–255

Sabbattini P, Canzonetta C, Sjoberg M, Nikic S, Georgiou A, Kemball-Cook G, Auner HW, Dillon N (2007) A novel role for the Aurora B kinase in epigenetic marking of silent chromatin in differentiated postmitotic cells. EMBO J 26:4657–4669

Schaefer A, Sampath SC, Intrator A, Min A, Gertler TS, Surmeier DJ, Tarakhovsky A, Greengard P (2009) Control of cognition and adaptive behavior by the GLP/G9a epigenetic suppressor complex. Neuron 64:678–691

Schiltz RL, Mizzen CA, Vassilev A, Cook RG, Allis CD, Nakatani Y (1999) Overlapping but distinct patterns of histone acetylation by the human coactivators p300 and PCAF within nucleosomal substrates. J Biol Chem 274:1189–1192

Sharrocks AD (2001) The ETS-domain transcription factor family. Nat Rev Mol Cell Biol 2:827–837

Shaw PE, Saxton J (2003) Ternary complex factors: prime nuclear targets for mitogen-activated protein kinases. Int J Biochem Cell Biol 35:1210–1226

Smeets T, Wolf OT, Giesbrecht T, Sijstermans K, Telgen S, Joels M (2009) Stress selectively and lastingly promotes learning of context-related high arousing information. Psychoneuroendocrinol 34:1152–1161

Strahl BD, Allis CD (2000) The language of covalent histone modifications. Nature 403:41–45

Sweatt JD (2004) Mitogen-activated protein kinases in synaptic plasticity and memory. Curr Opin Neurobiol 14:1–7

Treves A, Rolls ET (1994) Computational analysis of the role of the hippocampus in memory. Hippocampus 4:374–391

Tsankova NM, Kumar A, Nestler EJ (2004) Histone modifications at gene promoter regions in rat hippocampus after acute and chronic electroconvulsive seizures. J Neurosci 24:5603–5610

van Praag H, Christie BR, Sejnowski TJ, Gage FH (1999) Running enhances neurogenesis, learning and long-term potentiation in mice. Proc Natl Acad Sci USA 96:13427–13431

Veldhuis HD, De Korte CCMM, De Kloet ER (1985) Glucocorticoids facilitate the retention of acquired immobility during forced swimming. Eur J Pharmacol 115:211–217

Vicent GP, Ballare C, Silvina Nacht A, Clausell J, Subtil-Rodriquez A, Quiles I, Jordan A, Beato M (2006) Induction of progesterone target genes requires activation of Erk and Msk kinases and phosphorylation of histone H3. Mol Cell 24:367–381

West AP (1990) Neurobehavioral studies of forced swimming: the role of learning and memory in the forced swim test. Prog Neuropsychopharmacol Biol Psychiatry 14:863–877

Witter MP (2007) The perforant path: projections from the entorhinal cortex to the dentate gyrus. Prog Brain Res 163:43–61

Yang SH, Jaffray E, Hay RT, Sharrocks AD (2003a) Dynamic interplay of the SUMO and ERK pathways in regulating Elk-1 transcriptional activity. Mol Cell 12:63–74

Yang SH, Sharrocks AD, Whitmarsh AJ (2003b) Transcriptional regulation by the MAP kinase signaling cascades. Gene 320:3–21

Yordy JS, Muise-Helmericks RC (2000) Signal transduction and the Ets family of transcription factors. Oncogene 19:6503–6513

Glossary

5-Aza-2-deoxy-cytidine (Decitabin) A cytosine in which the 5 carbon of the cytosine ring has been replaced with nitrogen. Decitabone is exclusively incorporated in DNA inhibiting mammalian *DNA methyltransferases*.

5-Azacytidine (AZA) A cytidine RNA analog in which the 5 carbon of the cytosine ring has been replaced with nitrogen. 5-Azacytidine can be incorporated in RNA and after metabolic activation also in DNA, where it functions as an inhibitor of mammalian *DNA methyltransferases*.

Acetylation The introduction, via an enzymatic reaction, of an acetyl group to an organic compound, for instance to *histones* or other proteins.

Adrenocorticotropin hormone (ACTH) A polypeptide tropic hormone secreted by the anterior pituitary gland in response to biological stress.

Agouti gene The murine agouti gene (A) controls fur color through the deposition of yellow pigment in developing hairs. Several variants of the gene exist, and for one of these (Agouti Variable Yellow, A^{vy}) the expression levels can be heritably modified by *DNA methylation*.

Alleles Different variants or copies of a gene. For most genes on the chromosomes, there are two copies: one copy inherited from the mother and the other from the father. The DNA sequence of each of these copies may be different because of genetic polymorphisms.

Angelman syndrome (AS) A rare pediatric diseases caused by chromosomal aberrations or epigenetic inactivation of genes on the maternal chromosome 15.

Anxiety disorders Disorders with different forms of abnormal and pathological fear and anxiety.

Assisted reproduction technologies (ART) The combination of approaches that are being applied in the fertility clinic, including *IVF* and *ICSI*.

ATRX Alpha-thalassemia/mental retardation syndrome X-linked (ATRX) is a protein that belongs to the switch/sucrose nonfermentable (SWI/SNF) family of chromatin remodeling proteins, which facilitate gene expression by allowing

A. Petronis and J. Mill (eds.), *Brain, Behavior and Epigenetics*,
Epigenetics and Human Health, DOI 10.1007/978-3-642-17426-1,
© Springer-Verlag Berlin Heidelberg 2011

transcription factors to gain access to their targets in chromatin. Mutations in the ATRX gene alter DNA methylation and have been associated with an X-linked mental retardation syndrome that is often accompanied by alpha-thalassemia (ATRX) syndrome.

Autism   A neuropsychiatric disorder characterized by impaired social interaction and communication, and by restricted and repetitive behavior.

Bipolar disorder (BPD)   A psychiatric disease defined by the presence of one or more episodes of abnormally elevated energy levels, cognition, and mood with or without one or more depressive episodes.

Bisulfite genomic sequencing   A procedure in which sodium bisulfite is used to deaminate cytosine to uracil in genomic DNA. Conditions are chosen so that 5-methylcytosine is not changed. PCR amplification and subsequent DNA sequencing reveal the exact position of cytosines which are methylated in genomic DNA.

Bivalent chromatin   A chromatin region that is modified by a combination of histone modifications such that it represses gene transcription, but at the same time retains the potential of acquiring gene expression.

Brain-derived neurotrophic factor (BDNF)   A protein which acts on certain neurons of the central and peripheral nervous system, supporting the survival of neurons and encouraging the growth and differentiation of new neurons and synapses.

Brno nomenclature   Regulation of the nomenclature of specific histone modifications formulated at the Brno meeting of the NoE in 2004. Rules are <Histone><amino acid position><modification type><type of modification>. Example: H3K4me3 = trimethylated lysine-4 on histone H3.

Bromo domain   Protein motif found in a variety of nuclear proteins including transcription factors and HATs involved in transcriptional activation. Bromo domains bind to histone tails carrying acetylated lysine residues.

CBP   CREB-binding protein involved in transcriptional regulation often associating with histone acetyltransferases such as p300.

Cell fate   The programmed path of differentiation of a cell. Although all cells have the same DNA, their cell fate can be different. For instance, some cells develop into brain, whereas others are the precursors of blood. Cell fate is determined in part by the organization of *chromatin* – DNA and the histone proteins – in the nucleus.

Cellular Memory (epigenetic)   Specific active and repressive organizations of chromatin can be maintained from one cell to its daughter cells. This is called *epigenetic inheritance* and ensures that specific states of gene expression are inherited over many cell generations.

Cerebellum   Region of the brain that plays a role in motor control, as well as language, attention, and some elements of emotion.

Cerebral cortex   A sheet of neural tissue covering the mammalian cerebrum.

ChIP   See *chromatin immunoprecipitation.*

ChIP-chip   After chromatin immunoprecipitation, DNA is purified from the immunoprecipitated chromatin fraction and hybridized on arrays of short DNA fragments representing specific regions of the genome.

ChIP-seq   Sequencing of the totality of DNA fragments obtained by ChIP using next-generation sequencing to quantify patterns of enrichment across the genome.

Chromatid   In each somatic cell generation, the genomic DNA is replicated in order to make two copies of each individual chromosome. During M phase of the cell cycle, these copies – called chromatids – are microscopically visible one next to the other, before they get distributed to the daughter cells.

Chromatin immunoprecipitation (ChIP)   This is a method for examining protein–DNA interactions occurring in the cell. DNA-binding proteins are cross-linked to the DNA and enriched using antibodies with specific affinity to particular (histone) proteins or covalent modifications on proteins. After ChIP, the genomic DNA is purified from the chromatin fragments brought down by the antiserum and analyzed by qPCR, microarray (ChIP-chip), or next-generation sequencing (ChIP-seq).

Chromatin remodeling   Locally, the organization and compaction of chromatin can be altered by different enzymatic machineries. This is called chromatin remodeling. Several chromatin remodeling proteins move *nucleosomes* along the DNA and require ATP for their action.

Chromatin   The nucleo-protein-complex constituting the chromosomes in eukaryotic cells. Structural organization of chromatin is complex and involves different levels of compaction. The lowest level of compaction is represented by an extended array of *nucleosomes.*

Chromo domain (chromatin organization modifier domain)   Protein–protein interaction motif first identified in *Drosophila melanogaster HP1* and *polycomb group proteins*. Also found in other nuclear proteins involved in transcriptional silencing and heterochromatin formation. Chromo domains consist of approximately 50 amino acids and bind to histone tails that are methylated at certain lysine residues.

Chromosomal domain   In higher eukaryotes, it is often observed that in a specific cell type, chromatin is organized (e.g., by *histone methylation*) the same way across hundreds to thousands of kilobases of DNA. These "chromosomal domains" can comprise multiple genes that are similarly expressed. Some chromosomal domains are controlled by *genomic imprinting*.

Corticotropin releasing hormone (CRH)   A polypeptide hormone and neurotransmitter involved in the stress response.

CpG dinucleotide   A cytosine followed by a guanine in the sequence of bases of the DNA. *Cytosine methylation* in mammals occurs primarily at CpG dinucleotides.

CpG island   A small stretch of DNA, of several hundred up to several kilobases in size, that is particularly rich in *CpG dinucleotides* and is also relatively enriched in cytosines and guanines. Most CpG islands comprise promoter sequences that drive the expression of genes.

CREB   cAMP response element-binding protein, a transcriptional activator for many immediate early genes.

Cytosine methylation   In mammals, DNA methylation occurs at cytosines that are part of *CpG dinucleotides*. As a consequence of the palindromic nature of the CpG sequence, methylation is symmetrical, i.e., affects both strands of DNA at a methylated target site. When present at promoters, it is usually associated with transcriptional repression.

Deacetylation   The removal of acetyl groups from proteins. Deacetylation of histones is often associated with gene repression and is mediated by histone deacetylases (HDACs).

"de novo" DNA methylation   The addition of methyl groups to a stretch of DNA which is not yet methylated (acquisition of "new" DNA methylation).

Dentate gyrus   Part of the hippocampal formation believed to contribute to memory formation and other brain functions.

Disomy   The occurrence in the cell of two copies of a chromosome, or part of a chromosome, that are identical and of the same parental origin (uniparental disomy).

DNA methyltransferase   Enzyme which puts new (*de novo*) *methylation* onto the DNA, or which maintains existing patterns of DNA methylation.

DNA demethylation   Removal of methyl groups from DNA. This can occur "actively," i.e., by an enzymatically mediated process, or "passively," when methylation is not maintained after DNA replication.

DNA methylation   A biochemical modification of DNA resulting from addition of a methyl group to either adenine or cytosine bases. In mammals, methylation is essentially confined to cytosines that are in *CpG dinucleotides*. Methyl groups can be removed from DNA by DNA demethylation.

Dopamine   A catecholamine neurotransmitter that has an important role in cognitive function, voluntary movement, reward, motivation, and prolactin production.

Dosage compensation   The X-chromosome is present in two copies in the one sex, and in one copy in the other. Dosage compensation ensures that in spite of the copy number difference, X-linked genes are expressed at the same level in males and females. In mammals, dosage compensation occurs by inactivation of one of the X-chromosomes in females.

Embryonic stem (ES) cells   Cultured cells obtained from the inner cell mass of the blastocyst, and for human ES cells, possibly also from the epiblast. These cells are totipotent; they can be differentiated into all different somatic cell lineages. ES-like cells can be obtained by dedifferentiation in vitro of somatic cells (see *iPS cells*).

Endocrine disruptor   A chemical component which can have an antagonistic effect on the action of a hormone (such as on estrogen) to which it resembles structurally. Some pesticides act as endocrine disruptors and have been found in animal studies to have adverse effects on development, and for some, to induce altered *DNA methylation* at specific loci. A well-characterized endocrine disruptor is *Bisphenol-A*, a chemical used for the productions of certain plastics.

Enhancer   A small, specialized sequence of DNA which, when recognized by specific regulatory proteins, can enhance the activity of the promoter of a gene(s) located in close vicinity.

Epi-alleles   Copies of a DNA sequence or a gene which differ in their epigenetic and/or expression states without the occurrence of a genetic mutation.

Epigenesis   The development of an organism from fertilization through a sequence of steps leading to a gradual increase in complexity through differentiation of cells and formation of organs.

Epigenetic code   Patterns of DNA methylation and histone modifications can modify the way genes on the chromosomes are expressed. This has led to the idea that combinations of epigenetic modifications can constitute a code on top of the genetic code which modulates gene expression.

Epigenetic inheritance   The somatic inheritance, or inheritance through the germ line, of epigenetic information (changes that affect gene function, without the occurrence of an alteration in the DNA sequence).

Epigenetic marks   Regional modifications of DNA and chromatin proteins, including *DNA methylation* and histone methylation, that can be maintained from one cell generation to the next and which may affect the way genes are expressed.

Epigenetic reprogramming   The resetting of *epigenetic marks* on the genome so that these become like those of another cell type, or of another developmental stage. Epigenetic reprogramming occurs for instance in *primordial germ cells* to bring them back in a "ground state". Epigenetic reprogramming and dedifferentiation also occur after *somatic cell nuclear transfer*.

Epigenetics   The study of heritable changes in gene function that arise without an apparent change in the genomic DNA sequence. Epigenetic mechanisms are involved in the formation and maintenance of cell lineages during development, and, in mammals, in *X-inactivation* and *genomic imprinting*, and are frequently perturbed in diseases.

Epigenome   The epigenome is the overall epigenetic state of a particular cell. In the developing embryo, each cell type has a different epigenome. Epigenome maps represent the presence of DNA methylation, histone modification, and other chromatin modifications along the chromosomes.

Epigenotype   The totality of epigenetic marks that are found along the DNA sequence of the genome in a particular cell lineage or at a particular developmental stage.

Epimutation   A change in the normal epigenetic marking of a gene or a regulatory DNA sequence (e.g., a change in DNA methylation) which affects gene expression.

Escape of X-inactivation   Regions and genes on the X-chromosomes which are not affected by the dosage compensation/X-inactivation mechanism and remain active on both X-chromosomes in females.

Euchromatin   A type of chromatin which is lightly staining when observed through the microscope at interphase. Euchromatic *chromosomal domains* are loosely compacted and relatively rich in genes. The opposite type of chromatin organization is *heterochromatin.*

Folate   A methyl donor obtained primarily from the diet involved in nucleotide synthesis and methylation reactions, including DNA methylation.

FRAXA   Fragile X mental retardation syndrome involving genetic (CCG repeat expansion) and epigenetic (DNA methylation) changes at the FRM1 gene promoter.

GABA γ-Aminobutyric acid, or the chief inhibitory neurotransmitter in the mammalian central nervous system.

GABAergic inhibitory neurotransmission   Neuronal signaling resulting from the binding of GABA to GABA receptors that decreases the probability of a target cell firing an action potential.

GAD67   Glutamate decarboxylase (also known as GAD1), an enzyme, which is responsible for catalyzing the production of γ-aminobutyric acid from L-glutamic acid.

Genome-wide association study (GWAS)   An examination of all or most of the genes in groups of individuals different for some specific trait or disease in order to identify DNA sequence-based factors that contribute to the origin of such phenotypes.

Genomic imprinting   An epigenetic phenomenon which affects a small subset of genes in the genome and results in mono-allelic gene expression in a parent-of-origin dependent way (for a given pair of alleles uniformly either the maternally or paternally derived copy is active).

Glucocorticoids   Steroid hormones that bind to the glucocorticoid receptor and affect immunological functions, metabolic processes, and responses to stress.

Glutamatergic excitatory neurotransmission   Neuronal signaling resulting from the binding of glutamate to glutamate receptors that increases the probability of a target cell firing an action potential.

GR/receptor   The glucocorticoid receptor (GR), encoded by the gene NR3C1, is the receptor that glucocorticoids, such as cortisol, bind to. The GR regulates genes that modulate development, metabolism, immune functions, and responses to stress.

Heterochromatin   A type of chromatin which is darkly staining when observed through the microscope at interphase. Heterochromatic chromosomal domains, found in all cell types, are highly compacted, rich in repeat sequences, and show little or no gene expression. Extended regions of heterochromatin are found close to centromeres and at telomeres.

Hippocampus   A region of the brain belonging to the limbic system that plays a role in long-term memory and spatial navigation.

Histone acetylation   Posttranslational modification of the ε-amino group of lysine residues in histones catalyzed by a family of enzymes called *histone acetyltransferases (HATs)*. Acetylation contributes to the formation of decondensed, transcriptionally permissive chromatin structures and facilitates interaction with proteins containing *bromo domains*.

Histone acetyltransferase (HAT)   An enzyme that acetylates (specific) lysine amino acids on histone proteins.

Histone code   Theory that distinct chromatin states of condensation and function are marked by specific histone modifications or specific combinatorial codes (see also epigenetic code).

Histone deacetylase (HDAC)   An enzyme that removes acetyl groups from histone proteins. This increases the positive charge of histones and enhances their attraction to the negatively charged phosphate groups in DNA.

Histone methylation   Posttranslational methylation of amino acid residues in histones catalyzed by *histone methyltransferases (HMTs)*. Histone methylation is found at arginine as mono- or dimethylation and lysine as mono-, di-, or trimethylation. Modifications are described depending on the position and type of methylation (mono-, di-, and trimethylation) according to the *Brno nomenclature*. Different types of methylation can be found in either open transcriptionally active or silent (repressive) chromatin (*histone code*). Methylated lysine residues are recognized by proteins containing *chromo domains*.

Histone methyltransferase (HMT)   Enzymes catalyzing the transfer of methyl groups from *S*-adenosyl-methionine (SAM) to lysine or arginine residues in histones.

Histone variants   Variants of canonical histones with distinct amino acid changes accumulating at distinct chromatin regions associated with transcriptional control or silencing.

Histone-demethylase (HDM)   Proteins catalyzing the active enzymatic removal of methyl groups from either lysine or arginine residues of histones. Prominent examples are LSD1 and Jumonji proteins.

Hypothalamic–pituitary–adrenal axis (HPA)   A complex interaction between the hypothalamus, pituitary, and adrenal glands that functions to control the stress response and many bodily processes.

Hypothalamus   A portion of the brain that links the nervous system to the endocrine system via the pituitary gland and controls body temperature, hunger, thirst, sleep, and circadian cycles.

Imprinted genes   Genes that show a parent-of-origin specific gene expression pattern controlled by epigenetic marks that originate from the germ line.

Imprinted X-inactivation   Preferential inactivation of the paternal X-chromosome in rodents (presumably also humans) during early embryogenesis and in the placenta of mammals.

Imprinting control region (ICR)   Region that shows germ line derived parent-of-origin dependent epigenetic marking which controls the imprinted expression of neighboring imprinted genes.

Imprinting   See *genomic imprinting*

In vitro fertilization (IVF)   Fertilization of a surgically retrieved oocyte in the laboratory, followed by a short period of in vitro cultivation before the embryo is transferred back into the uterus to allow development to term.

Induced pluripotent stem cells (iPS)   Cells derived from differentiated somatic cells by in vitro reprogramming. Reprogramming is triggered by the activation of pluripotency factor genes and cultivation in ES-cell medium. iPS cells are capable to generate all cell types of an embryo.

Intracytoplasmic sperm injection (ICSI)   Capillary mediated injection of a single sperm into the cytoplasm of an oocyte followed by activation to promote directed fertilization.

Intrauterine environment   The collective conditions affecting a fetus in the uterus.

Isoschizomers   Restriction enzymes from different bacteria which recognize the same target sequence in DNA. Often these enzymes respond differently to methylation of bases within their target sequence, which may make them important tools in DNA-methylation analysis. Thus, *Msp*I cuts both CCGG and C5mCGG, whereas *Hpa*II cuts only the unmethylated sequence.

Kinship theory of imprinting   An evolutionary theory, which attempts to explain the origin and evolution of imprinted genes.

LINE elements   Long interspersed (repetitive) elements dispersed among the human/mammalian genome. LINE elements are usually transcriptional silent and marked by DNA methylation.

Long-term potentiation (LTP)   A persistent, activity-dependent form of synaptic enhancement of neuron that is a model for certain types of long-term memory.

Major depression   A mental disorder characterized by low mood accompanied by low self-esteem, suicidal thought, and loss of interest or pleasure in normally enjoyable activities.

MAPK/ERK signaling   Signaling pathway in the cell, which consists of many proteins, including mitogen-activated protein kinase (MAPK, originally called ERK) that communicates signals from the cell surface to nucleus, affecting the levels and activities of transcription factors and gene expression.

Maternal effects   Long-term effects on the development of the embryo triggered by factors in the cytoplasm of the oocyte.

MeCP2   Methyl-CpG-binding protein 2 encodes a protein that is essential for the normal function of nerve cells; mutations in this gene cause Rett syndrome.

Methyl-binding domain (MBD)   Protein domain in Methyl-CpG-binding proteins (MBPs) responsible for recognizing and binding to methylated cytosine residues in DNA. Proteins containing MBDs form a specific family of proteins with various molecular functions.

Methyl-CpG-binding proteins (MBPs)   Proteins containing domains (such as MBD) binding to 5-methyl-cytosine in the context of CpG dinucleotides. MBPs mostly act as mediators for molecular functions such as transcriptional control or DNA repair.

Monozygotic twins   Twins developed from one zygote that splits and forms two embryos (also known as identical twins).

MTHFR   Methyl tetrahydrofolate reductase – a key enzyme in the folate (see above)-S-adenosylmethionine (SAM, see below) pathway.

Myelin   An electrically insulating material covering the axons on neurons.

Neuronal plasticity   The ability of the brain to change as a result of one's experience.

NMDA/receptor   The N-methyl-D-aspartate receptor is an ionotropic glutamate receptor that stimulates intracellular signaling cascades that affect gene transcription, synaptic plasticity, and learning and memory.

Noncoding RNA (ncRNA)   RNA transcripts that do not code for a protein. ncRNA generation frequently involves RNA processing.

Non-Mendelian inheritance   Inheritance of genetic traits that do not follow Mendelian rules and/or cannot be explained in simple mathematically modeled traits

Nucleolus   Specific compartments within the nucleus formed by rDNA repeat domains. Nucleoli are marked by specific heterochromatic structures and active gene expression.

Nucleosome   Fundamental organizational unit of chromatin consisting of 147 base pairs of DNA wound around a histone octamer.

Oligodendrocyte   A type of neuroglia that insulates axons in the CNS.

Paraventricular nucleus (PVN)   A neuronal nucleus in the hypothalamus containing neurons that are activated by stressful or physiological changes.

Pituitary   An endocrine gland protruding from the hypothalamus that secretes six hormones involved in homeostasis of an organism.

PKA   Cyclic adenosine monophosphate (cAMP)-protein kinase A. In LTP PKA is involved in memory consolidation.

Polyamines   A group of organic compounds that are composed of carbon, nitrogen, and hydrogen, and that have two or more amino groups.

Polycomb group proteins   Epigenetic regulator proteins forming multiprotein complexes (PRCs = polycomb repressive complexes). Polycomb group proteins possess enzymatic properties to control the maintenance of a suppressed state of developmentally regulated genes, mainly through histone methylation and ubiquitination.

Position effect variegation (PEV)   Cell/tissue specific variability of gene expression controlled by the temporal inheritance of certain epigenetic states. PEV is a consequence of variable formation of heterochromatin across the respective gene. A classical example of PEV is found in the certain mutations leading to variegated eye pigmentation in *Drosophila* eyes.

Prader–Willi syndrome (PWS)   A rare pediatric disease caused by chromosomal aberrations or epigenetic misregulation of genes on the paternal chromosome 15.

Protamines   Small, arginine-rich proteins that replace histones late in the haploid phase of spermatogenesis (during *spermiogenesis*). They are thought to be essential for sperm head condensation and DNA stabilization. After fertilization protamines are removed from paternal chromosomes in the mammalian zygote.

Psychosis   An abnormal condition of the mind, described as involving a loss of contact with reality.

Reelin   A protein that regulates neuronal migration in the developing brain and also performs various important functions (synaptic plasticity, dendrite development, adult neurogenesis) in the adult brain.

RNA interference (RNAi)   Posttranscriptional regulatory effects on mRNAs (control of translation or stability) triggered by processed ds and ss small RNA (si-, mi-, and pi-RNAs) molecules. Effects are propagated by enzymatic complexes such as RISC containing the small RNAs bound by Argonaute proteins.

Rubinstein–Taybi syndrome (RTS)   A disorder caused by mutations in the CREBBP gene, characterized by short stature, moderate to severe learning difficulties, distinctive facial features, and broad thumbs and first toes.

S-Adenosyl methionine (SAM)   A cofactor for all DNA (DNMTs) and histone methyltransferases (HMTs) providing the methyl group added to either cytosines (DNA) or histones (arginine or lysine).

S-Adenosylhomocysteine (SAH)   Hydrolyzed product formed after the methylation reaction catalyzed by DNA and *histone methyltransferases* using SAM as methyl group donor. SAH is a competitive inhibitor of SAM for most methyltransferases.

SAHA   Suberoylanilide hydroxamic acid, an inhibitor of certain histone deacetylases, leading to enhanced levels of histone acetylation. See also *TSA*.

Schizophrenia   A mental disorder characterized by disintegration of thought processes and of emotional responsiveness, involving hallucinations, paranoia, delusions, or disorganized speech and thinking.

Serotonin   A neurotransmitter produced in the brain that regulates mood, appetite, sleep, and impulse control. It is also known to influence the functioning of the cardiovascular, renal, immune, and gastrointestinal systems.

SET domain   A domain found in virtually all lysine-specific *histone methyltransferases (HMTs)*. A protein–protein interaction domain required for HMT activity and modulation of chromatin structure, frequently associated with cysteine-rich Pre-SET and Post-SET domains.

Silencer   Element in the DNA to which proteins bind that inhibits transcription of a nearby promoter. Silencer elements are recognized and bound by silencer proteins.

siRNAs   Small interfering RNAs, RNAs in the size range of 21–24 nucleotides derived from double-stranded long RNAs cleaved by Dicer. siRNAs are incorporated into the RISC complex to be targeted to complementary RNAs to promote cleavage of these mRNAs.

Skewing of X-chromosome inactivation   Unbalanced inactivation of X-chromosomes in females resulting in different effects of X-linked genetic difference such as recessive mutations.

snoRNAs   Small nucleolar RNAs involved in processing of small RNAs such as ribosomal RNAs.

Social environment   Social milieu – the people and institutions – with whom the person interacts.

Somatic cell nuclear transfer (SCNT)   Transfer of the nucleus of a somatic cell into an enucleated oocyte using a glass capillary to form an SCNT-zygote. After activation of the zygote the genome of the nucleus derived from the somatic cells becomes reprogrammed to start development.

Spermatogonia   Immature diploid sperm cells which develop into mature spermatozoa (sperm). Major epigenetic changes occur in spermatogonic cells.

Stem cell   Noncommitted cell which has the capacity to self renew and divide many times giving rise to daughter cells which maintain the stem cell function. Stem cells have the property to differentiate into specialized cells.

Sumoylation   Addition of a Small Ubiquitin-like Modifier or SUMO group to histone residues associated with transcriptional repression.

Totipotency   Capacity of stem cells to produce all cell types required to form a mammalian embryo, i.e., embryonic and extraembryonic cells (see *Pluripotency*). Totipotent cells are formed during the first cleavages of the embryo.

Trithorax group proteins   Proteins containing a thritorax-like bromo domain: They are usually involved in recognizing histone modifications marking transcriptionally active regions and contribute to maintenance of activity.

TSA   Trichostatin-A, an inhibitor of certain types of histone deacetylases.

Turner syndrome   A disorder affecting women which is caused by a chromosomal abnormality in which all or part of one of the X-chromosome is absent.

X-chromosome inactivation   Epigenetically controlled form of *dosage compensation* in female mammals resulting in transcriptional silencing of genes on surplus X-chromosomes. X-chromosome inactivation is triggered by the noncoding RNA Xist and manifested by various epigenetic modifications including histone methylation, histone deacetylation, and DNA methylation.

XIC   X-inactivation center. Region at which the XIST-mediated inactivation starts. Allelic changes/differences in the XIC may lead to skewed inactivation.

XIST   X-inactive specific transcript. The mammalian XIST gene codes for a nonprotein coding RNA that coats the inactive X-chromosome.

Zebularine   1-β-D-Ribofuranosyl-2(1H)-pyrimidinone, a cytosine analog that can be incorporated in RNA and in DNA, where it has DNA-methylation inhibitor effects.

Index

A

Abuse, 185–189, 192, 194, 198, 199
Acoustic startle reflex, 79
Agouti, 102
Allelic expression imbalance ratios, 132
Alzheimer's disease, 246, 254, 255
Androgen receptor, 125, 133
Angelman, 82
Anxiety, 292, 296, 297
ATRX, 133, 135
Attachment, 143–161
Autism, 77, 135, 136, 147, 154, 157–160
5-Aza–2-deoxycytidine, 257

B

Barr body, 121
BDNF, 80
Bereavement, 77
Bipolar disorder, 41–46, 85, 135
Birth weight, 76
Boundary, 130

C

Cancer, 248, 250
CBP. *See* CREB-binding protein (CBP)
c-Fos, 289–297
ChIP. *See* Chromatin immunoprecipitation (ChIP)
Choline, 79
Chromatin, 5–7, 9–14, 123, 270, 274, 279–281
Chromatin immunoprecipitation (ChIP), 134, 291
Chromatin remodeling, 37
Chromatin structure, 212–214, 218, 225
Chromium(III), 88
Clozapine, 11, 12, 14
Coadaptation, 170, 171
Cognitive disorders, 245–260

Comet assay, 87
Conditioned place paradigm (CPP), 257
CpG dinucleotides, 119
CpG islands, 123
CREB-binding protein (CBP), 250–252, 256, 259
Cycle of violence, 132
Cyclin-dependent kinase (Cdk), 254

D

Delusional disorders, 78
Dendritic spine, 252, 258
Dentate gyrus, 289–297
Depression, suicide, 49–63
Diabetes, 76
Diet, 101
Differentially methylated regions, 81
DNA methylation, 8, 41–46, 51, 55, 56, 60–62, 100
    tissue-specific, 105
Dopamine, 104
Dopamine 3, 83
Drug addiction, 246, 252, 257–258
Dry cleaner, 89
Duchenne muscular dystrophy, 123

E

Early-life adversity, 50–54
Electroconvulsive treatment, 278–280
Elk–1, 294–297
Embryogenesis, 83
Environment, 51, 52, 56, 63
    intratuterine, 75, 76, 79, 80
Environmental exposure, 104
Epidemiology, 105
Epigenetic mechanisms, 73
    DNA methylation, 72, 75, 80, 83
        gene-specific hypermethylation, 86

DNA methylation (*cont.*)
        global hypomethylation, 86
  DNA methyltransferases, 88
  histone modifications, 72
  RNA-associated silencing, 72
  siRNAs, 72
Epigenetics, 49–63, 98, 185–199
  DNA demethylation, 217–219, 227, 228
  DNA methylation, 211–217, 225–228
  pathway, 100
  study design, 106
ERK, 293–297
Ethnic minority status, 107
Exploratory behavior, 88
Exposure therapy, 253, 257, 258, 260
Expression microarrays, 125
Extinction, 246, 253, 257, 258, 260

F
Family, twin, and adoption studies, 73
  dizygotic, 74
  familial aggregation, 74
  monozygotic, 74
  twin pairs
    concordance, 74, 85
    discordant, 75, 85
    dizygotic, 74
    monozygotic, 74, 75, 85, 86
    pairwise concordance, 74
Famine, 76, 77
Fear conditioning, 250–255, 258, 259
Fecundability, 87
Fertility, 87
Fetal growth, 76
FG–7142, 292
FMR1
  CGG repeats, 129, 130
  CGG trinucleotide repeat, 129
Folate, 79, 100
Fragile X, 123
Fragile X mental retardation protein, 130
Fragile X syndrome (FXS), 129, 256, 257

G
GABA, 290, 292–293, 297
GABA A, 83
Gene–environment correlation, 106
Gene–environment interaction, 104
Genetic code, human variability, 71
Genomic imprinting, 42, 44, 145–150, 157, 158
Gestation, 102
Glucocorticoid, 288, 291–292, 294–297
Glucocorticoid receptor, 291–292, 294–297

Glucose–6-phosphate dehydrogenase (G6PD), 124
Glutamic acid decarboxylase, 10

H
Haemophilia, 123
HDAC. *See* Histone deacetylase (HDAC) inhibitors
HDAC1, 247–249, 258, 259
HDAC2, 247, 249, 258–260
Hemorrhage, 79
Hippocampus, 250–254
  CA1, 79
  cell differentiation, 80
  cell proliferation, 80
  cell survival, 80
  dentate gyrus, 79
  5-HT1A, 80
Histone, 1–14, 245–260, 288–297
Histone acetylation, 246, 247, 249–253, 255–257, 259, 270–275, 278–281, 295
Histone acetyltransferase (HAT), 246, 247, 250–252, 256
  CREB-binding protein (CBP), 272–274, 280
  p300, 272–274, 280
  PCAF, 272, 273, 280
Histone code, 247, 249
Histone deacetylases (HDAC), 45, 245–260
  HDAC1, 273–275, 280
  HDAC2, 273, 274, 277, 280
  inhibitors, 245–260
Histone H3 phosphoacetylation, 292, 295
Histone methylation, 274, 275, 279–281, 296, 297
Histone modifications, 51, 60, 61, 63
Histone phosphorylation, 275, 280, 288, 289, 293, 294, 297
Histone variant
  histone H3.3, 275, 276
  histone H2A.Z, 276
Homocysteine, 101
Hormones
  corticotropin-releasing hormone (CRH), 76, 77
  cortisol, 76
  glucocorticoid hormone, 76
  glucocorticoids, 76
Human genome project, 71
Huntington's disease (HD), 246, 255, 256
Hydroxymethylcytosine, 46
Hypoxia, 79

I

ICD. *See* International Classification
    of Diseases (ICD)
ICD–10, 78
Immigrants, 107
    age at migration, 108
Imprinting, 81
    erasure, 82
    establishment, 82
    insulin-like growth factor 2, 83
    loss of imprinting, 82
    maintenance, 82
Inactivation centre (XIC), 120
Incidence, 73, 78
Inflammation, 112
Insulin-like growth factor 2, 81, 82
International Classification of Diseases
    (ICD), 78
Intragenomic conflict, 171, 179
    conflict, 170

J

Jerusalem Perinatal Study, 78, 79, 87

L

Lead, 87–89
Learning, 288, 290, 296, 297
Life course, 111
LINE–1 hypothesis, 124
Long interspersed nuclear elements
    (LINEs), 45
Long-term potentiation (LTP), 251–253,
    256, 259
    early phase long-term potentiation (E-
        LTP), 269
    late phase long-term potentiation (L-LTP),
        269, 277
Lysine deacetylases, 249

M

Major depression, 288, 297
Manual extraction, 79
Maternal, 187–192, 194, 195, 198
Maternal behavior
    glucocorticoid receptor (GR) expression,
        222–226, 229
    licking and grooming (LG) and arched-
        back nursing (ABN) posture,
        223–229
    neuroendocrine and hypothalamic-
        pituitary-adrenal (HPA) stress
        responses, 223–224
Maternal care, 110

Maternal infection, 76
Maternal nutrition/diet effects,
    gestational stress, 223–225
Maternal sepsis, 79
Mechanisms, 83
Memory, 246, 250–256, 258–260, 287–297
    long-term memory, 268–270, 272, 278
    short-term memory, 268, 273
Metabolic syndrome, 14
Methionine, 101
Methyl-CpG-binding protein 2 (MECP2), 133
Migration, 107
Mitogen-activated protein kinase (MAPK),
    250–252
Monoamine, 176
    dopaminergic, 174, 175
    noradrenergic, 174, 175
    serotonergic, 174, 175
    serotonin, 175
Monoamine oxidases, 132
Monoaminergic
    dopamine, 175
    noradrenaline, 175
Monozygotic twins, 42–44
Morbidity, 73
Morris water maze, 288, 290, 296
Motor activity, 79
MSK, 293–295
Mutations, de novo, 83

N

NASCAR, 89
Negative symptoms, 73
Neglect, 185–189, 192, 199
Neural tube defects, 79, 99, 103
Neurodegenerative disorders, 246, 254–256,
    260
Neurodevelopment, 99, 104, 189
Neuronal alpha tubulin, 134
Next-generation sequencing, 46
Nicotinamide, 247, 255, 257
Nitric oxide, 259
NMDA receptors. *See* N-methyl-D-aspartate
    (NMDA) receptors
N-methyl-D-aspartate (NMDA) receptors,
    250, 251, 259, 291–297
Nonaffective psychoses, 78
Non-coding RNAs (microRNA), histone
    modification, 212, 213
Nonhistone proteins, 249, 251, 256, 259, 260
Novelty seeking, 88
Nuclear actor-kappa-B (NF-κβ), 259
Nucleosome, 5, 6, 8, 9, 246, 247, 249

Nutrition, 75
  supplementation, 79

O
Obstetric complications, 79
Oogonia, 83

P
p300, 251, 256, 260
Parental origin effects, 44
Parenting, 185, 187, 188, 192, 199
Paternal age, 73, 81–83, 86
Paternal age-related schizophrenia, 86
Phenylbutyrate, 248, 256, 257
Physical activity, 88
Placenta, 83
Polycomb group proteins, 123
Positive symptoms, 73
Postmortem brain, 44–46
Postnatal cross-fostering and hypothalamic-
      pituitary-adrenal (HPA) stress
      responses, 224
Posttraumatic stress disorder (PTSD), 288, 297
Prader–Willi syndrome (PWS), 82, 176, 179
  serotonin, 173, 174, 177
Preeclampsia, 76, 79
Premutations, 130
Prenatal famine, 99
Prepulse inhibition, 79
Preterm birth, 76
Prevalence, 73
Prodromal period, 73
Protamines, 87, 88
Pseudoautosomal regions, 124
Psychiatric disorder, 24
Psychosis, 73, 75
PTSD. *See* Posttraumatic stress disorder
    (PTSD)

Q
Quantitative trait loci (QTL), 123

R
Regulation, 23–37
Rett syndrome (RTT), 134
Rubinstein–Taybi syndrome (RTS), 246, 256

S
S-adenosyl methionine (SAM), 45, 46
Schizoaffective disorders, 78
Schizophrenia, 2–14, 98, 135, 154–160
  biological mechanism, 112
  environmental causes, 98

epigenetic changes, 104
etiology, 99
incidence, 108
Schizophrenia-related disorders, 78
Schizotypal disorder, 78
Serotonin 2A, 83
Signaling, 288, 291–297
Silencing, 123
Single-and double-strand breaks, 87
Single nucleotide polymorphisms (SNPs),
    4, 79, 136
S-nitrosylation, 259
Social brain, 143–161
Social context, 109
Social defeat, 111
Sodium butyrate, 248, 252–257, 259
Somatic cell hybrids, 125
Spatial learning, 88
Sperm, 86–88
Spermatogenesis, 83, 120
Spermatogonia, 83
Sperm chromatin, 87
Steroid sulphatase, 125
Stress, 76, 78–80, 110, 288, 293
    Arab/Israeli six day war, 77
Structural maintenance of chromosomes, 126
Suberoylanilide hydroxamic acid (SAHA),
    248, 252, 255, 256, 258
Superior temporal gyrus, 85
Synaptic plasticity, 246, 251–253, 256–259
Synaptogenesis, 252, 258, 259

T
Tetrachloroethylene, 89
Tetraethyl lead, 89
Time-to-pregnancy, 87
Toxic-gain-of-function, 130
Transcription start sites, 6, 7, 9, 11
Transgenerational, 186, 197–198
Trauma, 77
Trichostatin A, 248, 250, 252–253,
    255–257, 259
Trithorax group protein, 123
Trophoblast, 119
Tubala, 134
Turner's syndrome, 84, 85, 129, 133

U
UTX, 126

V
Valproate, 248, 249, 252, 253, 255

W
War, 77
White matter neurons, 3

X
X-chromosome, 86
    dosage compensation, 85
    maternal, 84, 85
    paternal, 84, 85

random inactivation, 85
    skewed X-chromosome inactivation, 85
X-chromosome inactivation, 42–44
X-inactivation, 120, 121, 123, 124, 135, 136
X-linked mental retardation, 126
X-linked retardation syndromes, 85
X^p/X^m, 121, 125